The Clinician's Handbook for Dental Sleep Medicine

Second Edition

The Clinician's Handbook for
Dental Sleep Medicine

SECOND EDITION

Steve Carstensen, DDS
Ken Berley, DDS, JD

QUINTESSENCE PUBLISHING

Berlin | Chicago | Tokyo
Barcelona | London | Milan | Paris | Prague | Seoul | Warsaw
Beijing | Istanbul | Sao Paulo | Sydney | Zagreb

One book, one tree: In support of reforestation worldwide and to address the climate crisis, for every book sold Quintessence Publishing will plant a tree (https://onetreeplanted.org/).

Library of Congress Cataloging-in-Publication Data

Names: Berley, Ken, author. | Carstensen, Stephen, author.
Title: The clinician's handbook for dental sleep medicine / Stephen Carstensen and Ken Berley.
Description: Second. | Batavia, IL : Quintessence Publishing Co. Inc., [2024] | Ken Berley was the first-named author on the previous edition. | Includes bibliographical references and index. | Summary: "Oral appliance therapy results in much better therapy adherence than CPAP for patients with obstructive sleep apnea. This new update of the bestselling title is the how-to guide for incorporating dental sleep medicine into an existing dental practice and includes advice on examination, appliance selection, follow-up care, complications, legal issues, and medical insurance and Medicare"-- Provided by publisher.
Identifiers: LCCN 2024019946 | ISBN 9781647241964 (paperback)
Subjects: MESH: Sleep Apnea Syndromes--therapy | Sleep Bruxism--therapy | Dentistry--methods
Classification: LCC RC737.5 | NLM WL 115 | DDC 616.2/09--dc23/eng/20240524
LC record available at https://lccn.loc.gov/2024019946

QUINTESSENCE PUBLISHING USA

Quintessence Publishing Co, Inc
411 N Raddant Road
Batavia, IL 60510
www.quintessence-publishing.com

5 4 3 2 1

Editor: Kristen Clark
Production: Angelina Schmelter
Design: Sue Zubek

Printed in the USA

Dedications

The impact of dentistry in health care is growing rapidly. I am dedicated to supporting the health care professionals who choose to push beyond their basic education to learn more about the impact they can have on community health. Those brave enough to say "yes" to opportunities can make a true difference in the lives of those who trust them. This approach would not be possible without the mentors who provided me with opportunities to grow—Dr L.D. Pankey, Dr Keith Thornton, Midge Carstensen, RDH, and countless others who have participated in reducing barriers to health at all stages of life. I hope every reader of this book is as fortunate as I am to have such strong support.

—Steve Carstensen, DDS

I would like to dedicate this book to my father, James A. Berley, who had undiagnosed OSA and died as a result of a stroke in the middle of the night. His death led directly to this book and changed my life. Also, I would like to dedicate this book to my wife, Patty Berley, RDA, who has stood by me through thick and thin, even when I was unworthy of her love.

—Ken Berley, DDS, JD

Contents

Preface

Life is short. Before you know it, you will be looking at your professional life in the rear-view mirror trying to figure out how you spent the time you were given. How did it go so fast? As Benjamin Franklin said, "You may delay, but time will not." Now, in the sunset of my professional career, the thing that I am most proud of is that I committed to the screening and treatment of sleep-disordered breathing (SDB) early in my professional career. I sincerely derive comfort from the fact that my professional efforts have resulted in an improved quality of life for thousands of my patients. As I have said in many of my lectures, on a good day as a dentist I may be able to save a tooth or improve a smile. On a good day as a dental sleep medicine (DSM) practitioner, I may be able to save a patient's life. I am very proud that I have helped so many patients sleep. While the dental health of our patients is vitally important, nothing is more important than air. Without that, life doesn't exist.

With the rise of DSM, dentists are in a unique position to modify the anatomy of the upper airway and improve a patient's oxygen levels during sleep. The simple act of advancing or supporting the mandible during sleep can change the lives of millions of patients who are struggling. When we advance a patient's mandible, nocturnal arousals and sleep fragmentations are diminished because the airway is patent. The patient enjoys more restful sleep and an improved quality of life.

SDB and obstructive sleep apnea (OSA), which is a subset of SDB, are true epidemics in this country. Simply defined, SDB is difficulty maintaining a patent airway during sleep. The symptoms range from simple snoring to prolonged and complete closure of the patient's airway. The patient's tongue and soft palate are typically the culprits responsible for nocturnal airway resistance. But when we advance the mandible, the tongue and hyoid bone are placed under tension, which decreases resistance and reduces the likelihood of complete or partial airway closure.

Epidemiologists estimate that more than 200 million Americans snore nightly and at least 52 million have clinically significant OSA. That means that up to 50% of the adults and 10% of the children you see each day in your dental office likely have some degree of SDB. SDB and OSA are directly associated with hypertension, coronary artery disease, stroke, diabetes mellitus, dementia, and early death. SDB results in the activation of the sympathetic nervous system, resulting in the release of adrenaline and cortisol. When released as a result of the patient's struggle to breathe, adrenaline initiates a "fight or flight" sympathetic response. During sleep, our body is supposed to be resting and repairing, not fighting for oxygen. Opening a patient's airway with a mandibular advancement device (MAD) can change their life. Nothing that you do as a health care professional will be more impactful for your patients.

DSM was introduced approximately 40 years ago in an effort to advance the use of MADs as a treatment alternative to continuous positive airway pressure (CPAP). Now, after 40 years of growth and growing pains, oral appliance therapy (OAT) is an accepted alternative to CPAP and is the first-line treatment for SDB/OSA, with reimbursement available under most medical insurance policies and Medicare. While CPAP remains the first choice of treatment for the majority of physicians, the percentage of physicians who regularly recommend OAT for their patients with SDB/OSA is growing rapidly. This shift toward OAT as the therapy of choice has resulted in an explosion in the field of DSM. Now, over 30% of all dentists provide some level of OAT to their patients, and the number of full-time DSM practitioners is growing each year. With the acceptance of DSM as an effective treatment and the expansion of medical insurance reimbursement, the addition of DSM into a general dental practice can result in significant financial gain.

There are a number of dental professional service organizations that foster and support DSM, with the American Academy of Dental Sleep Medicine (AADSM) being the largest. All of the service organizations provide various levels of training and credentialing; however, the AADSM offers diplomate certification, which is generally recognized as the highest level of training and credentialing available. With that said, readers should be aware that no significant financial investment is needed in order to provide OAT and treat OSA. You do not have to enroll in an expensive program or purchase costly equipment to treat your patients. After reading and implementing the information and techniques discussed in this handbook, you will have the knowledge and techniques necessary to successfully practice DSM. Do not be deceived into thinking that you need to spend thousands of dollars to get your DSM practice started. That is not necessary. All you need is information and a true desire to help your patients live better lives.

You have my congratulations on your decision to treat your patients' SDB; you will not regret adding DSM to your practice. Thank you for allowing Steve and me the opportunity to instruct, assist, and inspire you in your pledge to treat your OSA patients. Please don't get discouraged as you begin. Find the CPAP failures that are currently experienced by patients in your practice and start by treating them. Learn and repeat!

Respectfully,
Ken Berley, *DDS, JD*

Acknowledgments

We would like to thank the team at Quintessence Publishing and Kristen Clark, our editor, for their guidance and assistance in the development of this handbook. Also, a big thank you to our families and friends who have tolerated and supported us throughout this process. Your understanding has been invaluable.

Contributors

Patty Berley, RDA

Karen Parker Davidson, DHA, MSA, MEd, MSN, RN
Adjunct Professor
Department of Public Health
School of Health Sciences
Liberty University
Lynchburg, Virginia

Adjunct Professor
Division of Health Administration
School of Health Sciences
Central Michigan University
Mount Pleasant, Michigan

Bill Esser, PT

Brad Gilden, DPT
Private Practice
Old Greenwich, Connecticut
New York City, New York

Patrick McKeown
Founder
Oxygen Advantage

Director of Education and Training
Buteyko Clinic International
Galway, Ireland

Joy L. Moeller, RDH, BS
Private Practice
Palisades, California

Klaus Vogt, Prof Dr, Dr med
Guest Professor
Faculty of Medicine
University of Latvia
Riga, Latvia

MedTecResearch
Krakow am See, Germany

Samantha Weaver, MS, CCC-SLP
Director
Academy of Orofacial Myofunctional Therapy

Private Practice
Palisades, California

Innocent sleep. Sleep that soothes away all our worries. Sleep that puts each day to rest. Sleep that relieves the weary laborer and heals hurt minds. Sleep, the main course in life's feast, and the most nourishing.

—*William Shakespeare, Macbeth*

1

Clinical Guide for the Practice of Dental Sleep Medicine

The Sleep Deprivation Epidemic

An old Irish proverb says, "A good laugh and a long sleep are the best cures in the doctor's book." It is easy to champion the physical, mental, and social benefits of a good night's sleep. Sleep is mandatory for life. Humans can live approximately 4 days without water and 40 days without food but cease to function normally after missing a single night of sleep. Missing sleep for 10 days can be lethal. Even the early Greeks and Romans worshiped Hypnos and Somnus, their gods of sleep. We are all aware that every human must achieve a certain quality and quantity of sleep to function normally, but sadly, millions of individuals across the globe are unable to achieve a good night's sleep. For these individuals, life can be a real struggle. A simple task can turn into an adventure without adequate sleep. Despite all the medical and social advances of modern society, good sleep has never been harder to achieve.

We struggle with sleep for many reasons. People face various social, environmental, and physiologic barriers when attempting to sleep. Frequently, sleep quality is sabotaged by lifestyle decisions—the self-inflicted consequences of daily choices. Attempting to sleep in a noisy, hot, or bright environment is common. Too many people live sedentary lives with insufficient exercise, and sleeping is much more difficult if we are not physically tired. A great American weekend is now defined by watching football on the couch or binge-watching the latest Netflix release. Alcohol consumption, which significantly exacerbates sleep-disordered breathing, is also at an all-time high. We are hyperconnected with a growing array of computer-driven screens and glowing devices. The blue light emitted from many screens stimulates serotonin production and contributes to insomnia. Our technologic advances have given us the ability to work anywhere on the face of the planet at any time during the day or night, and we can stay in constant contact with anyone in the world. The health-conscious person striving for a good night's sleep must be very disciplined in light of this sensory onslaught.

In addition to the societal and entertainment choices that rob us of sleep, our ability to sleep is directly affected by certain physical characteristics and anatomical deficiencies. First and foremost, the human ability for complex vocalization and speech has created an anatomical weakness—a smaller maxillofacial complex and subsequently a decreased airway diameter. The airway from the hard palate to the top of the trachea is collapsible, with collapse typically manifested during the deeper levels of sleep. If the airway is restricted, or collapses completely, the increased respiratory effort required to breathe can lead to arousals and other physical consequences. Airflow is restricted, and blood oxygen/carbon dioxide levels become unbalanced. The repeated cycle of airway restriction/collapse and recovery to resume breathing has many names. *Sleep-related breathing disorder* (SRBD) is the general term, with *obstructive sleep apnea* (OSA) being the most consequential subset.

In addition to the anatomical component of OSA, Western civilization has adopted a fast food and microwave meal–style of living. Poor diet has resulted in rampant obesity in the United States, and OSA is closely linked to obesity and diabetes mellitus. These diseases are almost inseparable and have long-term health consequences. As patients become larger, fat deposits in the base of the tongue and the lateral walls of the airway are enlarged, reducing the cross-sectional area of the oropharyngeal lumen and making it more likely to collapse. Therefore, obesity greatly contributes to or exacerbates OSA. According to the Centers for Disease Control and Prevention (CDC), approximately 65% of Americans are overweight or obese. In many states, more than 35% of the population is obese, with the percentages rising each year (Fig 1-1). Obesity hypoventilation syndrome (OHS) is a severe disease state, and over 90% of patients diagnosed with it have OSA.[2]

Finally, OSA appears to have some roots in the Western practice of bottle-feeding and the use of pacifiers and sippy cups. Nonproductive suckling may result in craniofacial respiratory complex collapse (CFRC) and increased dental crowding in children, exacerbating childhood sleep disorders.[3]

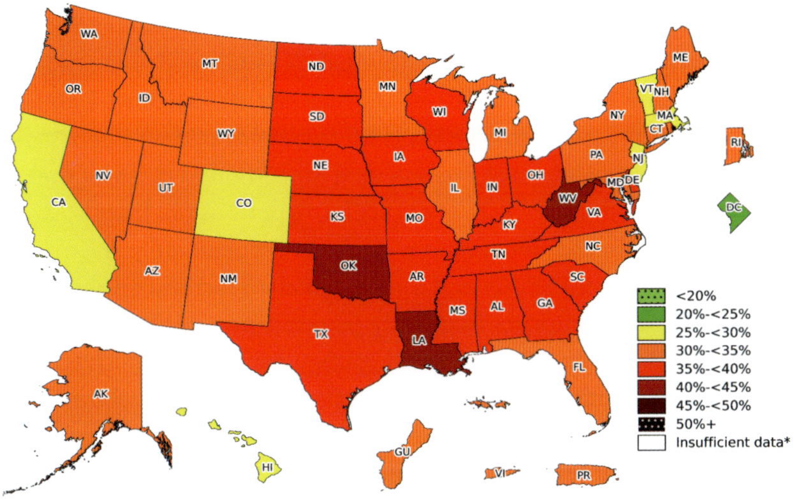

Fig 1-1 2022 obesity map. (Reprinted with permission from the CDC Behavioral Risk Factor Surveillance System.[1])

This coalition of factors, including a smaller orofacial complex, increased BMI, an aging population, and decreased levels of exercise, has resulted in an explosion of OSA in the United States. Often, individuals with OSA are unaware that they have difficulty breathing during sleep, and it is most commonly recognized as a problem by family members or bed partners who observe the individual during obstructive episodes. Individuals who sleep alone may be unaware of the condition because no one is present to poke them in the ribs. OSA patients may seek medical care for symptoms of fatigue or daytime sleepiness, but not all patients exhibit excessive daytime sleepiness (EDS). Sadly, OSA may remain undetected for years or even decades because patients become conditioned to the daytime sleepiness and fatigue associated with significant levels of sleep disturbance.

Lack of adequate air leads to a cascade of devastating physical and emotional consequences. Restricted airway function affects our ability to sleep and can give rise to insomnia, an altered arousal threshold, asphyxia, hypoxemia, hypercapnia, and sleep fragmentation. Increased respiratory effort and airway collapse can lead to EDS and contribute to a host of comorbid diseases.

The Rise Of Dental Sleep Medicine

This is an exciting time to be a dentist. The field of dental sleep medicine (DSM) is exploding. This is primarily because the majority of individuals with sleep disorders do not present to physicians for treatment of their sleep issues.[4] Instead, people typically seek medical care for comorbid diseases that are directly associated with SRBDs, in particular, hypertension, fatigue, stroke, cardiovascular disease, and diabetes mellitus. Unfortunately, most physicians do not screen for SRDBs, and the precipitating factors contributing to the patient's chief complaint frequently go undiagnosed.[5] However, many patients suffering from SRBDs also seek routine dental care, which provides knowledgeable dentists with a screening opportunity. Dentists who are properly trained to recognize the signs and symptoms of SRBDs can potentially provide life-saving referrals and oral appliance therapy (OAT) to sleep-deprived patients. Patients with SRBDs exhibit identifiable intraoral signs and symptoms, as well as physical and social symptoms.

DSM was founded on the principle that the mandible can be moved and supported to maintain an open airway during sleep. The tongue is attached anteriorly to the genial tubercles on the lingual aspect, and if the mandible is protruded with a mandibular advancement device (MAD), the tongue is advanced. This opens the airway and minimizes airway restriction. MADs work in the same manner as the head tilt, chin lift, jaw thrust maneuver used to open the airway in CPR. The simple act of holding the mandible in a stable or slightly protruded position during sleep may be adequate to prevent or mitigate the physiologic consequences of airway obstruction and resultant nocturnal hypoxemia. There is an ever-increasing number of MADs being cleared by the FDA to treat SRBDs, including snoring and OSA, and properly trained dentists are integral partners in the treatment of SRBDs.

Although still in its infancy, DSM is the fastest-growing discipline in dentistry. Screening and treating patients with SRBDs can greatly improve their health and generate a significant source of income for your dental practice.

Terminology

This section explains some useful terminology in the field of DSM.

Apnea

Apnea literally means "without air." An apnea is identified during a sleep study when the patient's airflow peak signal drops by ≥ 90% compared to the pre-event baseline for at least 10 seconds as measured using an oronasal

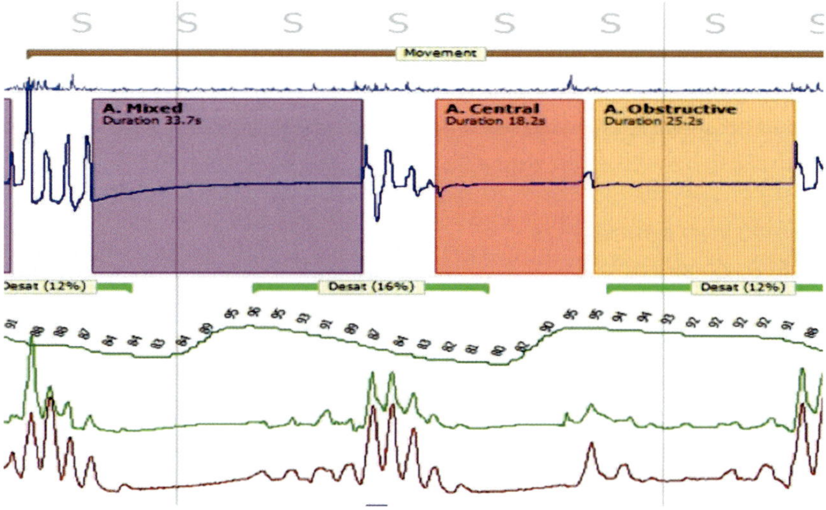

Fig 1-2 Screenshot of a home sleep apnea test (HSAT) indicating the different types of apneas. While the patient is in the supine position (S), the first event is scored as a mixed event because the respiratory effort belt signals are flat (no effort) for more than half of the event. Recovery breaths follow the mixed apnea, where the patient is gasping for breath. Then the next two events are scored as a central for 18.2 seconds, a small breath, then an obstructive event where the patient is trying to breathe but no air is entering the lungs. Notice that a desaturation follows each of the events.

thermal signal, positive airway pressure (PAP) device flow, or an alternative apnea sensor. There is no requirement for desaturation or arousal. Apneas can be classified as obstructive, central, or mixed, depending on the patient's respiratory effort during the event. If the patient is trying to breathe and cannot, the event is classified as obstructive. If the patient is not trying to breathe, the event is designated as central apnea. A mixed apnea is a combination of obstructive and central apnea, where the event is more central than obstructive (Fig 1-2).

Arousal

An arousal is a sudden change from a deeper level of sleep to a lighter level of sleep. Patients usually do not awaken and are unaware of the arousal, but daytime sleepiness and fatigue are common symptoms of frequent arousals.

Arousals are classified as respiratory arousals and environmental arousals. Respiratory arousals are caused by any respiratory event and are directly related to the patient's effort to breathe. As oxygen levels decrease and carbon dioxide levels rise during an apnea or hypopnea event, chemosensors in the brain arouse motor pathways to restore airway function and normal respiration. Treatment of respiratory arousals can improve daytime symptoms. Environmental arousals occur as a result of non-respiratory stimuli. Many things can cause a patient to arouse during sleep. Anything from noise from a TV left on at night to the temperature in the bedroom or air quality and light control can be associated with a disruptive sleep environment.

Home sleep apnea tests

Frequently, home sleep apnea tests (HSATs) are used to diagnose OSA. However, HSATs typically cannot fully measure the quality and quantity of sleep. HSATs measure different bodily metrics, such as respiratory activity and breathing patterns. Common metrics measured during an HSAT include the following:

- Respiratory activity, breathing patterns, and chest motion
- Heart rate and blood oxygen level
- Actigraphy, or nocturnal movement and motor activity
- Sleep position and position changes
- Snoring events and intensity

Hypopnea

Hypopnea is a drop in peak signal excursion of at least 30% compared to the pre-event baseline for at least 10 seconds measured using nasal pressure (recommended sensor), PAP device flow, or an alternative hypopnea sensor. Additionally, to qualify as a hypopnea, the event must involve at least 3% oxygen desaturation from the pre-event baseline OR the event must be associated with a cortical electroencephalogram (EEG) arousal[6] (Fig 1-3).

Alternatively, Centers for Medicaid and Medicare Services (CMS) defines a hypopnea as a drop in peak signal excursion by at least 30% compared to the pre-event baseline for at least 10 seconds measured using nasal pressure (recommended sensor), PAP device flow, or an alternative hypopnea sensor AND oxygen desaturation of at least 4% from the pre-event baseline. Scoring hypopnea using a 4% desaturation is a Medicare requirement. When treating a Medicare patient, make sure that the appropriate scoring parameters were used by the sleep lab or the patient will not qualify for benefits under Medicare.

Polysomnography

A polysomnogram (PSG), also called an in-lab sleep study, is a continuous recording of specific physiologic markers and variables over a full night of

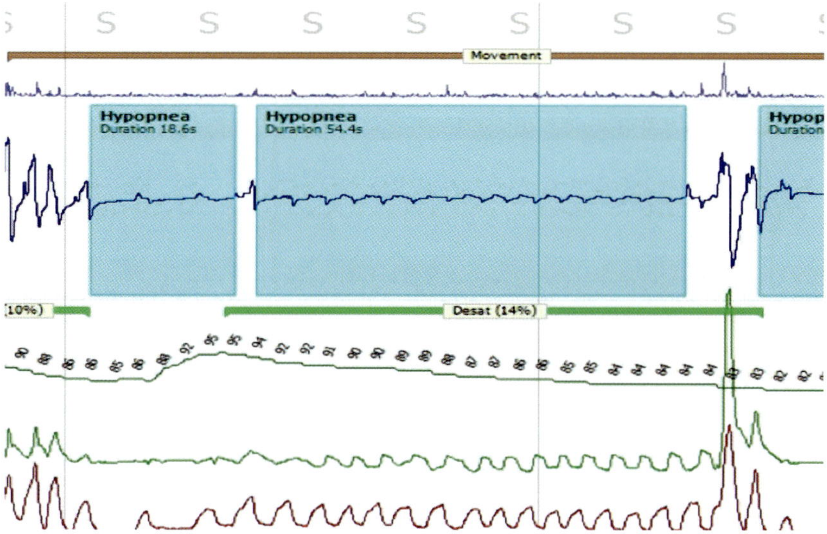

Fig 1-3 Screenshot of HSAT indicating hypopneas. Notice that the patient's airflow is not a flat line. Air is entering the lungs, but the volume is reduced to the point that the patient's blood SaO_2 is not maintained. The decreased airflow results in a 14% desaturation. At all times during the event, the patient is attempting to breathe but is unable to adequately maintain oxygen levels.

sleep that helps to identify and diagnose various sleep disorders (Fig 1-4). Typically, a PSG records the following parameters:

- Brainwaves (via EEG)
- Blood oxygen levels
- Eye movements (via electrooculogram [EOG])
- Muscle tone (via electromyogram [EMG])
- Respiratory activity, breathing patterns, and chest motion (via nasal flow sensor and effort belts around the chest)
- Heart rate (via electrocardiogram [ECG])
- Leg movements (via EMG)
- Snoring
- Sleep position

Respiratory disturbance index

The respiratory disturbance index (RDI) is calculated as the number of respiratory events (apneas, hypopneas, and respiratory effort–related arousals [RERAs]) divided by the number of hours of sleep documented during a PSG study.

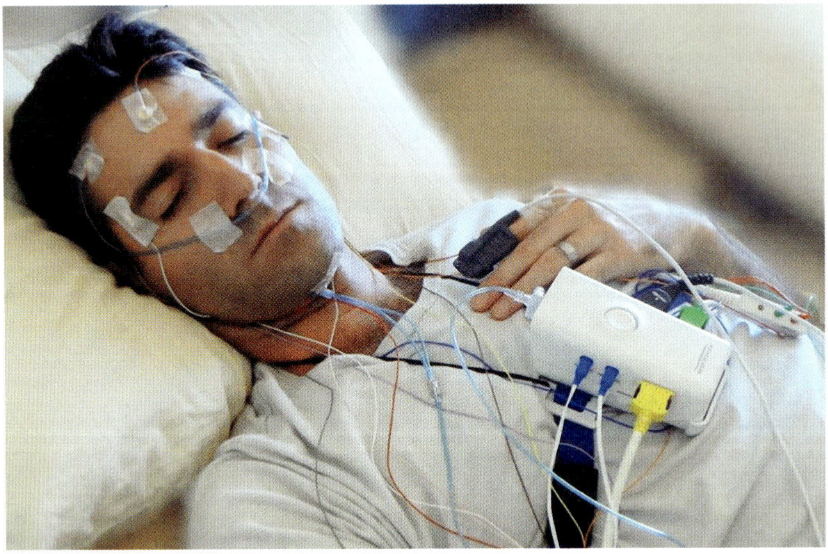

Fig 1-4 Patient during a PSG.

Respiratory effort–related arousal

Respiratory effort–related arousal (RERA) is not always scored during a sleep test. It is defined as a sequence of breaths lasting at least 10 seconds and characterized by increasing respiratory effort or by flattening of the inspiratory portion of the flow signal, leading to an arousal from sleep. The sequence of breaths does not include apneas or hypopneas. Because the definition of a hypopnea has never been consistent and is more frequently revised than other sleep breathing parameters, RERA is not typically used to describe SRBDs but may be useful for informing clinicians about sleep fragmentation.

Snoring

Snoring is traditionally defined as breathing during sleep with a rough, hoarse noise due to vibration of the soft palate and tongue. It is helpful to separate patients who simply make a snoring noise from patients whose snoring results in a RERA. For the purposes of this text, the authors refer to snoring as any respiratory-related noise made during sleep that does not result in an arousal. Respiratory noises and events that result in an arousal, but do not qualify as an apnea or hypopnea, are referred to as a RERA. It should be noted that loud snoring is the most common symptom of a patient with OSA.

Overview of Sleep-Related Breathing Disorders

SRBD, also known as *sleep-disordered breathing* (SDB), is a collection of conditions or disorders where patients suffer from the consequences of restricted breathing and/or reduced oxygenation during sleep. Although OSA is generally referred to as SRBD, SRBD is a much broader term that includes a spectrum of breathing anomalies, ranging from chronic or habitual snoring (resulting in airflow limitations) to upper airway resistance syndrome (UARS), OSA, central and complex apnea, and in some cases, Cheyne-Stokes respiration and obesity hypoventilation syndrome. Although OHS is not a true sleep disorder, patients with very severe OSA who are morbidly obese frequently suffer from daytime hypoventilation, which can be mitigated with the use of a single-arch temporomandibular joint (TMJ) splint that encourages the patient to function with their mandible protruded during the daytime. The amount of protrusion built into the daytime splint varies with the severity of the patient's condition. Patients with severe OHS use continuous positive airway pressure (CPAP) and a MAD during sleep.

SRBD symptoms routinely become more severe and complex with age, and the consequences of the resultant sleep fragmentation and oxygen desaturation can be deadly. SRBDs make maintaining oxygenation during sleep difficult as a result of repeated upper airway restriction and resistance during sleep that causes recurrent nocturnal asphyxia, fragmented sleep, fatigue, daytime sleepiness, major fluctuations in blood pressure, and increased sympathetic nervous system activity.[7] An aging population and skyrocketing obesity further contribute to SRBDs. As we age, the airway often becomes smaller, due to increased fat deposits, and more collapsible, secondary to hormonal changes. A patient who has been diagnosed with OSA is at increased risk for hypertension, stroke, diabetes mellitus, and heart attack, as well as early mortality. The physiologic changes associated with SRBDs can be devastating to a patient's ability to stay oxygenated during sleep. This is particularly impactful when a patient has a compromised immune system.

The various airway conditions associated with SRBDs include, but are not limited to, respiratory noise, snoring, flow limitations, RERAs, UARS, hypopneas, OSA, OSA syndrome (OSAS), mixed sleep apnea, and central sleep apnea. The risk factors and underlying pathophysiologic mechanisms of these disorders have both overlapping and unique features.

Figure 1-5 shows the continuum of sleep disorders, progressing from a baby making a "cute noise" when sleeping all the way to apneas, where the airway is totally obstructed. Each level represents a higher degree of collapse with increasingly serious consequences. Although SRBDs cannot be accurately represented as a true progression (snoring does not inevitably result in OSA), it is important to see that every diagnosis lies within a larger scope of poor airway function.

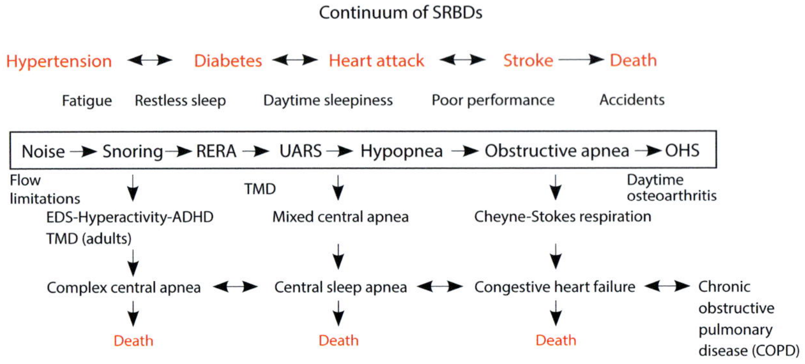

Fig 1-5 Continuum of sleep disorders and related conditions.

Once a patient starts experiencing hypopneas and apneas, medical insurance may provide benefits. The last stage of SRBDs is when patients have difficulty maintaining an open airway during the daytime. OHS is common in morbidly obese patients with BMIs greater than 45. Therapies for OHS may include a TMJ mandibular advancement (Gelb) splint, portable oxygen, and weight loss therapy. A daytime advancement splint is simply one of the many tools which can help these patients stay adequately oxygenated during the day. The ultimate goal is weight loss, which will likely include bariatric surgery. OHS involves autonomic nervous system dysfunction and is not well managed in the dental office. Patients with OHS are commonly treated with multiple therapies by collaborating health care providers.

Obstructive sleep apnea

Common symptoms of OSA include the following[8]:

- Unexplained daytime sleepiness
- Loud snoring with periods of silence followed by gasps as breathing resumes
- Attention deficit and/or hyperactivity in children
- Trouble concentrating; mood changes such as irritability, anxiety, treatment-resistant depression, and forgetfulness
- Temporomandibular disorder symptoms, sleep bruxism
- Decreased sex drive, sexual dysfunction, and heavy night sweats
- Restless leg syndrome/periodic limb movements
- Restless or fragmented sleep and lack of dreams

- Increased heart rate and/or blood pressure (systemic hypertension), ischemic heart disease, congestive heart failure
- Decline in performance at work
- Dry mouth/throat sensations upon awakening
- Fatigue
- Gastroesophageal reflux disease (GERD)
- Impaired cognition (memory and concentration)
- Insomnia and parasomnias (confused arousals and sleep-related eating disorders)
- Morning headaches
- Nocturia

Other medical problems common in patients with OSA include stroke or other ischemic cerebrovascular disease, erectile dysfunction, diabetes mellitus, and/or insulin resistance. Patients with OSA may also experience unexplained weight gain. Drowsiness in the daytime can result in increased industrial and automobile accidents. Some research links OSA to cognitive decline such as dementia.[9]

Risk factors for OSA are listed here:

- Family history of OSA
- Male sex (for adults): male-female ratio of 3:1
- Menopausal state in women: Hormone replacement therapy decreases the risk for OSA in postmenopausal patients.
- Age: OSA risk increases with age but plateaus after middle age (50 to 55 years of age).
- Obesity or excessive body weight:
  - 70% of patients with OSA are overweight or obese.
  - The prevalence of OSA increases in direct proportion to total weight.
  - The association between BMI and OSA is weaker in the Asian population.
  - A 10% increase in weight is associated with a sixfold increase in risk for OSA.
  - Central obesity found within the waist and hips results in a greater risk of OSA than general obesity.
  - The risk for OSA is greater if the patient's waist is greater than 40 inches for men and 36 inches for women.
  - Obesity increases the risk for OSA by decreasing the pharyngeal diameter due to fat deposition; reducing lung volume, resulting in the loss of caudal traction in the upper airway, which increases the risk for oxygen desaturation; and reducing upper airway muscle tone and neuromuscular control.

- Snoring
- Craniofacial dystrophy and oropharyngeal anatomical factors:
  - Increased neck size (greater than 17 inches in men and 16 inches in women)
  - Long face syndrome
  - Nasal narrowing and congestion
  - Macroglossia (enlarged tongue)
  - Elongated soft palate and enlarged uvula
  - Narrow dental arches and vaulted palate
  - Enlarged tonsils and adenoids, especially in children
  - Lingual and palatal tori
  - Narrow lateral pharyngeal wall distance (generally the lateral upper airway dimension is more important than the anteroposterior dimension in the predictive risk of OSA)
  - Midface hypoplasia, retrognathia, micrognathia, or mandibular hypoplasia
  - Caudal displacement of the hyoid bone
- Ethnicity: Africans, Asians, Pacific Islanders, and Hispanics have a greater risk for developing OSA than Caucasians.
- Smoking and alcohol use
- Medications: Using muscle relaxants, sedatives, anesthetics, or opioid analgesics increases the Apnea-Hypopnea Index (AHI) and the risk for OSA.[9]

COVID-19 and SRBDs

Several articles published in 2021 confirm a direct correlation between the severity of a patient's SRBD and morbidity associated with COVID-19 infection. Patients with OSA experienced an approximately eight-fold increase in risk for COVID-19 infection compared to a population of similar age receiving care in a large, racially and socioeconomically diverse healthcare system. Among COVID-19 patients, OSA is associated with an increased risk of hospitalization and approximately double the risk of respiratory failure.[10] A patient with OSA is much more likely to have one of the serious comorbid diseases associated with COVID-19 mortality. Frequently, OSA patients are obese and have diabetes. Obese patients are disproportionately hospitalized and frequently placed on ventilators. This combination of comorbid diseases, coupled with an acute respiratory viral infection, can be deadly.

ADA policy statement on SRBDs

In 2017, the American Dental Association (ADA) voted to approve a policy statement on dentistry's role in the treatment of SRBDs.[11] This policy places the treatment of SRBDs firmly within the scope of practice of every dentist. While dentists are not obligated to provide treatment for SRBDs, they are encouraged to screen all patients for SRBDs and document the results in each patient's record. When the screening is positive, the patient must be informed of the possibility of an SRBD and referred to a sleep physician for appropriate diagnosis and therapy.

Respiratory Effort Explained

Any sound made during sleep is a sign of increased respiratory effort. As resistance increases, respiratory-related noise or snoring increases. Eventually, the effort is significant enough that the patient's arousal threshold is breached, and sleep is fragmented. Increased respiratory effort can be damaging to a growing child. The more a child struggles to breathe during sleep, the more disrupted or fragmented sleeping becomes. With increasing respiratory effort and sleep fragmentation, children will exhibit increasingly disruptive daytime behaviors and are frequently misdiagnosed as hyperactive. When children are tired, they can become aggressive and defiant. It takes a well-informed clinician to recognize that a sleep issue may be the underlying cause of observed behaviors.

In adults, respiratory-related noise, regardless of whether it causes patient arousal, is a sign of increased effort to maintain oxygenation during sleep. As resistance increases, typical snoring sounds are common. When resistance is accompanied by respiratory arousals, daytime symptoms are quick to follow. As the respiratory effort required to breathe continues to increase, susceptible individuals begin to display the menagerie of symptoms outlined in Fig 1-5.

Inspiration produces negative pressure, and the airway collapses. A partial collapse is called a *hypopnea,* and a complete collapse is called *apnea*. If a sleeping patient exhibits five or more hypopneas and/or apneas per hour, the SRBD is classified as OSA. A diagnosis of OSA from a sleep physician–interpreted sleep study may mean that medical insurance and Medicare will provide benefits for treatment. For sleep disorders that do not qualify as OSA, no insurance coverage is available.

There is no direct relationship between the severity of a patient's physical symptoms and the number of respiratory arousals and oxygen desaturations experienced during each night of sleep. Some people with low event counts have severe symptoms, whereas other patients with apneas and hypopneas affecting nearly every minute of sleep exhibit few subjective complaints. Although clinicians tend to focus on apneas and hypopneas, successful treatment of SRBDs is directly associated with reducing arousals and oxygen desaturations. These are the events that lead to fragmented sleep and sympathetic nervous system activation.

Diagnosis

OSA is diagnosed with an overnight sleep study that must be interpreted by a board-certified sleep physician. The overnight sleep study can be either a PSG, which is conducted by professionals in a specialized facility, or an HSAT (also called an HST), which is performed under the subject's control. Obviously, home testing is less costly, and therefore the popularity of PSG has diminished due to insurance restrictions. Either method is adequate to diagnose SRBDs, but PSG is considered the gold standard for testing.

PSG is performed in a sleep laboratory by a registered polysomnographic technologist (RPSGT). Among the numerous variables PSG records is EEG (brainwave activity). This allows the RPSGT to determine if a patient is actually asleep and identify (or score) sleep stages. This is very helpful for determining the severity of an SRBD. HSAT, on the other hand, is a limited channel test, with most devices incapable of recording EEG signals. Therefore, a sleep study conducted with HSAT often cannot produce sleep time data. This is a major disadvantage and may result in diagnostic inaccuracies.

All diagnostic sleep tests must be read and interpreted by a board-certified sleep physician, a medical doctor who has completed a 1-year fellowship in sleep medicine and passed a comprehensive board examination in the diagnosis and treatment of sleep disorders. Current classification systems include more than eighty sleep disorders, with OSA being only one subset.[12] Sleep medicine focuses on sleep, sleep disorders, and sleep-related conditions and is a subspecialty within several medical specialties, including neurology, pulmonology, internal medicine, family medicine, otolaryngology, pediatrics, and psychiatry.

For dentists treating OSA, the authors agree that it is generally easier to treat a patient who presents with hypopneas. Hypopnea is considered by some to be less severe than an apneic event; however, most researchers have determined that hypopneas have a "similar if not indistinguishable impact" on sleep fragmentation and health outcomes. Patients who primarily experience apneas present with a more significant closure of the airway, complicating treatment. Therefore, when a dentist is evaluating a sleep study, it is always helpful to determine the number of obstructive, hypopneas, and centrals that occurred during the sleep study, as each event responds differently to OAT.

Apnea-Hypopnea Index

The Apnea-Hypopnea Index (AHI) is calculated as the number of respiratory events (apneas, hypopneas) divided by the number of hours of sleep documented during a PSG study. It is important to distinguish whether all respiratory events are included (central and obstructive) or only obstructive events. Ideally, a total AHI inclusive of central and obstructive events is reported along with a separate total for central apnea index.

Respiratory event index

The respiratory event index (REI) is calculated as the number of respiratory events divided by the number of hours of *estimated* sleep using an HSAT. The recommended approach for estimating sleep time is by editing the periods when the participant is likely awake, as evidenced by artifact, movement, and characteristic changes in heart rate and breathing, from the total recording.

Because HSAT does not include EEG, it cannot precisely measure sleep time. AHI values for adults are classified as follows:

- Normal: AHI < 5
- Mild sleep apnea: 5–15 events per hour of sleep
- Moderate sleep apnea: 16–30 events per hour of sleep
- Severe sleep apnea: AHI > 30

For children, because of their different physiology, an AHI greater than 1 is considered abnormal.[13]

A patient's AHI is the most widely used marker to evaluate the severity of OSA, but other factors are just as important. These factors include the degree of daytime sleepiness, the nadir of oxygen saturation (SaO_2), the extent of sleep fragmentation, the presence of nocturnal arrhythmias, and comorbid cardiovascular and neurologic disorders.

DSM practitioners must be aware that multiple sleep studies will likely reveal significant night-to-night variability of the AHI in patients with OSA. Furthermore, PSG and HST, which are each subject to night-to-night variability, often provide disparate results for the same patient. There may be several reasons for this variability, including the use of alcohol, muscle relaxants, sedatives, or opioids; changes in the percentages of rapid eye movement (REM) sleep; variations in the amount of supine verses non-supine sleep; the degree of nasal resistance or congestion; and, over time, changes in weight and hormone levels. Clinicians should be careful to consider sleep test results derived by different means.

Oxygen desaturation index

The oxygen desaturation index (ODI) refers to the number of dips (3% or 4%; ODI3%, ODI4%) in SaO_2 relative to a local baseline per hour of sleep from an overnight sleep study. Unlike the AHI, the ODI is almost always automatically derived using analysis software. Software programs use various algorithms for averaging SaO_2 signals, defining local baseline SaO_2, requiring minimal durations of oxygen fall, and identifying and excluding artifacts. At sea level, a normal blood oxygen level (saturation) is usually 96% to 97%. Although there are no generally accepted classifications for the severity of oxygen desaturations, reductions to not less than 90% usually are considered mild, dips into the 80% to 89% range can be considered moderate, and levels below 80% are considered severe.

The criteria used to determine the index may vary depending on the scoring rules used. According to the 2007 guidelines from the American Academy of Sleep Medicine (AASM), any event with a 3% drop in blood oxygen level is counted toward the total. For example, a change from 95% to 92% would be a recordable event. However, Medicare and some other insurance companies require a 4% change for an event to be counted. When evaluating a sleep study, it is necessary to determine what parameters were used to score the study. This is especially pertinent when comparing studies taken at different times or with different equipment to determine improvement or worsening of OSA.

Sleep and breathing measurements beyond AHI

AHI was the first descriptor of OSA, but as an event count, it is limited in its usefulness. AHI does not correlate well with symptoms or all-cause mortality.[14] Neither does it resolve in a predictable way with any common treatment. All events that last 10 seconds or longer count only as one event. One author's father had apnea events ranging from 10 to 92 seconds, yet each counted as an individual, equal contribution to an overall severe AHI diagnosis. Many people with "mild" AHI by count suffer from significant disruptions to their health. Scientists and clinicians are deriving different markers from PSG data and exploring clinical applications. Soon, AHI will become one of many variables and not the sole determinant of disease burden. What you will learn in this text about defining OSA will always be useful, but the rapid growth of research and understanding will require changing terminology as new determinants of disease become more widely adopted.

Some examples of recently defined disease benchmarks include the following:

- Hypoxic burden—the frequency and severity of OSA related hypoxia[15]
- Arousal burden—EEG-based calculation of sleep fragmentation[16]
- Ventilatory burden—automated calculation of breathing volume during sleep[17]

OSA is a Medical Disease

OSA has been determined to be a medical disease by the AASM. It is currently the position of the AASM and the American Medical Association (AMA) that physicians are the only professionals qualified to order an overnight sleep test. However, the American Academy of Dental Sleep Medicine (AADSM) has recently issued a policy statement that states that it is within the scope of practice for a dentist who is well trained in the treatment of SRBDs to order an HSAT. Readers are advised to check their state's dental board for directions on the legality of ordering HSTs. As of this writing, it is universally agreed that a board-certified sleep physician is the only medical professional adequately trained to diagnose SRBDs. Therefore, a dentist must coordinate with a sleep physician to provide OAT, as all diagnoses and treatment planning for SRBDs/OSA should be provided by a sleep physician. The sleep physician controls the treatment of OSA and determines when OAT is appropriate for a patient.

Because OSA is a medical condition, OAT is filed on the patient's medical insurance or Medicare. Current Dental Terminology (CDT) codes for OAT have been provided by the ADA. However, as of this writing, no dental insurance carriers provide benefits for the treatment of OSA. The fact that most medical insurance policies and Medicare provide coverage presents a major opportunity to provide OAT without using your patient's dental insurance benefits. DSM practitioners must become proficient in filing medical insurance and Medicare claims to meet the demands of a significant number of patients in their communities.

Many dentists are now partnering with colleagues in sleep medicine to provide therapy for SRBD patients. SRBDs directly or indirectly affect many biologic systems within the human body; therefore, numerous medical disciplines are involved in the treatment of OSA's comorbid conditions. Dentists trained in DSM can be vital members of multidisciplinary teams of health care professionals working together to control this deadly disease and should develop an extensive physician-based referral practice.

Cost of Untreated and Undiagnosed OSA

During sleep, people should be quiescent. The parasympathetic nervous system should be in control, and blood pressure and heart rates should be at their lowest. Sleep should be a time of physical and mental repair. However, patients with OSA experience repeated sympathetic spikes throughout the night. Hypoxia (absence of oxygen supply) results in a sympathetic response and the resultant release of cortisol and adrenaline, which initiates a cascade of physiologic events known as the fight or flight response. This contributes to sleep disruption (fragmentation) and daytime sleepiness.

The carotid bodies are a small cluster of chemoreceptors and supporting cells located near the bifurcation of the carotid arteries. The carotid bodies detect changes in the oxygen/carbon dioxide (O_2/CO_2) composition of arterial blood. A decrease in the partial pressure of oxygen (PaO_2) and increase in partial pressure of carbon dioxide ($PaCO_2$) activates the sympathetic nervous system, which causes heart rate to elevate, blood pressure to increase, and respiratory effort to increase. The effect of these sympathetic episodes is an increase in chronic disease and shortened life expectancy in patients with untreated OSA. The consequences of untreated OSA include the following[9]:

- Increased mortality (particularly among young and middle-aged adults)
- Decreased SaO_2 and PaO_2 and increased $PaCO_2$ during sleep
- Increased systemic and pulmonary artery pressure: increased left ventricular and right ventricular output and increased pulmonary ventricular resistance
- Neurocognitive and psychiatric effects:
  - Depression and anxiety
  - Decreased quality of life
  - Decreased alertness and vigilance (likely the result of sleep fragmentation and hypoxemia)
  - Impairment of neurocognitive performance (executive function, learning, and memory)
- Sleep fragmentation/disturbance, which is often seen as excessive daytime sleepiness
- Cardiovascular effects:
  - Systemic hypertension (independent of obesity). Due to an increase in sympathetic nervous system activity, there is an increase in systolic and diastolic blood pressure, which does not fall during sleep. This is termed "non-dipping" and is emerging as a key indicator of increased cardiovascular risk.
  - The prevalence of OSA increases in drug-resistant hypertension:
    - Each additional apnea event per hour of sleep increases the odds of hypertension by about 1%.

    - Each 10% decrease in nocturnal SaO_2 increases the odds of hypertension by 13%.
    - Pulmonary hypertension (prevalence of 20% to 70% of OSA patients). PAP therapy has been shown to improve OSA-related pulmonary hypertension.
  - Coronary artery disease (nocturnal angina)
  - Sudden cardiac death (typically occurs between 12 and 6 am)
  - Congestive heart failure. There is an increased prevalence of congestive heart failure in patients with OSA due to compromised heart function with both systolic and diastolic dysfunction.
  - Cardiac arrhythmias. Sinus arrhythmias are most common, and there is an increase in atrial fibrillation. Apneic events result in a severe disruption to heart homeostasis.
  - Cerebrovascular disease. There is an increased risk of stroke in persons with OSA, an increased risk of mortality, and an increased risk of OSA following a stroke.
  - OSA is associated with an increase in carotid artery intima-media thickness (marker for atherosclerosis).
- Metabolic dysfunction:
  - Insulin resistance and altered glucose metabolism
  - Increased risk of type 2 diabetes mellitus
  - Increased serum level of leptin and ghrelin (key hormones controlling appetite and fat metabolism)
  - Metabolic syndrome (obesity, hypertension, insulin resistance, and dyslipidemia)
    - Two-thirds of children with OSA have metabolic syndrome.
    - One in four children with metabolic syndrome has OSA.
- Miscellaneous consequences:
  - Increased need for health care
  - Erectile dysfunction
  - GERD
  - Negative intrathoracic pressure

OSA, combined with societal pressures to voluntarily restrict sleep, has given birth to a generation of individuals who are dangerously sleepy.[18] Less than 15% of those suffering from OSA have been diagnosed, and of the millions of patients who have been diagnosed, less than 50% are compliant with CPAP therapy. The economic cost of unmanaged moderate to severe OSA in the United States is estimated to be as much as $165 billion annually.[18] This figure is skewed because it does not include the millions of patients suffering from

UARS who are frequently very sleepy and prone to accidents. For clarity, UARS is resistance to breathing during sleep that causes an arousal but does not fit the definition of OSA.

A Harvard study on SRBDs indicated that the average person with uncontrolled moderate to severe OSA personally spends between $4,000 and $6,000 each year as a direct result of untreated OSA. These costs come from job absenteeism, medical care, sleep aids, lost productivity, and accidents.[18]

Today, automobile and truck accidents attributed to excessive sleepiness are commonplace. A recent poll by the National Sleep Foundation found that 60% of adults admit to driving drowsy within the last year. Drowsy drivers are involved in more than 300,000 accidents each year, which result in over 6,000 deaths. Further, 4.5% of drivers surveyed admitted to nodding off or falling asleep while driving within the last month. Collision costs associated with drowsy driving are estimated to be $11.1 billion annually. The 2012 National Sleep Foundation poll found that 37.9% of adults in the US admitted to unintentionally falling asleep during the day at least once within the last month.

How Big Is the Problem?

Despite the severe societal and health consequences of SRBDs, a surprisingly small number of PSG studies have been conducted to determine the prevalence of OSA in the general population. It has been estimated that 20 million Americans suffer from moderate to severe OSA and that at least one person in five (65 million Americans) has mild OSA. In the late 1980s and early 1990s, three large cohort studies were performed in the United States: the Wisconsin Sleep Cohort,[19] the Sleep Heart Health Study,[20] and the Penn State Cohort.[21] Based primarily on these three studies, the prevalence of SRBDs was estimated to be between 6.5% and 9% in women and between 17% and 31% in men. However, these estimates were subsequently revised to 34% in men aged 30 to 70 years and 17% in women aged 30 to 70 years.[22] No matter the source, it is conservatively estimated that 52 million Americans have clinically significant OSA.[18]

In 2015, the HypnoLaus Study published in Lancet reported a significantly higher incidence of OSA.[23] In this study, 2,121 citizens of Lausanne, Switzerland, were diagnosed after a full-night PSG (via HSAT). Of the participants, 1,024 (48%) were men, and 1,097 (52%) were women. The median age of all participants was 57 years (interquartile range 49 to 68; range 40 to 85), and the mean BMI was 25.6 kg/m^2.

Figure 1-6 shows the prevalence of SRBDs according to clinically defined categories (mild, moderate, and severe) in the men and women who

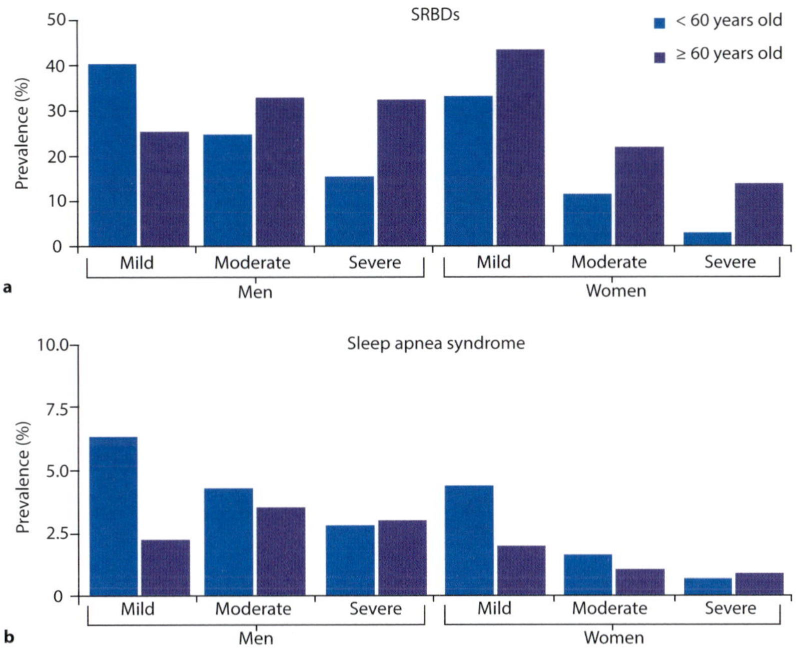

Fig 1-6 Prevalence of SRBDs and sleep apnea syndrome, according to age and sex, as reported by the HypnoLaus Study in 2015.[23] *(a)* A mild SRBD was defined as between 5 and 14 events per hour. Severe SRBD was defined as at least 30 events per hour. SRBD categories differed by age ($P < .0001$ in men and in women). *(b)* Mild sleep apnea syndrome was defined as between 5 and 14 events per hour and an Epworth score greater than 10, moderate sleep apnea syndrome was defined as between 15 and 19 events per hour and an Epworth score greater than 10, and severe sleep apnea syndrome was defined as at least 30 events per hour and an Epworth score greater than 10. Categories of sleep apnea syndrome differed by age ($P < .0001$ in men and $P < .001$ in women).

participated in the HypnoLaus Study. An AHI of five or more events per hour (mild to severe OSA) was recorded in 858 of the 1,024 men in the study (83.8% of the men [95% confidence interval: 81.4–86.0]!). In addition, 60.8% of the women had an AHI greater than 5. This study used new nasal pressure sensors able to detect small variations in airflow, whereas older studies used less sensitive thermistors. Additionally, the HypnoLaus Study employed the more liberal 2012 AASM definition of hypopnea (3% desaturation). However, neither the flow sensors nor the AASM scoring criterion fully explained these results. Participants in this study were otherwise healthy, non-obese (BMI 25.6) adults between 40 and 85 years old. And yet out of the 2,121 participants, 72% of them had an AHI greater than 5. Additional findings of this study indicated that an AHI greater than 20.6 events per hour was independently associated with the presence of hypertension, diabetes mellitus, metabolic syndrome, and depression.

The HypnoLaus study is not the only one to present proof that the incidence of OSA in the general population has been underestimated. In 2010, a study[24] from São Paulo, Brazil, including 1,042 participants (aged 20 to 80 years) found that 46.6% of men and 30.5% of women had an AHI greater than 5. This São Paulo study also used the new airflow sensors to measure nasal pressure and showed that 32.8% of participants had OSA syndrome. It should be noted that the nasal sensors used in these studies are currently the standard technique used in all modern clinical sleep laboratories.

Sadly, children are not immune to airway issues. It has been estimated that 10% of all children suffer from some form of SRBD. A recent study on SRBDs in children seeking orthodontic treatment found that "approximately 7% of adolescent orthodontic patients may be at significant risk for some form of sleep-disordered breathing."[25] Most of these patients exhibit pronounced snoring or wheezing during sleep. These children may exhibit craniofacial dystrophy, lymphatic hypertrophy in the form of enlarged tonsils or adenoids, narrow arches, and vaulted palates. Some, but not all, are obese.

Growth hormones are primarily released during sleep, so disrupted sleep may inhibit normal growth. Children with OSA frequently present with symptoms of bruxism, mouth breathing, tongue thrusting, and bedwetting and may be failing to thrive. These children frequently have an existing diagnosis of attention deficit hyperactivity disorder (ADHD), which is a mental disorder characterized by excessive activity, problems paying attention, or difficulty controlling inappropriate behavior. Children with airway issues often exhibit chronic fatigue, which displays as hyperactivity and frequently causes problems in school. Therapy for children with OSA can include adenotonsillectomy, CPAP, myofunctional appliance therapy, and maxillary expansion orthodontic therapy.[26]

Given the results of the epidemiologic studies on the prevalence of SRBDs, we can conservatively conclude that 25% or more of dental patients have OSA. It has been estimated that only 15% of patients who suffer from OSA have been diagnosed; therefore, OSA is a significant underdiagnosed and undertreated chronic disease in the United States. Now is the time for dentists to join our physician colleagues in tackling this devastating disease.

Why Are We So Sleepy?

There are many reasons people are sleepy, and not all are related to SRBDs. Insomnia is the most commonly diagnosed sleep disorder, mostly because non-sleep physicians are more comfortable making this diagnosis. However, it is frequently comorbid with OSA. Insomnia, also known as *sleeplessness*, is a disorder where patients have difficulty falling asleep or staying asleep as long as desired. Insomnia typically results in daytime sleepiness, low energy, irritability, and a depressed mood. It may result in an increased risk of motor vehicle accidents and problems focusing and learning. Insomnia can be short term, lasting for days or weeks, or long term, lasting for months or years. Conditions that frequently produce insomnia include OSA, psychologic stress, chronic pain, heart failure, hyperthyroidism, heartburn, restless leg syndrome, menopause, certain medications, and drugs such as caffeine, nicotine, and alcohol. Insomnia can also be directly associated with jet lag or working a night shift or swing shift. Diagnosis is based on history, sleep habits, and an examination to look for underlying causes. The definitive test for insomnia is a Multiple Sleep Latency Test performed in a sleep lab. It is expensive and burdensome and becoming less frequently performed. Screening may be performed with two questions: *(1)* Do you have trouble sleeping? *(2)* Do you have difficulty falling or staying asleep?

Americans seem to place a low priority on sleep. Our lifestyles glorify long hours of work and study in the pursuit of prosperity. Americans have bought into the cultural norm that sleep deprivation is an essential element in achieving success. These choices can lead to the most obvious symptom—excessive daytime sleepiness (EDS).

EDS is typically determined by the Epworth Sleepiness Scale (ESS). The ESS is widely used in the field of sleep medicine as a subjective measure of a patient's overall sleepiness. The test consists of a list of eight situations in which patients rate their tendency to become sleepy on a scale of 0 (no chance of dozing) to 3 (high chance of dozing). The scale estimates whether a patient is experiencing excessive sleepiness that may require medical attention.[25] Typically, a patient with OSAS has an AHI greater than 5 and an ESS of at least 10. Subsequent chapters discuss screening methods and the use of the ESS, and conscientious dental practitioners should be aware of the various causes of sleep deprivation and the resultant EDS. However, screening patient populations for OSA based on levels of sleepiness can be unproductive. Other methods of screening seem to result in better specificity.

CPAP Therapy: The Gold Standard?

CPAP has remained the gold standard for treating OSA for many years. CPAP works by administering a constant and continuous stream of air under pressure delivered through a mask (interface) worn over the nose or nose and mouth. The pressure is set to prevent collapse in the oropharynx from negative respiratory pressure. When used, CPAP is the most effective means of preventing closure of the airway, thus reducing AHI. However, adherence to therapy is a real problem.[27]

Medicare considers a patient to be compliant with CPAP when it is used 4 hours per night at least 5 nights per week. All CPAP devices record time of use and many other details of adherence to therapy. If patients sleep 8 hours per night for 7 nights (56 hours of sleep per week), patients minimally compliant with CPAP must use the CPAP machine for 20 hours per week to be 36% compliant (20/56 hours). If an OSA patient uses the CPAP machine 36% of the time, Medicare continues to pay for the machine, but imagine if patients brushed only a little over a third of their teeth—those teeth would be healthy, but what about the rest of the mouth?

Compliance with CPAP is unacceptably low, with many studies reporting ranges as low as 25% full compliance over 1 year. This lack of CPAP compliance is a depressing statistic. The health of millions of patients is dependent on a better solution. Lack of compliance is due to various issues, including but not limited to mask leakage, latex allergies, claustrophobia, sinus problems, sleep fragmentation due to mask- and pressure-related arousals, and the stigma of wearing the device. Patients with more severe OSA and more perceived symptoms (sleepiness, snoring, witnessed apnea) are also the most likely to adhere to therapy. Mild OSA, AHI with predominantly experienced hypopnea, and lack of perceived benefit correlate with early abandonment of CPAP therapy.

The treatment of OSA has been further complicated by an FDA Class 1 recall of Philips Respironics CPAPs, BiPAPs, respirators, and ventilators. Philips Respironics produced approximately 80% of CPAPs available in the United States, and the recall has greatly hampered the treatment of OSA, as CPAP is the first line of therapy prescribed by the vast majority of physicians. An FDA Class 1 recall is the most serious type of recall, indicating that the continued use of Philips Respironics CPAPs and BiPAPs could cause serious injuries or death. The CPAPs were recalled due to the breakdown of sound proofing insulation, which could be aspirated into the lungs of the user. As of this writing, hundreds of deaths have been attributed to this failure, and many patients are still waiting for a replacement CPAP.

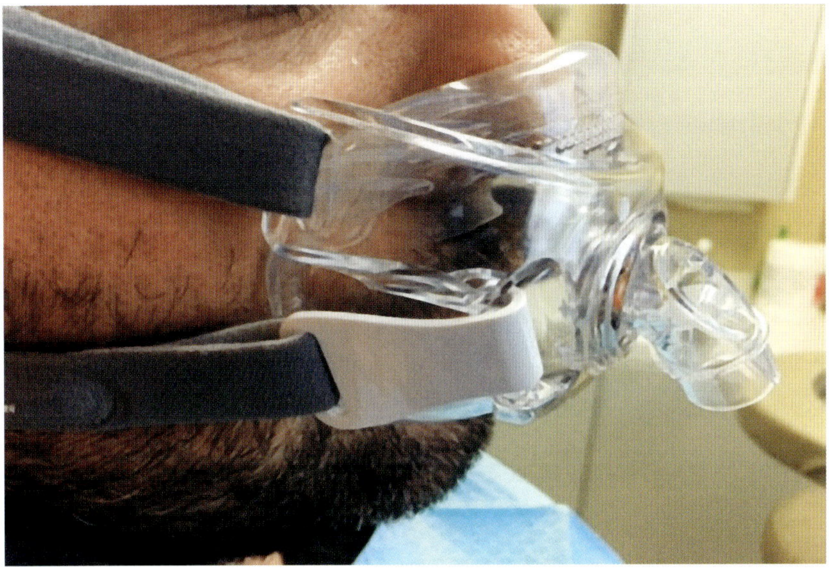

Fig 1-7 A patient is fitted for a MAD that will be used in combination with his CPAP machine. The MAD can be used when no electricity is available and allows for a reduction in air pressure.

Fortunately, CPAP is not the only treatment for SRBDs. By modifying or enlarging the upper airway with the assistance of surgery, orthodontics, or a MAD, nocturnal oxygenation can be maintained, thereby improving the quality and quantity of sleep. There is a significant opportunity for dentists to provide viable alternative therapy. OAT results in much better adherence to therapy than CPAP, although this is generally according to patient reports rather than objective data. MAD therapy may not be as efficacious in lowering AHI as CPAP, but increased compliance, in most cases, results in comparable therapeutic results[28] (Fig 1-7). There are many reasons patients prefer OAT to CPAP, but no therapy is universally accepted. The best choice of treatment is the one the patient will use to maintain an open airway during the largest percentage of sleep time.

References

1. Adult Obesity Maps. Centers for Disease Control and Prevention, 2023. https://www.cdc.gov/obesity/php/data-research/adult-obesity-prevalence-maps.html. Accessed 7 Feb 2024.
2. González BNO, Plascencia NR, Zapata JAP, et al. Obesity hypoventilation syndrome, literature review. Sleep Adv 2024;5:zpae033.

3. Schmid KM, Kugler R, Nalabothu P, Bosch C, Verna C. The effect of pacifier sucking on orofacial structures: A systematic literature review. Prog Orthod 2018;19:8.
4. Zahrin D. Delaying and seeking care for obstructive sleep apnea: The role of gender, family, and morality. Health (London) 2018;22:36–53.
5. Namen AM, Forest DJ, Huang KE, et al. Physicians report sleep apnea infrequently in older and older vulnerable adults. J Am Geriatr Soc 2017;65:2023–2028.
6. Ruehland WR, Rochford PD, O'Donoghue FJ, Pierce RJ, Singh P, Thornton AT. The new AASM criteria for scoring hypopneas: Impact on the apnea hypopnea index. Sleep 2009;32:150–157.
7. White DP. Sleep-related breathing disorder. 2. Pathophysiology of obstructive sleep apnoea. Thorax 1995;50:797–804.
8. Kryger MH, Roth T, Dement WC. Principles and Practice of Sleep Medicine, ed 6. Elsevier, 2017.
9. Lee-Chiong TL. Somnology 2: Learn Sleep Medicine in One Weekend. CreateSpace, 2011.
10. Mass M. Obstructive sleep apnea and risk of COVID-19 infection, hospitalization and respiratory failure. Sleep Breath 2021;25:1155–1157.
11. American Dental Association. The Role of Dentistry in the Treatment of Sleep Related Breathing Disorders. https://www.ada.org/-/media/project/ada-organization/ada/ada-org/files/resources/research/the-role-of-dentistry-in-sleep-related-breathing-disorders.pdf. Accessed 2 Feb 2024.
12. Obstructive sleep apnea syndrome. In: American Academy of Sleep Medicine. The International Classification of Sleep Disorders. American Academy of Sleep Medicine, 2001.
13. Berry RB, Gamalda CE, Harding SM, et al. AASM scoring manual version 2.2 updates: New chapters for scoring infant sleep staging and home sleep apnea testing. J Clin Sleep Med 2015;11:1253–1254.
14. Shahar E. Apnea-hypopnea index: Time to wake up. Nat Sci Sleep 2014;6:51–56.
15. Azarbarzin A, Sands SA, Stone KL, et al. The hypoxic burden of sleep apnoea predicts cardiovascular disease-related mortality: The Osteoporotic Fractures in Men Study and the Sleep Heart Health Study. Eur Heart J 2019;40:1149–1157 [erratum 2019;40:1157].
16. Shahrbabaki SS, Linz D, Hartmann S, Redline S, Baumert M. Sleep arousal burden is associated with long-term all-cause and cardiovascular mortality in 8001 community-dwelling older men and women. Eur Heart J 2021;42:2088–2099.
17. Parekh A, Kam K, Wickramaratne S, et al. Ventilatory burden as a measure of obstructive sleep apnea severity is predictive of cardiovascular and all-cause mortality. Am J Respir Crit Care Med 2023;208:1216–1226.
18. The Price of Fatigue: The Surprising Economic Costs of Unmanaged Sleep Apnea. The Harvard Medical School Division of Sleep Medicine, 2010. https://sleep.med.harvard.edu/what-we-do/public-policy-research. Accessed 2 Feb 2024.
19. Young T, Palta M, Dempsey J, Skatrud J, Weber S, Badr S. The occurrence of sleep-disordered breathing among middle-aged adults. N Engl J Med 1993;328:1230–1235.
20. Quan SF, Howard BV, Iber C, et al. The Sleep Heart Health Study: Design, rationale, and methods. Sleep 1997;20:1077–1085.
21. Bixler EO, Vgontzas AN, Lin HM. Prevalence of sleep related breathing disorders in women: Effects of gender. Am J Respir Crit Care Med 2001;163:608–613.
22. Peppard PE, Young T, Barnet JH, Palta M, Hagen EW, Hla KM. Increased prevalence of sleep related breathing disorders in adults. Am J Epidemiol 2013;177:1006–1014.
23. Heinzer R, Vat S, Marques-Vidal P, et al. Prevalence of sleep related breathing disorders in the general population: The HypnoLaus study. Lancet Respir Med 2015;3:310–318.
24. Tufik S, Santos-Silva R, Taddei JA, Bittencourt LR. Obstructive sleep apnea syndrome in the Sao Paulo epidemiologic sleep study. Sleep Med 2010;11:441–446.
25. Rohra AK Jr, Demko CA, Hans MG, Rosen C, Palomo JM. Sleep disordered breathing in children seeking orthodontic care. Am J Orthod Dentofacial Orthop 2018;154:65–71.
26. Moreira GA, Pradella-Hallinan M. Sleepiness in children: An update. Sleep Med Clin 2017;12:407–413.

27. Gulati A, Ali M, Davies M, Quinnell T, Smith I. A prospective observational study to evaluate the effect of social and personality factors on continuous positive airway pressure (CPAP) compliance in obstructive sleep apnoea syndrome. BMC Pulm Med 2017;17:56.
28. Sharples LD, Clutterbuck-James AL, Glover MJ, et al. Meta-analysis of randomized controlled trials of oral mandibular advancement devices and continuous positive airway pressure for obstructive sleep apnoea-hypopnoea. Sleep Med Rev 2016;27:108–124

Sleep is that golden chain that ties health and our bodies together.

—Thomas Dekker

2

An Overview of Sleep and Sleep Disorders

Sleep can be defined as a naturally recurring periodic suspension or alteration of consciousness during which the body and nervous system are restored. Sleep is characterized by an inhibition of sensory input, an inhibition of voluntary skeletal muscle activity, and a marked reduction of metabolic processes. Sleep is a rapidly reversible state of sensory reduction and stereotypic posture. During sleep there is a significant reduction in the individual's ability to respond to external stimuli.[1]

Because breathing disorders were first identified during sleep, and that is when the airway is unprotected, they were labeled as a type of sleep disorder and studied by both neurologists and pulmonologists. This chapter primarily considers the neurologic implications of sleep-related breathing disorders (SRBDs). Primary care dentists do not need to become brain scientists or lung experts to fulfill their role in treating these disorders, but a working knowledge of both subjects helps for communicating with colleagues in medicine.

Why Do We Sleep?

Until technologic advances allowed for more specific information to be gathered about what happens during sleep, scientists and physicians knew very little about sleep. Physiologists can now track changes in the immune system, brain activity, hormone production, and mitochondrial activity, along with countless other details associated with a rhythm that generally follows a light/

dark cycle. By studying brainwave details, fluid circulation changes, blood flow clues, the anatomy, and a myriad of other data together with advanced imaging such as functional MRI, neuroscientists have now unlocked many (though far from most) of the mysteries of brain function.

Many features of sleep appear to have a purpose. It has been shown that nearly every animal species, including one-celled organisms, has a cycle that can be detected as a waxing and waning of physiologic processes. As the complexity of the organism increases, this cycle becomes more recognizable as what we think of as sleep. This cycle varies widely depending on the living conditions of the species. For example, marine mammals would drown if their brains were not programmed to bring them to the surface for respiration periodically. To enable this activity while still allowing the brain to rest and regenerate, half the marine mammal brain is asleep at a time, switching partway through the rest period. Other animal species retain optic input in one half of the brain to keep an eye out for predators while the other half of the brain's visual cortex shuts down, also reversing during the quiescent period.[2] Humans have a recognizable quiescent period labeled sleep, during which the cortex of the brain is insulated from most somatic and sensory input. These inputs remain vital to the autonomic nervous system (ANS), however, and are critical to homeostasis. The filter between the ANS and the subcortical and cortical regions is the limbic system.

Functions of sleep

Sleep provides the brain and body time for many critical functions free from the need to maintain homeostasis in response to the activities of wakefulness. Sleep is both a function of the brain and a function for the brain. It is generated and maintained by central neural networks using specific neurotransmitters in distinct areas of the brain and is central to the development and optimal operation of the brain. Deep sleep is required for the removal of metabolic toxins generated during wakefulness, as well as for protective and adaptive behavior and immune defense.

The human body physically restores itself during sleep. During sleep, most of the systems in the body are in an anabolic state of repair.[3] This directly contributes to healing and restoration of the immune, skeletal, nervous, and muscular systems. Additionally, the healing processes that occur during sleep include the removal of waste products that build up during periods of activity. Physical restoration and healing appear to take place primarily during slow-wave (non–rapid eye movement [NREM] stage 3 [N3]) sleep, during which body temperature, heart rate, and brain oxygen consumption decrease. Evidence is

TABLE 2-1 How much sleep people really need

Age	Sleep need
Newborns (0–2 months)	12–18 hours
Infants (3–11 months)	14–15 hours
Toddlers (1–3 years)	12–14 hours
Preschoolers (3–5 years)	11–13 hours
School-age children (5–10 years)	10–11 hours
Preteens and teens (10–17 years)	8.5–9.25 hours
Adults	7–9 hours

(Data from National Sleep Foundation.[3])

mounting that neurologic repair may occur primarily during rapid eye movement (REM) sleep. What can be definitively stated is that it is vitally important for patients to achieve deeper levels of sleep and allow the natural circadian rhythm to flow without interruption.

Dreaming

Numerous theories have been hypothesized to explain the mechanism and function of dreaming. Dreaming can occur in any stage of sleep, but dreams seem to be more vivid and violent during REM sleep. Dreams may be generated by the random firing of neurons in the cerebral cortex during this period. The use of antidepressants, acetaminophen, ibuprofen, or alcoholic beverages may result in the suppression of dreams, whereas the use of melatonin may result in an increase in dreams. SRBDs are most commonly manifested during REM sleep due to atonia of the airway-protective muscles. A very common quality of life improvement reported in our practices is for patients to say, "I'm dreaming again!" when an SRBD is reduced or eliminated. Presumably, this is because the patient's REM periods are becoming more common and memory consolidation is more effective.

Sleep time

Sleep is deemed to be adequate when there is no daytime sleepiness or dysfunction without a known cause. Many patients voluntarily restrict sleep time as a lifestyle choice. A careful history can help set proper expectations for any therapy associated with sleep. No matter how well an oral device protects the airway, if a patient is not spending sufficient time asleep, some symptoms will persist. The amount of sleep needed varies by age, diminishing as people get older (Table 2-1). Mature adults generally spend less time in deeper levels of sleep, and their sleep tends to be more fragmented. However, in general, adults should strive for 8 hours of sleep each night. Researchers have determined that sleeping 7 to 8 hours each night is directly related to increased life expectancy and improved cardiac health.[4] Though some individuals claim that they can function well on 5 hours of sleep or less, research has not proven this to be true. Neurocognitive deficits seem to increase proportionally with increased sleep deprivation,[5] which is particularly worrisome when considering the trucking and commercial airline industries.[6]

Sleep Stages

Building on the discovery of electrical signals in the brains of animals, Hans Berger, a German scientist, recorded the first electrical signals in human brains in 1924, and by 1934 he had invented the electroencephalogram (EEG), a device that changed neurology forever.[2] Scientists used EEGs to test humans at all times of the day and night, resulting in the identification of characteristic brainwaves that directly correlate with certain physiologic states. Combining EEG frequencies and amplitude with observed physical characteristics (eg, eye movements, paralysis, blood pressure, heart rate, respiration, and temperature) resulted in the discovery and definition of the various sleep stages. While circadian rhythms have been described in both plants and animals since ancient times, with the discovery of the EEG, it became possible to accurately measure brain activity associated with distinct circadian disruption. The measurable effects of light and darkness on sleep patterns began to emerge. With this improved ability to describe normal sleep patterns, the ability to identify sleep disorders became the foundation of sleep medicine as a subspecialty.

A brainwave is the summation of the electrical activity of numerous neurons. Rapid fluctuations of voltage occur between various parts of the brain, and their frequency, amplitude, and shape can be described. EEGs can be used to record this electrical activity and the action potentials during sleep. Each stage of sleep has a recognizable wave pattern that can be used to assess the patient's level of consciousness or depth of sleep.

Sleep occurs in repeating cycles known as REM and non-REM, and specific body activities are characteristically found in these distinct stages. The scientific definitions of these states rely on the electrical signals. Some technologies, including consumer sleep devices and professional, FDA-cleared testing systems, use surrogate electrical signal patterns. Algorithms using other, more easily obtained biodata have been built to describe sleep states without the need for surface electrodes on the head. This enhanced technology reduces the barriers to testing, which is beneficial for improving population health.

Non-REM

Non-REM (NREM), sleep is further divided into N1, N2, and N3 stages, which are defined entirely by brainwave changes. Other physiologic features are common to each stage, but the only way to label any patient's sleep pattern with precision is to know the brainwave pattern; this is what sleep technologists and sleep physicians are trained to look for. Sleep stages are determined by the frequency of the predominant wave pattern in any time segment, or epoch, of the recordings during sleep.

N1

N1 is a transition from wakefulness to sleep. Alpha waves observed during wakefulness diminish, and a mixed pattern emerges. Muscle activity diminishes (as recorded via electromyogram [EMG]), and ocular activity (as recorded via electrooculogram [EOG]) begins to show a slow-rolling eye movement pattern. N1 sleep occupies 3% to 8% of normal sleep time. During N1 sleep, patients maintain some awareness of their surroundings and, if awakened during this stage, may think that they were never asleep.

N1 can be characterized by hypnagogic sensations that consist of an array of neurologic and sensory experiences as a direct response to sleep initiation or awakening from sleep. These neurologic effects can range from mild or barely perceptible imagery to vivid hallucinations. Additionally, there can be motor responses in the form of hypnic jerks, or "sleep starts," and a sense of falling. These are involuntary twitches involving few or many muscle groups that frequently cause the patient to arouse during sleep initiation. There is a sympathetic nervous system surge—a transient rapid heartbeat, quickened breathing, sweating, and a spike in blood pressure. They can be worrisome to the person and to the bed partner but do not represent any known pathology, and there is no need for treatment other than reassurance.

N2

N2 is the beginning of true sleep, making up between 45% and 55% of sleep time. During this stage, eye movements diminish and brainwaves become slower. There are also brief bursts of rapid brain activity called sleep spindles. EMG activity is diminished. The patient loses all sense of his or her surroundings and is more difficult to arouse. Sleep is now controlled by the parasympathetic nervous system, which results in a decrease in core body temperature, blood pressure, and heart rate. The brain is preparing itself for deeper sleep.

N3

N3 is deep sleep, or the period during which delta waves occur. Delta waves are a type of high-amplitude brainwave found in humans with a frequency of 1 to 4 hertz (Hz) that are thought to emerge from the thalamus. During N3 sleep, delta waves make up more than 20% of EEG activity, with limited EOG activity. It should be noted that N3 designates a combination of the older labels of sleep stages 3 and 4, referring to sleep during which all the brainwaves are high amplitude and low frequency.

N3 makes up between 15% and 20% of total sleep time, and the majority of N3 sleep occurs during the first 3 hours of sleep. Muscle tone is decreased even more than during N2. People in N3 sleep are difficult to wake up. When aroused from N3 sleep, they may be groggy and disoriented for several minutes.

N3 is the stage during which most growth hormones are released, making it imperative that children receive significant amounts of N3 sleep. Some researchers hypothesize that the body repairs itself during N3 sleep. Deep sleep is important for a patient to feel refreshed in the morning. If insufficient time is spent in N3, sleep will not feel satisfying. As we age, the total amount of N3 sleep we receive is markedly reduced, and N1 is alternatively increased. This may partially explain why elderly patients have difficulty maintaining sleep.

REM

"Eye pops" or rapid eye jerks are the most identifiable characteristic of REM sleep. When brainwave patterns were correlated with these observations, the science of sleep medicine was born. During REM sleep, the brain is nearly as active as during wakefulness; it takes a trained observer of the two EEG signals to distinguish them when placed side by side. Besides the ocular motion, the other defining characteristic of REM sleep is body paralysis. Patients experiencing REM sleep undergo paralysis (muscle atonia) of the larger muscle groups. The diaphragm, heart, and a few vital sphincters are unaffected, but skeletal and smooth muscle tone is nearly extinguished by inhibitory signals within the motor nerve centers in the central nervous system.[3] REM sleep is characterized by low-voltage, mixed-frequency EEG waves, with possible saw-toothed theta activity. Each REM session should have at least one identifiable instance of rapid eye movement. Some researchers believe that the brain and nervous system repair themselves during REM sleep.

Reading Sleep Studies

This section helps sleep dentists understand what is measured during polysomnography (PSG) in a sleep lab. These data are usually unavailable from

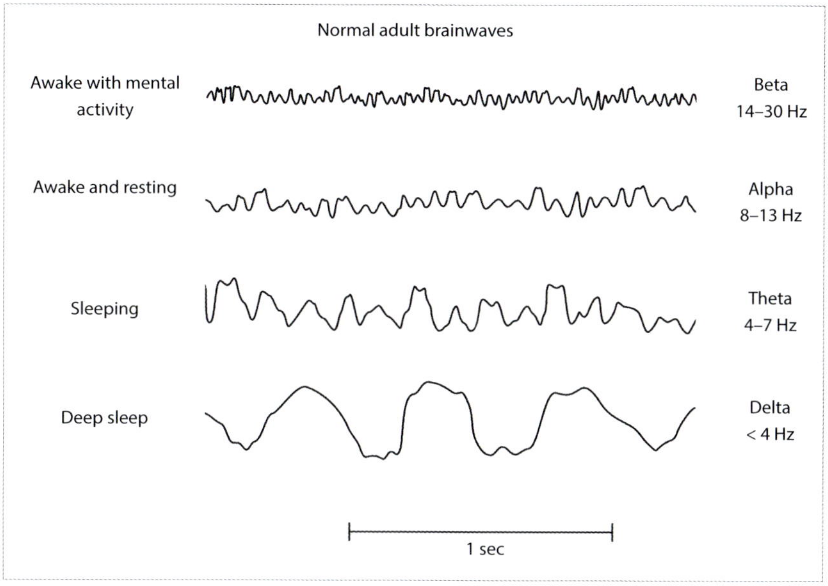

Fig 2-1 EEG activity during sleep and wakefulness.

most home sleep apnea tests (HSATs), but dentists may have reason to read a detailed sleep study or get involved in a conversation with a registered polysomnographic technologist (RPSGT) or sleep physician. By arming themselves with a working knowledge of sleep study details, dentists can establish themselves as credible and interested colleagues.

EEG wave frequencies

Basic EEG wave frequencies during sleep and wakefulness are measured in Hz (Fig 2-1):

- Delta waves (< 4 Hz): Patient is in N3 sleep, increased amplitude (> 75 µV), decreased frequency
- Theta waves (4–7 Hz): N1 to N3 and REM sleep
- Alpha waves (8–13 Hz): Patient awake with eyes closed, amplitude < 50 µV
- Beta waves (> 13 Hz): Patient awake and alert, decreased amplitude, increased frequency

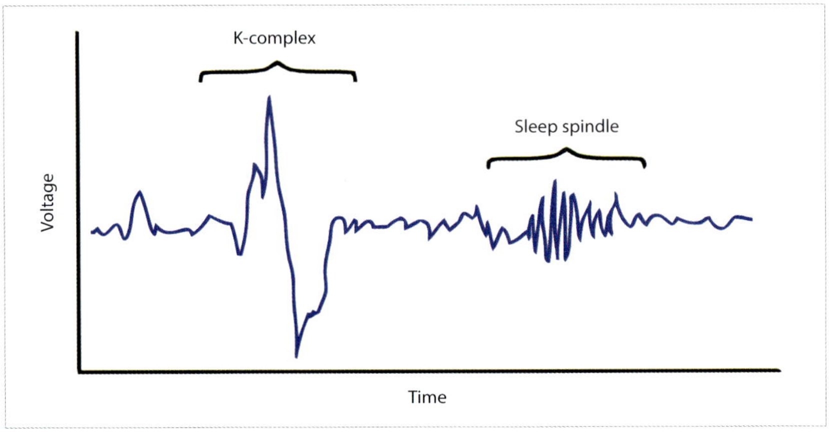

Fig 2-2 Example of a K-complex and a sleep spindle during N2 sleep, when eye movement stops and brainwaves become slower.

- EEG waveforms:
  - K-complex: Present in N2 sleep (Fig 2-2); increased amplitude, biphasic wave (an initial sharp negative deflection immediately followed by a positive high-voltage slow wave) with duration of ≥ 2 Hz; seen in the central and frontal leads
  - Saw-toothed waves: Present in REM sleep; theta waves with a notched waveform; prominent in vertex and frontal leads
  - Sleep spindles: Seen in N2 and N3 sleep (see Fig 2-2); brief oscillations with a frequency of 12–14 Hz lasting 0.5–1.5 seconds with an amplitude of < 50 μV; "pseudospindles" or "drug spindles" related to benzodiazepine, alcohol, or barbiturate use can be distinguished due to a higher frequency (≥ 15 Hz)

Scoring sleep stages

PSG data are divided into 30-second time periods or epochs. Each epoch is assigned a single sleep stage that makes up the majority or greatest percentage of the epoch (Fig 2-3).

STAGE W: WAKE

- > 50% of the epoch has alpha EEG waves over the occipital region with the patient's eyes closed.
- High chin EMG tone.

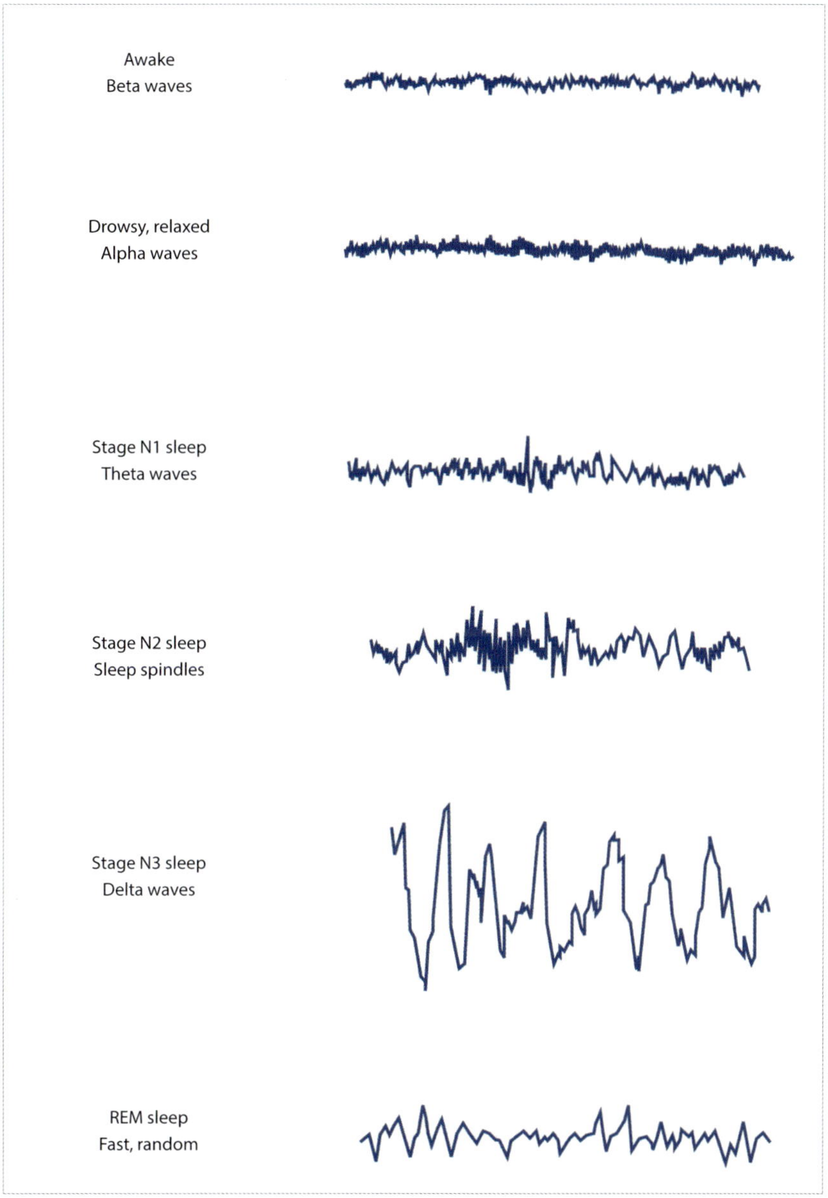

Fig 2-3 Sleep stage waves.

- During the transition from wake to N1 sleep, rolling eye movements, also referred to as reading eye movements, are common (conjugate slow movement followed by a rapid movement in the opposite direction).

STAGE N1

- Alpha waves are replaced by low-amplitude, mixed-frequency (4–7 Hz) waves that occupy > 50% of the epoch.
- Absence of K-complexes and sleep spindles.
- Tonic chin EMG levels are typically lower than during relaxed wakefulness.

STAGE N2

- The start of stage N2 is defined by the presence of K-complexes (not associated with arousals) or sleep spindles during the first half of the epoch or during the last half of the previous epoch if the criteria for stage N3 are absent (see Fig 2-2).
- The continuation of stage N2 is defined by the presence of low-amplitude, mixed-frequency EEG rhythms and the epoch containing, or being preceded by, K-complexes or sleep spindles.
- Scoring of stage N2 is terminated when the epoch is scored as W, N3, or REM or when arousals or major body movements are followed by N1 (low-amplitude, mixed-frequency EEG).

STAGE N3

- ≥ 20% of the epoch (≥ 6 seconds) is occupied by slow-wave (0.5–2 Hz and > 75 μV) EEG activity over the frontal regions.

STAGE R: REM

- Presence of the following:
  - EEG: Low-amplitude, mixed-frequency activity
  - EOG: Rapid eye movement
  - Chin EMG: Low tone (lowest level in the study or at least no higher than the other sleep stages)
- REM sleep can be either tonic (without rapid eye movements or muscle twitches) or phasic (with rapid eye movements and muscle twitches).

A hypnogram is a pictorial representation of the stages of sleep that occur during an overnight PSG (Fig 2-4). The time of sleep is represented on the horizontal *x*-axis running from sleep onset on the left until the patient awakens on the far right. The vertical *y*-axis shows which stage of sleep the patient was in at any given time during the night. The sleep stages represented are wake (W), stage 1 (N1), stage 2 (N2), stage 3 (N3), and REM. Hypnograms are routinely included on all PSGs.

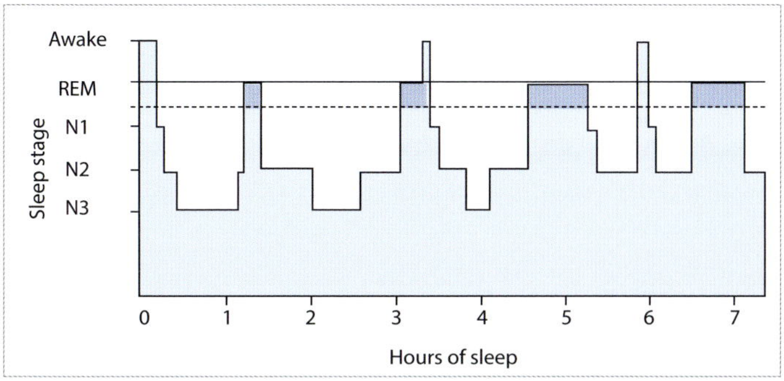

Fig 2-4 Hypnogram illustrating the stages of sleep experienced over the course of an overnight PSG.

By accepting these scientifically defined stages as the medical norm, disease is identified when signals fall outside the agreed upon parameters. Because these data are used to define normal sleep, any sleep testing technology that cannot determine whether a patient is asleep (eg, HSAT, pulse oximetry, and consumer wearable devices) cannot provide an Apnea-Hypopnea Index (AHI) with the same accuracy as an in-lab PSG. Current at-home testing employs questionable labels of sleep time and staging using nonstandard definitions. This can lead to confusion between medical professionals and scientists during research or even when discussing clinical findings for patient care decisions. Recent studies have also shown night-to-night variability in sleep data measurements that must be considered when assessing sleep parameters for diagnosis and treatment efficacy. Any one single night in a sleep lab or at home may not be representative of the general quality of sleep and sleep breathing the patient experiences. Clinicians must keep this in mind when using home-based measurements.

Sleep and Wake Neurotransmitters

Sleep and wake states are controlled by certain wake- and sleep-promoting neurotransmitters. The main wake-promoting neurotransmitters include serotonin, norepinephrine, hypocretin (orexin), glutamate, acetylcholine, dopamine, and histamine. The main sleep-promoting neurotransmitters include acetylcholine (wake and REM neurotransmitter), melatonin, glycine, galanin, gamma-aminobutyric acid (GABA), adenosine, growth hormone, interleukin-1β

(IL-1β), nitric oxide, prostaglandin D2 (PGD2), tumor necrosis factor α (TNF-α), and vasoactive intestinal peptide. Acetylcholine is the main REM sleep neurotransmitter, and GABA is the main NREM neurotransmitter. The inhibition or secretion of the appropriate neurotransmitter promotes either wakefulness or sleep/sedation. For example, adenosine is a sleep neurotransmitter whose levels progressively increase during sustained wake periods, contributing to the sleep drive part of the circadian rhythm. Caffeine is an adenosine receptor blocker, which results in increased wakefulness and decreased EEG slow-wave activity during sleep. Diphenhydramine is a first-generation histamine-1 receptor blocker that results in sleepiness and mild sedation. There are many examples of how sleep and wake neurotransmitters are inhibited or potentiated to achieve physiologic outcomes.[7]

Sleep Disorders and Airway Management

The *International Classification of Sleep Disorders*[8] describes the various diagnoses available to physicians when evaluating a given patient. Now in its third edition (*ICSD-3*), this classification includes dozens of distinct labels to be applied to a set of clinical findings and patient presentations. Dentists involved in sleep medicine treat two of these conditions directly: obstructive sleep apnea (OSA) and a movement disorder called sleep bruxism. Of course, this dental treatment is not curative but rather management, as most therapy is not aimed at the etiology but rather at the clinical expression of the problem. A critical part of OSA management is airway therapy. Ongoing clinical observation and emerging scientific studies are also documenting the expanded usefulness of maintaining an open airway in the presence of other sleep diseases, so airway therapy may become a recognized part of treatment of other *ICSD-3* diseases.

To date, the predominant choice for airway therapy in the United States is positive airway pressure (PAP) in its various forms. Physicians diagnose sleep-disordered breathing (SDB) and prescribe PAP therapy, and they rely on dentists for the fabrication of custom mandibular advancement devices (MADs). Any dentist interested in providing this therapy is expected to be well trained on airway issues, including the anatomy, physiology, response, and resolution of tissues under stress. Although these subjects are covered in dental school, practicing dentists often have not thought about the anatomy of the upper airway in many years or have avoided patients with temporomandibular disorders. It is incumbent upon dental professionals, however, to be able to think three-dimensionally about the area they are treating and to be ready to manage airway and stomatognathic complications that might arise.

Fig 2-5 Nasal endoscopy.

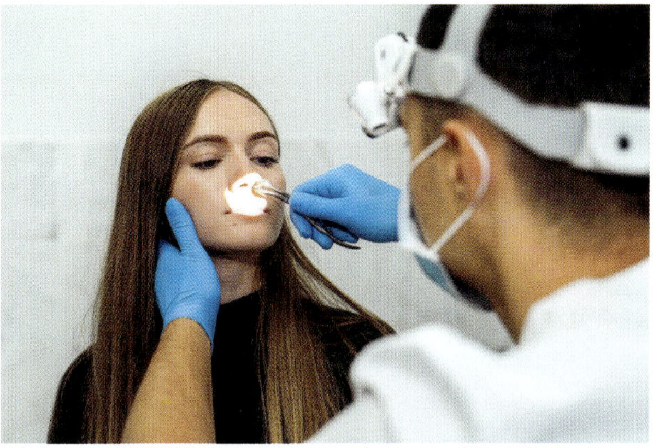

Airway anatomy

The nasal airway, from the external nasal valve (nares) to the top of the palate, is a complex area that is generally unaffected by normal respiratory pressure changes after growth completion. Before the onset of puberty, breathing patterns and airflow have profound influences on the shape of the growing skeletal structure of the craniofacial respiratory complex. Airflow through the nasal airway can be restricted by tissue changes, such as with allergic rhinitis, or improved by mechanical dilators, decongestants, and surgery. Because the nasal mucosa and the underlying tissues do not move in the same way as the more flexible oropharynx, however, the nasal airway retains a mostly constant lumen and functional anatomy.

Airflow through the nose can be measured using rhinomanometry. This easy-to-use device provides a graphical representation of inhalation and exhalation patterns. Data from rhinomanometry is used to establish a nasal phenotype. Understanding nasal function is very useful when determining the appropriate therapy or discussing results (see chapter 16).

The epiglottis can become a source of airway obstruction when it is malformed, has a neuromuscular deficit that affects its position and function, or is pushed out of place. Larger nearby tissues, such as a tumor, hypertrophic lingual tonsils, or the base of the tongue if it is oversized or pushed into the airway due to malformed craniofacial bones, can distort the resting posture or function of the epiglottis. Epiglottal dysfunction is relatively easy to spot with a nasal endoscope, but it is usually discovered only when other treatments are inexplicably insufficient and an ear, nose, and throat (ENT) physician is consulted (Fig 2-5). Because the larynx and trachea are rigid, respiratory pressure changes do not affect their lumens.

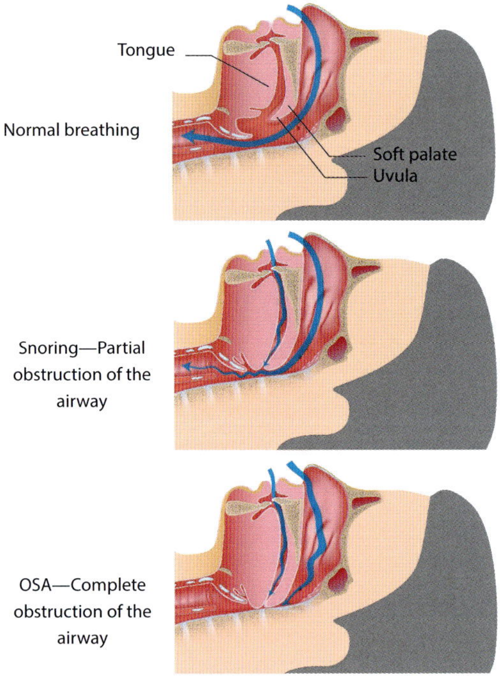

Fig 2-6 Illustration of the airway during normal breathing, snoring, and OSA.

Between the soft palate and the epiglottis lies the oropharynx, bordered on the dorsal by the spine and posterior pharyngeal muscles. These muscles are thin and attached somewhat firmly to the spine. The ventral two-thirds of the lumen of the oropharynx is made up of mucosa backed with muscle, fascia, and ligaments. The collapsible oropharynx is both a defining feature of the human—allowing for traits such as speech and emotional expression—and a specific weakness of the respiratory system. In susceptible individuals, the pressure changes of respiration create a narrowing or complete obstruction of the oropharynx. The negative pressure required to close the airway is the critical closing pressure (Pcrit). This can be measured using special equipment but is rarely done in clinical practice. Despite being a free-moving bone, the mandible is connected, directly or indirectly, to all the tissues of the oropharynx. When a person lies down to sleep in the supine position, gravity can draw the mandible down and back, diminishing mechanical support of these tissues. During REM sleep, further loss of muscle tone reduces the dilator effect of airway muscles, requiring less and less inspiratory pressure-drop to pull the walls of the oropharynx together, causing hypopnea, a reduction in airflow, or apnea, cessation of air movement altogether (Fig 2-6). When the body's normal respiration results in oropharyngeal collapse with complete occlusion, this is termed OSA.[4]

MADs use the mandible as a handle to support the ventral oropharyngeal tissues against the collapsing forces generated by respiratory effort. These devices are provided by trained dentists, who are the only medical professionals qualified to evaluate the patient's oral health to determine the appropriateness of this treatment and minimize the potential side effects of oral appliance therapy (OAT).

Sleep disorders

Physicians recognize another state of respiratory disturbance called central sleep apnea (CSA), in which there is no action by the diaphragm or other respiratory muscles. This lack of muscle function represents a respiratory control system deficit rather than a mechanical one. Because the oropharynx may be open or closed, MAD therapy is not indicated for the treatment of CSA. Interestingly, however, because most patients are diagnosed with both CSA and OSA, treating the OSA with MAD therapy also generally results in fewer CSA events scored on follow-up sleep tests.[9] The reasons for this are incompletely understood but are probably related to variations in chemosensitivity to blood carbon dioxide levels in regulatory centers of the central nervous system. CSA events sometimes increase with PAP therapy, a condition called *complex sleep apnea*. This lack of uniform response by patients to therapy is common in sleep medicine, and clinicians must carefully observe treatment outcomes and be ready to change strategies if indicated.

Another sleep-related problem is insomnia. Insomnia includes difficulty falling asleep, difficulty maintaining sleep through the whole night, or just a sense of poor sleep quality, which is typical of many sleep disturbances. Roughly 35% of the US population reports trouble sleeping, but fewer than 1% of those surveyed saw a physician specifically for sleep problems, so the actual number is difficult to state. Many dental patients take prescriptions or over-the-counter medications for sleep.[10] Because sleep quality is generally not included in a dental health history, patients may think any sleep-related complaints are irrelevant; however, asking patients questions about their sleep quality along with the details of their medication history can often lead to the discovery of insomnia complaints. Insomnia is treated by medications, counseling by professionals trained in cognitive behavioral therapy for insomnia (CBT-I), and even with online apps. These online resources are valuable tools for the dentist to suggest.[11] Clinical reports abound where treating an SRBD resulted in fewer complaints of insomnia. The scientific link, however, remains unproven, and patients should not be led to expect this quality of life improvement. In any case, insomnia with an SRBD diagnosis has a name: comorbid insomnia and sleep apnea (COMISA). COMISA is so common that dentists should include questions about insomnia persistence on follow-up assessments with the relevant patients.

When sleep is not quiescent, observation and/or testing can reveal sleep events that lead to a diagnosis falling within one of the many other *ICSD-3* designations, generally labeled *parasomnias*. Parasomnias are in a large category of disorders that include events from NREM sleep, REM sleep, and those unrelated to any specific sleep stage. These events may be neurologic, such as nightmares, or involve movement disorders like sleepwalking. They may involve potentially dangerous acts that stem from REM sleep behavior disorder. The fact that many patients with an SRBD also have parasomnia complaints underscores the value of a collaborative approach to therapy. Managing the airway has no direct effect on the expression of a parasomnia, but removing the sleep disturbance effect of an SRBD often allows the patient's other problems to diminish. This is not always the case, so diligent and detailed history-taking and follow-up is always crucial to therapy.

It is important to realize that there is a medical definition for sleep bruxism and that treatment is performed with MAD therapy and opening the airway. The current consensus between interested clinicians and scientists is that sleep bruxism has a heterogeneous etiology and responds to many types of therapy with unstable resolution. Patients may enjoy many nights with no extra muscle activity only to find themselves wakening with symptoms again, often with no clear triggering event. People with a history of sleep bruxism will be matched better to certain types of MADs than others.

Each of these disturbances to the normal pattern of sleep may produce symptoms in any given patient, some more so than others. Clinicians involved in managing sleep quality must recognize that when sleep is disrupted (whether by an obstructive event, leg movement disorder, or other parasomnia), patients may know only that they have trouble sleeping. If their goal is to improve sleep quality, care teams must identify their individual pathology, called a *phenotype*.

Advances in science are providing more precise ways of labeling sleep disruptions and directing clinicians to recommend more appropriate therapy. The longer a sleep disturbance goes on, the longer normal sleep patterns are disrupted, which may result in the need to not only remove the source of the disturbance but also perform specific procedures to reverse the disruption. In other words, what begins as an upper airway closing problem can reset sleep centers of the brain and produce more than one disruption to homeostasis. CBT-I and coaching about sleep hygiene are often helpful.

Conclusion

Sleep is an endlessly complex part of normal human physiology, with variations so numerous that it is safe to say no two people sleep exactly alike. Any medical professional looking to engage in the treatment of sleep-related disorders is encouraged to learn more about how dental sleep medicine fits into the vast field of sleep medicine. An accessible companion to this text is *Sleep Medicine for Dentists: An Evidence Based Overview,* Second Edition, edited by Giles J. Lavigne, Peter A. Cistulli, and Michael T. Smith (Quintessence, 2020). For more in-depth information, we highly recommend *Principles and Practice of Sleep Medicine,* Seventh Edition, edited by Meir Kryger, Thomas Roth, and William C. Dement (Elsevier, 2022). It is a frequently cited resource in this book and other sleep literature and is updated occasionally with the most current research. *Empowered Sleep Apnea: A Handbook for Patients and the People Who Care about Them* by David E. McCarty and Ellen Stothard (BookBaby, 2022) has valuable information presented in a storytelling style that is very useful for team and patient communication..

References

1. Office of Communications and Public Liaison, National Institute of Neurological Disorders and Stroke. Brain Basics: Understanding Sleep [publication 08-3440-c]. National Institutes of Health, 2017.
2. Kryger MH, Roth T, Dement WC. Principles and Practice of Sleep Medicine, ed 6. Elsevier, 2017.
3. National Sleep Foundation. Sleep-Wake Cycle: Its Physiology and Impact on Health. National Sleep Foundation, 2006.
4. Patel SR, Ayas NT, Malhotra MR, et al. A prospective study of sleep duration and mortality risk in women. Sleep 2004;27:440–444.
5. Gastaut H. The Abnormalities of Sleep in Man. Aulo Gaggi, 1968.
6. O'Hagan AD, Issartel J, McGinley E, Warrington G. A pilot study exploring the effects of sleep deprivation on analogue measures of pilot competencies. Aerosp Med Hum Perform 2018;89:609–615.
7. Swartz BE. The advantages of digital over analog recording techniques. Electroencephalogr Clin Neurophysiol 1998;106:113–117.
8. International Classification of Sleep Disorders, ed 3. American Academy of Sleep Medicine, 2014.
9. Kuzniar TJ, Kovacevic-Ristanovic R, Freedom T. Complex sleep apnea unmasked by the use of mandibular advancement device. Sleep Breath 2011;15:249–252.
10. Walker M. Why We Sleep: Penguin, 2017.
11. Lee-Chiong TL. Sleep Medicine Essentials. Wiley, 2010.

The link between insufficient sleep and chronic disease is now so strong that the Centers for Disease Control and Prevention (CDC) has declared insufficient sleep a public health epidemic.

—Matthew Walker

3

Dental Sleep Medicine Protocols and Practice

Practice Development

Developing a successful dental sleep medicine (DSM) practice depends on many things. Most practitioners new to the field tend to concentrate on aggressive obstructive sleep apnea (OSA) screening techniques that are designed to identify every patient with a potential sleep-related breathing disorder (SRBD) in their practice. However, while screening your present dental population is important, developing a referral-based practice is by far the most important component of building a successful DSM practice. This is because your dental practice has a limited number of patients who suffer from SRBDs. If you do not establish a physician referral network, your DSM practice will collapse after your current patient base and their friends and family have been treated. Dentists need a steady stream of freshly diagnosed patients who need treatment, and that means local sleep doctors must know who you are and why they should trust you. Physician referrals are the only way to sustain a long-term DSM practice.

Going by often-quoted statistics, most practices have between 100 and 250 current patients who have a nocturnal airway issue. These patients are an excellent place to begin your practice and gain clinical confidence, and this first cohort of patients can be the foundation for long-term success. You already have a relationship, there is professional trust, and following successful treatment, they are often eager to promote your practice. Frequently, patients introduced to oral appliance therapy (OAT) by their dentists become enthusiastic ambassadors. The most common reason stated for this is, "No one ever told me about oral devices before." The dentist is seen as a caring hero, and the patient wants to share the story. While it's excellent for them to talk to friends and family about the care they received, what really helps is for them to take that message back to the diagnosing physician. When that doctor hears how great the patient's sleep has become, they may think of OAT and that dentist for their other patients. Asking for referrals, online reviews, and even short video testimonials for the practice's social media are key parts of growing your DSM practice.

Developing a physician referral base is difficult and time-consuming. There are many techniques for establishing a referral relationship with sleep physicians and primary care physicians (PCPs), but no single technique works universally. Most dentists start the process by sending their local physicians a letter introducing OAT as an alternative to continuous positive airway pressure (CPAP). Included with the letter are brochures, office prescription forms to be used by the referring physician, research articles on OAT, and an offer to meet the physician personally to discuss OAT. The success of these types of letters varies greatly. You won't find a sleep physician who is unfamiliar with OAT or who has not fielded many calls and letters from dentists offering to help. Unless you have a location remote enough to have few competitive dentists nearby, you must find a way to differentiate yourself. As you discover patients in your practice who have been diagnosed but are not in treatment, you can ask them about how the sleep physician approached treatment options. Did they discuss various ways of keeping the airway open or only CPAP? Did they suggest the patient ask their own dentist for OAT or was a list of vetted practices provided? Did it seem they were open to keeping the patient's wishes in mind or did their attitude imply that their medical expertise was the most important thing? Stories from patients will help you understand your local sleep physician and form a strategy for relationship building.

You may ask around a bit and find a PCP or ear, nose, and throat (ENT) specialist who has taken an interest in sleep and feels that board-certified sleep physicians are not necessary for many patients. They can become great allies in helping more people in the community. Keep in mind that any trained physician can order a sleep test, make a diagnosis, and prescribe therapy. They have scope of practice rules just like dentists and they can take continuing education courses to learn more about sleep to widen their scope of practice.

The American Academy of Sleep Medicine (AASM) insists that only their board can provide credentials for diagnostic services, but that is the trade organization's point of view—not a legal position. Taking a prescription from a physician who is not board certified in sleep medicine does not place dentists at any risk. The same is true for cardiologists, OB/GYNs, internal medicine physicians, and others, though most of them are reluctant to "cross the line" into another specialty area and do not top DSM referral lists. Several ENTs and a few PCPs feel qualified in our service area.

When introducing yourself to the local physician community, make sure to personalize your introductory letters. Don't just switch out physician names. Putting time and effort into getting to know physicians has the same effect as getting to know your patients before handing them a detailed treatment plan; it opens their minds to consider this new relationship that is being offered. Once the letter has been sent, most dentists follow up with a phone call and/or a personal visit to the office. The goal is to become friends with your referring physicians and nurse practitioners. Chances are, they have someone in their service area they already trust, and once that decision is made, physicians are unlikely to keep "finding another sleep dentist" at the top of their minds in day-to-day clinical work. Sometimes it is simply a matter of being in the right place at the right time if a physician's last patient or two were unhappy with the OAT they received from the previously vetted dentist. Or maybe one of your mutual patients had nothing but great things to say about the care they received in your office.

If there are two or three dentists you know with non-overlapping patient bases, you may consider hiring a marketing person to sell physicians on all of your practices, with patients directed to any member of the consortium. Some device manufacturers employ representatives to increase physician awareness of OAT; getting to know these representatives can help a great deal.

Once your local physicians realize that you can solve their patient CPAP noncompliance issue, they may begin to refer some of their CPAP failures to your office for alternative therapy. If you do not get a chance to personally meet with some of your local physicians, it is most effective to ask how you can best help them successfully treat their patients and how to easily communicate with their office. For example, some physicians do not want to use a referral form like those commonly employed between general dentists and their dental specialist colleagues. Their notes are already in their electronic health records, and your paper form is inconvenient for them.

Not surprisingly, physicians are hesitant to refer patients until they are assured that you are following appropriate protocols and getting good treatment results. Physicians want you to follow AASM and American Academy of Dental Sleep Medicine (AADSM) practice parameters. If you choose to attain recognition from the American Board of Dental Sleep Medicine, add that to all your correspondence. One bit of caution here: Check with your state regulations for what you are allowed to say about yourself, lest you are thought to be misleading the public. This is especially important if you choose to limit your practice to sleep services.

At the same time you are busy developing a referral practice, your office should employ screening tools to evaluate your current patient base for any patients with sleep-disordered breathing (SDB). There are several screening tools that can be used to assess a patient's risk of SDB. Patients will present with certain physical, social, nocturnal, and daytime symptoms that can be used to evaluate whether they should be referred to a sleep physician. The Epworth Sleepiness Scale (ESS), the Berlin Sleep Questionnaire, and the STOP-BANG questionnaire are frequently used to evaluate undiagnosed patients. The American Dental Association (ADA) policy statement on SDB emphasizes the responsibility placed on all dentists to screen all patients for SDB.[1]

Epworth Sleepiness Scale

The ESS is an eight-item questionnaire that measures a person's general propensity to fall asleep in the following situations:

1. Sitting and reading
2. Watching television
3. Sitting inactive in a public place (eg, a theater or a meeting)
4. As a passenger in a car for 1 hour without a break
5. Lying down to rest in the afternoon
6. Sitting and talking to someone
7. Sitting quietly after lunch without drinking alcohol
8. Stopped in a car for a few minutes in traffic

Each item is scored based on the chances of dozing: 0 (never), 1 (slight chance), 2 (moderate chance), or 3 (high chance). Aggregate scores under 10 are considered normal, and anything over 10 indicates that sleepiness is excessive, and a sleep specialist referral is recommended. Patients with OSA have higher ESS scores, and these scores improve with effective treatment.[2] This subjective assessment is highly influenced by the patient's self-image and possibly by employment status, quality of life issues, and other factors. While the scores are proven to be clinically valid, dentists should also consider other details the patient may share, if given the opportunity. On the other hand, a simple screening tool like this, provided without much explanation, can give clinicians valuable insight into the patient's state of mind concerning their sleep health. As you get to know the patient better and obtain other data such as sleep study results, keep in mind how they filled out the ESS as a data point for their ability to self-assess and their willingness to be honest about symptoms. Occasionally, it is valuable to enlist the patient's partner to fill out their "observational" ESS. This method is not validated but can be useful in the overall care plan.

Protocols for the Treatment of OSA

AADSM and AASM practice parameters

The ADA and the AADSM have issued protocols for the treatment of SDB by general dentists. These protocols are intended to be a guide for the treatment of OSA by general dentists.

The AADSM, primarily a dentist organization, and the AASM, mostly consisting of physicians but also including PhD researchers and dentists, have actively pursued uniformity in the practice of DSM and have published protocols and practice parameters for OAT. While many sleep physicians still follow the original 2005 *AASM Practice Parameters*, those parameters were updated in 2015 (Box 3-1).

BOX 3-1 AADSM/AASM practice parameters for the treatment of OSA and snoring with OAT

- **We recommend that sleep physicians prescribe oral appliances, rather than no therapy, for adult patients who request treatment of primary snoring (without OSA).**
- When OAT is prescribed by a sleep physician for an adult patient with OSA, we suggest that qualified dentists use custom, titratable appliances rather than non-custom oral devices.
- **We recommend that sleep physicians consider prescription of oral appliances, rather than no treatment, for adult patients with OSA who are intolerant of CPAP therapy or prefer alternative treatment.**
- We suggest that qualified dentists provide oversight, rather than no follow-up, of OAT in adult patients with OSA to survey for dental-related side effects or occlusal changes and reduce their incidence.
- We suggest that sleep physicians conduct follow-up sleep testing to improve or confirm treatment efficacy, rather than conduct follow-up without sleep testing, for patients fitted with oral appliances.
- We suggest that sleep physicians and qualified dentists instruct adult patients treated with oral appliances for OSA to return for periodic office visits, as opposed to no follow-up, with a qualified dentist and a sleep physician.

Bold text indicates a standard; nonbold text indicates a guideline. (Adapted from Ramar et al.[3])

In 2022, the AADSM published their own updated set of standards for OAT in adults with SDB: "Dental Sleep Medicine Standards for Screening, Treating, and Management of Sleep-Related Breathing Disorders in Adults Using Oral Appliance Therapy,"[4] summarized here with permission. Here, the term *qualified dentist* (QD) is used to indicate dentists who have completed some or all training from AADSM's Mastery curriculum. To ensure high-quality patient care is provided, screening, treatment, and management of patients with OSA or snoring should adhere to standards of care in an ethical and medicolegal framework, including following best practices for informed consent, risk management, quality assurance, and record keeping. Patient care should be delivered within the scope of the QD's competence in a patient-centered environment that recognizes the diversity of patient populations.

1. A patient may initiate a visit to the QD, who provides a screening consultation that may include a review of the chief complaint(s), a clinical assessment of oral/craniofacial risk factors, and validated questionnaire(s). In 2017, the ADA established a policy that all dentists should screen patients.
2. If appropriate and in accordance with applicable laws, a home sleep apnea test (HSAT) may be ordered and administered by the QD, or the patient may be referred to a medical provider for sleep testing.
3. The patient must be referred to a medical provider, who is responsible for diagnosing OSA and/or other sleep-related conditions. Alternatively, the medical provider may refer a diagnosed patient from their practice directly to the QD.
4. Prior to commencing OAT, the QD should determine whether the patient is a candidate for OAT and select a suitable appliance through a comprehensive DSM examination that reviews oral/craniofacial condition risks and predictive factors for successful OAT. This examination should include informed consent and financial arrangements necessary to commence OAT.
5. Upon patient acceptance of the treatment plan, relevant dental records and imaging may be obtained to determine the appropriate oral appliance within the context of the patient's oral presentation.
6. Upon resolution of the signs and symptoms of OSA, the QD may elect to use pulse oximetry or HSAT, in accordance with applicable laws, to aid in identifying the appropriate therapeutic position of the appliance.
7. Ultimately, the patient is referred to the medical provider for verification of treatment efficacy and long-term follow-up. If signs and symptoms do not resolve and treatment modifications do not lead to resolution, the patient should be referred to the medical provider for adjunct treatment or treatment alternatives.

Patient outcomes are optimized when medical and dental providers work together at every appropriate opportunity with shared goals and open communication.

Even since this article was updated in 2022, details have changed between adoption by the AADSM Board of Directors and this writing. Dentists treating SDB in adults are urged to consult this full paper as they continually update their knowledge of this clinical field (see chapter 10 for more details).

ADA policy statement on the role of dentistry in the treatment of SRBDs

SRBDs are characterized by disruptions in normal breathing patterns. They are potentially serious medical conditions caused by anatomical airway collapse and altered respiratory control mechanisms. Common SRBDs include snoring, upper airway resistance syndrome (UARS), and OSA. OSA has been associated with metabolic, cardiovascular, respiratory, and dental diseases, as well as others. In children, undiagnosed and/or untreated OSA can be associated with cardiovascular problems, impaired growth, and learning and behavioral problems.

Dentists play an essential role in the multidisciplinary care of patients with certain SRBDs and are well positioned to identify patients who are at greater risk for SRBDs. SRBDs can be caused by a number of multifactorial medical issues and are therefore best treated through a collaborative model. Working in conjunction with colleagues in medicine, dentists have various methods available for mitigating these disorders. In children, the dentist's recognition of suboptimal early craniofacial growth and development or other risk factors may lead to medical referral or orthodontic/orthopedic intervention to treat and/or prevent SRBDs. Various surgical modalities exist to treat SRBDs. Custom-made, titratable oral appliances can improve SRBDs in adult patients compared to no therapy or placebo devices, and OAT can improve OSA in adult patients, especially those who are intolerant of CPAP. Dentists are the only health care providers with the knowledge and expertise to provide OAT.

The dentist's role in the treatment of SRBDs includes the following:

1. Dentists are encouraged to screen patients for SRBDs as part of a comprehensive medical and dental history to recognize symptoms such as sleepiness, choking, snoring, or witnessed apneas and to evaluate for risk factors such as obesity, retrognathia, or hypertension. These patients should be referred as needed to the appropriate physicians for proper diagnosis.
2. In children, screening through history and clinical examination may identify signs and symptoms of deficient growth and development or other risk factors that may lead to airway issues. If a risk for SRBDs is determined, intervention through medical/dental referral or evidence-based treatment

may be appropriate to help treat the SRBD and/or develop an optimal physiologic airway and breathing pattern.

3. OAT is an appropriate treatment for mild and moderate sleep apnea and for severe sleep apnea when CPAP is not tolerated by the patient.
4. When OAT is prescribed by a physician through written or electronic order for an adult patient with OSA, a dentist should evaluate the patient for the appropriateness of fabricating a suitable oral appliance. If deemed appropriate, a dentist should fabricate an oral appliance.
5. Dentists should obtain appropriate patient consent for treatment that reviews the treatment plan and any potential side effects of using OAT and expected appliance longevity.
6. Dentists treating SRBDs with OAT should be capable of recognizing and managing the potential side effects through treatment or proper referral.
7. Dentists who provide OAT to patients should monitor and adjust the oral appliance for treatment efficacy as needed or at least annually. As titration of oral appliances has been shown to affect the overall success and final outcome of treatment, unattended cardiorespiratory or portable monitors may be used by the dentist to help define the optimal target position of the mandible. A dentist trained in the use of these portable monitoring devices may assess the objective interim results for the purposes of oral appliance titration.
8. Surgical procedures may be considered as a secondary treatment for OSA when CPAP or OAT is inadequate or not tolerated. In select cases, such as patients with concomitant dentofacial deformities, surgical intervention may be considered as a primary treatment.
9. Dentists treating SRBDs should continually update their knowledge and training with DSM continuing education.
10. Dentists should maintain regular communication with the patient's referring physician and other health care providers to update them on the patient's treatment progress and any recommended follow-up treatment.
11. Follow-up sleep testing by a physician should be conducted to evaluate the improvement or confirm the treatment efficacy for OSA, especially if the patient develops recurring OSA-relevant symptoms or comorbidities.

Discussion

The major difference between the ADA statement and the AADSM protocols is that the ADA represents all dentists, not just those who have elected to be involved in a specific segment of the profession. This makes the ADA statement more applicable to daily dental practice. Additionally, HSAT usage by dentists is controversial. As stated earlier, establishing a good referral base takes years. Therefore, to jumpstart their DSM practices, some dentists have made the decision to circumvent protocols and not refer their screened SRBD patients. Although it is generally accepted that a dentist *cannot* diagnose OSA, many dentists are frustrated that they do not have the ability to treat their own patients without a sleep physician being involved in diagnosing and prescribing OAT. To make matters worse, some sleep physicians are adamantly opposed to any treatment other than CPAP. Surveys have found many reasons for this opposition, including the following:

- CPAP is reliable and is obtained by a simple prescription without the need to engage any other professionals.
- Mandibular advancement device (MAD) therapy is less effective than CPAP at reducing the Apnea-Hypopnea Index (AHI) to normal levels for most patients.
- Physicians are unaware of the true incidence of oral device side effects and think they are more common and troublesome than what is found in most trained dental practices.
- Many dentists do not file medical insurance.
- Many dentists do not file (participate) with Medicare.
- Dentists are not proficient at communicating with referring physicians.
- Many dentists who are filing medical insurance are not in network, and therefore patients frequently have a large out-of-pocket expense for treatment.
- Many dentists do not follow AASM/AADSM treatment protocols.
- Some dentists refuse to refer screened patients to a sleep physician for consultation, thereby cutting the sleep physician out of the treatment.

This lack of connection between dentists and sleep physicians has, in some cases, resulted in dentists referring their patients to a local sleep physician who then refuses to allow the referring dentist to participate in the treatment of their OSA dental patients. Occasionally, sleep physicians will not write prescriptions for OAT, even if their patients are completely nonadherent to CPAP. Unfortunately, this resistance to OAT has resulted in many dentists resorting to using HSAT devices for diagnosis via a physician connected to the HSAT company or source. This eliminates the possibility of referring their screened dental patients to a local sleep physician who is opposed to OAT. Instead, these dentists ask the patient's PCP to sign the prescription for OAT based on the diagnosis by the telehealth physician (see chapter 10).

The COVID-19 pandemic produced a strong shift toward telemedicine, including for sleep medicine. With parity in payment systems between face-to-face clinical appointments and telehealth visits, patient preferences have strongly moved to online care. This enables good medical care while avoiding many of the constraints of the past. Telehealth physicians are responsible for the medical side of patient care, including arranging for CPAP therapy or polysomnography (PSG) testing, just as if the patient were being seen in a local clinic. Once the patient begins OAT, the dentist can use telemedicine to manage the patient during therapy as well, with the patient returning to the office only for evaluation of the device and for annual visits with orofacial examinations.

The HSAT protocol has sparked a heated debate that has gone on for years. The AASM has opined that a dentist who orders a sleep study or owns HSAT equipment is practicing medicine without a medical license, which can be a criminal offense in some states. Sadly, some dentists have been reported to their state dental and medical boards for using HSAT devices and remote sleep physicians to diagnose OSA. To further complicate things, although most PCPs have limited knowledge of SDBs and may not be the most appropriate health care professionals to monitor OSA patients, many DSM practitioners use PCPs as a source for their MAD prescriptions and letters of medical necessity (LOMNs) when necessary.

No state legislation or board of dental examiners has sanctioned the diagnosis of OSA by a dentist. A few states have taken the position that HSAT use by a dentist for any reason is unlawful. Regulations are constantly changing, and readers should review their state regulations to determine if there are any prohibitions to using HSAT in their state. The AADSM website maintains up-to-date information on these changing state regulations. Additionally, it is wise to discuss HSAT use with all referring physicians to determine their preferences. The best route is to create a culture of trust between the physician and the dentist so that each patient can receive appropriate treatment. Some patients should be seen by only the medical doctor, whereas others can be managed quite effectively by the trained dental provider.

The authors strongly support the ADA policy statement. We believe that it is vitally important for local sleep physicians to be involved in the diagnosis of patients. We also believe that it is unwise for a dentist to use HSAT to circumvent local sleep physician involvement. However, we think that every office participating in OAT should have the ability to determine if patient devices are adequately titrated. Therefore, we believe that HSAT use during the titration of a MAD is a vital part of fulfilling the intent of the prescription signed by the physician. Years of experience have shown that a practitioner cannot successfully determine whether a MAD is adequately titrated by subjective symptom improvement alone. We routinely use HSAT and pulse oximetry to assist in appliance titration.

Although oversight from a local sleep physician is ideal, there are areas of the country where the closest sleep physician is a significant drive away. With the introduction of the AADSM policy statement on the use of HSAT, dentists are now free to facilitate testing for OSA. Distant location of the closest sleep physician is one reason, but there are a number of other reasons why dentists might not want to send a patient for an overnight study. This is particularly true in the case of a patient who exhibits few or no signs of OSA but presents with temporomandibular disorder (TMD) symptoms. Given that a significant percentage of patients with TMD also have an SRBD, it is helpful to screen/test these patients before initiating TMD therapy, as research has shown that a TMD splint can exacerbate OSA.[5] While it is true that these patients could be referred to a sleep physician simply based on the fact that they present with myofascial pain, in today's environment of high medical insurance deductibles, patients tend to refuse referrals to sleep physicians in the absence of SRBD symptoms. Additionally, because many of these patients are younger, nonobese females, it may be impossible to qualify them for an overnight PSG. In our offices, if screening indicates a risk of a sleep-related problem, overnight oximetry screening, at a minimum, is appropriate and indicated. The authors use both local and telehealth physician services, depending on patient preferences. Some people want to stick with their medical provider group, others want service as soon as possible. Insurance coverage is usually not a factor, as telehealth companies have enrolled in most major medical plans. Insurance benefits, protocols, and choices are covered in chapter 11.

Another factor to consider when submitting HSAT to medical billing is any policy limiting how many tests the patient can have covered, like calendar restrictions on radiographs in the dental office. Even submitting a test that has zero payable amount resets the clock and can result in denial of a claim from another provider's office, ultimately costing the patient more out-of-pocket expense.

The decision to use telemedicine and/or in-office HSAT testing should be based on the needs and the size of each individual DSM practice. Interestingly enough, one of the authors (Ken Berley) has a 99% physician referral DSM practice in Arkansas and a 75% telemedicine/in-office HSAT practice in Utah. The decision to develop the diverse practice models was strictly based on the time and effort required to develop a physician referral practice. It can take many years to entice enough physician referrals to have a busy DSM practice. With telemedicine and HSAT testing, any well-trained dentist can launch a DSM practice.

Obstacles to Overcome

Sleep physicians are not trained to take impressions of the teeth, handle the complications of OAT, or evaluate whether a patient's dentition is healthy enough to support a MAD. DSM professionals are the only healthcare providers qualified to provide MADs. When DSM clinicians joined the sleep community, there was significant disagreement regarding the protocol for the treatment of OSA patients by dentists. Sleep medicine is governed and controlled by the AASM, and physicians practicing in the field of sleep wanted to make sure that all patients being treated for SRBDs were diagnosed and monitored by a board-certified sleep physician. To help accomplish this goal of physician oversight, MADs were classified as durable medical equipment (DME). DMEs are reusable pieces of medical equipment, such as wheelchairs, walkers, crutches, and hospital beds, that are used in a patient's home to improve quality of life. For a patient to qualify to receive a piece of DME (eg, an oral appliance), a physician must diagnose a condition that can be improved by it. Then the physician writes a prescription for the DME and provides the patient an LOMN to present to the treating dentist. Therefore, dentists who practice DSM technically are considered DME providers, though at the same time are required to use doctor skills to evaluate oral health and choose the appliance most suited to the patient. This strange arrangement is why DSM providers need a prescription from the treating physician and an LOMN to file medical insurance or Medicare for OAT.

Effectiveness of therapy

With hour-by-hour comparison, CPAP is more effective than MAD therapy at maintaining an open airway and eliminating desaturations. This comparison results in CPAP being universally preferred by physicians. Therefore, it is not uncommon for a dentist to refer a screened dental patient to a sleep physician, who then diagnoses the patient with mild apnea and prescribes a CPAP rather than a MAD. CPAP uses air pressure to stent open the collapsible portions of the airway, using a mask, or "interface," that covers the nose, mouth, or both together. The mask is connected by a flexible hose to a flow generator that blows air at a constant level of pressure. The air pressure is adjustable depending on the amount needed to prevent collapse during respiration. This is like blowing up a balloon. If enough pressure is applied, the airway will open. Most CPAP devices prescribed today are auto-adjusting. The flow generator continually monitors breathing and adjusts the pressure within parameters set by the prescribing physician so that the airway stays open in every body position and sleep stage. This ability to self-adjust makes autoPAP a very effective tool for treating SRBDs. The question is whether the patient can sleep with the mask and air pressure.

Unfortunately, many studies show that most CPAP patients do not use therapy all night. This has resulted in a less-than-ideal definition of successful CPAP therapy. Success is defined by sleep physicians and Medicare as wearing the CPAP device for only 4 hours per night for 5 nights per week.[6] The reasoning for the lenient success definition is due to very poor patient adherence to therapy. On the other hand, most patients who wear a MAD report using it all night for most nights. It is important to note that in the few studies where the objectively measured use of MADs was compared to patient reports, general agreement between the measurements was found. There are no widespread patient population studies that show consistent full-night adherence to CPAP therapy by an overwhelming number of subjects.

Noncompliance with CPAP and compliance with MAD therapy opens the door for OAT as an alternative to CPAP or to be used in combination therapy. Using CPAP with a MAD at the same time has two distinct advantages. First, less CPAP pressure is necessary to open the patient's airway when the mandible is prevented from falling back or open. Second, the MAD is still functional when the CPAP is removed in the middle of the night. This strategy is particularly helpful in patients with high BMIs and an elevated AHI. Unfortunately, most insurance benefits for DME allow for only one therapy to be covered. CPAP machines have continuing costs of use (eg, replacement hoses and masks), so it's generally better for the patient to add OAT out of pocket.

Another form of combination therapy involves the patient using CPAP at home and OAT while traveling. This is because there is typically greater symptom relief with CPAP but reluctance to deal with the troubles of packing the CPAP for a trip. Rather than go without any treatment—risking socially unpopular snoring (the main reason stated in some offices)—the patient puts up with slightly less effective treatment for a short time. If the patient has significant cardiovascular comorbid risk, the dentist should consult with the medical care team before endorsing any time away from CPAP.

MEAN DISEASE ALLEVIATION

When comparing the success of CPAP versus OAT, it is helpful to apply the concept of mean disease alleviation.[7] Mean disease alleviation takes into consideration the efficacy of each therapy, as well as the length of wear. The effectiveness of each therapy is calculated by the product of the adjusted compliance and therapeutic efficacy divided by 100. For example:

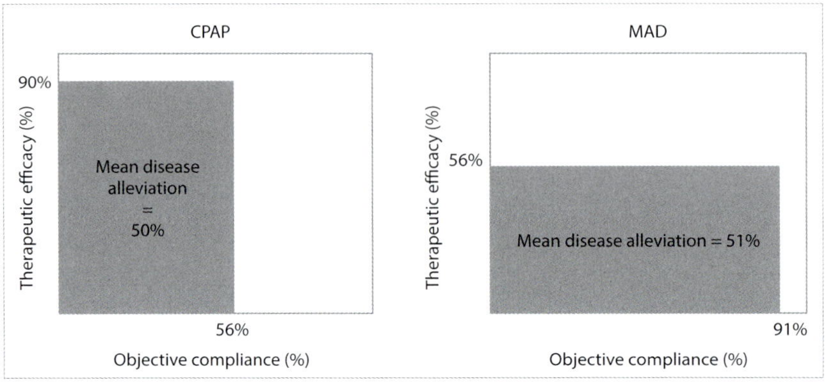

Fig 3-1 Mean disease alleviation.

- Patient X has a baseline AHI of 50.
- When using a CPAP, this AHI decreases to 5 (therapeutic efficacy = 90%).
- When using an oral appliance, this AHI decreases to 10 (therapeutic efficacy = 80%).
- The patient wears his CPAP an average of 4 hours per night out of 8 total sleep hours (objective compliance = 50%).
- The patient wears his oral appliance an average of 6 hours per night out of 8 total sleep hours (objective compliance = 75%).
- Mean disease alleviation with CPAP = (50 × 90)/100 = 45% of the total disease is eliminated.
- Mean disease alleviation with OAT = (75 × 80)/100 = 60% of the total disease is eliminated.

Using this example, the hypothetical patient's OSA was reduced by 60% when using MAD therapy and by 45% using CPAP therapy. Therefore, mean disease alleviation calculations may be a better way to evaluate the comparative effectiveness of MAD therapy (Fig 3-1).[8]

Snoring appliances

It is important for dentists who are new to the practice of DSM to understand that they should not immediately fabricate snoring appliances for patients who exhibit snoring symptoms. About 70% of these patients likely have OSA. Patients with significant snoring must be tested and diagnosed by a sleep physician. Only if the patient is found to *not* have OSA is a MAD truly a "snoring appliance."

Medical insurance and Medicare

Filing medical insurance can be a major obstacle for new DSM practitioners. Although filing for medical coverage is not difficult, it is significantly different than filing dental insurance. As a general principle, the authors recommend that dentists employ a medical insurance billing company during the first year of providing OAT. This will eliminate some of the stress placed on your office staff. It is very important for DSM practitioners to be enrolled as a Medicare DME "non-participating" provider. Physicians want you to be able to file Medicare. As a non-participating enrolled provider you can choose, on a case-by-case basis, to either accept the Medicare allowable or balance bill your full fee.

For a dentist to be successful in DSM, the office team must become competent in necessary details of medical insurance and Medicare (see chapter 11). Many patients will not accept treatment if the dental office is unable or unwilling to file with their health insurance. The authors feel people are justified in expecting benefits from policies they pay for, and refusing to participate with health insurance imposes the dentist's choices on that expectation. Additionally, physicians are hesitant to refer OSA patients to an office that cannot maximize a patient's health insurance coverage and minimize their out-of-pocket expense. Because tens of millions of people in the United States suffer from SRBDs, any reduction in barriers to treatment improves community health.

Insurance information and benefits should be confirmed prior to the initial examination or consultation so that financial discussions are productive. Asking a patient to send a photograph of both sides of their medical insurance card prior to the appointment is an efficient way to get started. The authors have tried systems where coverage details are gathered in advance, so plan limits, policies, and deductibles can be investigated prior to the visit, and systems where such things are delayed until after the consultation when the patient is deemed to be a good candidate for OAT and agrees to treatment. If the data is available at the examination/consultation appointment, treatment acceptance is far higher than if the patient must wait out a delay. By the time the office team calls the patient with benefit news for a financial discussion, enthusiasm for the treatment may have waned. Gathering data first requires some investment of team resources with the risk that some patients will say "no." Waiting to discuss finances until a later phone call carries the cost of the examination visit plus the administrative time, with a greater risk of "no."

Most medical insurance companies routinely require preauthorization or precertification before OAT is initiated. If you choose to provide your patients with only an itemized statement and suggest that they initiate a claim after treatment delivery, they risk being denied the coverage they otherwise could have had with the preauthorization. Obtaining the precertification number comprises the bulk of predelivery administrative time. A medical billing company includes this service in the fee you pay them, avoiding the cost of arranging these details with dental administrative team members.

Blue Cross Blue Shield and some other medical insurance companies restrict coverage if the patient has periodontal disease or temporomandibular joint dysfunction but do not provide definitions in medical policies, leaving it up to the dentist to determine if there is a clinical contraindication for OAT. This requirement is another reason that only qualified dentists can provide MADs. Physicians are not trained to assess these conditions and cannot certify safety for the patients.

Another detail to keep in mind is that Medicare and some commercial insurance plans cover only those appliances that appear on a list called PDAC—Pricing, Data Analysis, and Coding of HCPCS Level II DMEPOS Codes. Knowing this in advance allows dentists to choose whether a device on the list is the best fit for the patient or if another must be chosen. Providing a non-PDAC device for a patient with this restriction is allowed clinically but cannot be submitted for benefits. This requires careful communication with the patient. Details about consulting the PDAC list are included in chapter 11.

Documentation necessary for treatment

When an OSA patient is referred to a dentist for OAT, the office staff should ensure that all the appropriate documentation is received with the referral. If the referral is from a sleep physician, it will likely include a copy of the sleep study and the sleep physician's interpretation or diagnosis. A detail that has been used to deny coverage is the necessity of a physician encounter prior to the sleep study; insurance companies want evidence that the physician thought the test was medically necessary. The chart notes relevant to the study may or may not be included. Because these chart notes are necessary for a complete history of the patient's OSA and comorbid diseases, it is important to request them and for the dentist to review the data. Often patients with an AHI < 15 must have a documented comorbid disease, such as cardiovascular risk or mood disorders, to qualify for treatment of their OSA. Medical policies are available online and should be consulted for lists of qualifying comorbidities if your patient is diagnosed with an AHI between 5 and 15. These conditions must appear in the physician's signed encounter notes to satisfy qualifying requirements.

If a referral is received from a PCP, sleep tests and other documentation may be missing. Therefore, your office may be required to track down the necessary records. In the authors' opinion, prudent practitioners will not make a MAD without reviewing the diagnostic study and the sleep physician's interpretation. Dental practitioners need to have a firm understanding of the severity of the disease before initiating OAT. The advent of precision medicine means that therapy teams must study test results. Emerging data is showing that the details of the SRBD, such as the ratio between the number of apnea and hypopnea events, might indicate different therapy.[9] A patient with mostly apnea events may need more protrusion than a patient who experiences only hypopneas and whose airway stays open. The dentist may choose different devices based on this analysis.

In addition to the sleep study, you will need a signed prescription for a MAD (E0486) and an LOMN from the referring physician. These documents do not have to be separate from the medical encounter note and are often contained within the "Plan" or "Interpretation" section near the end of the note. The prescription should be clearly stated in a detailed written order: "Patient unable to tolerate CPAP for OSA, G47.33" is an LOMN. Most physicians are used to the requirements for these details and will need little prompting by your administrative staff. If the required language is missing, create a simple document with the necessary declarations and fax it to the physician for signature. The referral should include the patient's contact information for your staff to reach out to the patient.

After the dental staff has assembled the necessary documentation, and if the patient is not a member of your dental practice, it is beneficial to have a well-trained staff member contact the patient to review his or her dental history and get information on the patient's current dentist. During that conversation, questions should be asked about the dental health of the patient. Patients who have not had a dental examination and cleaning within the last year should be instructed to have a checkup with their existing dentist.

Dental health requirements

No research has been conducted in DSM to establish the number of teeth necessary to safely conduct OAT. It has been hypothesized that 8 to 10 teeth per arch, distributed evenly, are necessary, but that restriction is purely anecdotal. The more teeth the patient has, the better. Remember that many patients have no real alternative to OAT; therefore, if the authors can devise a way to stabilize the mandible forward, we generally do. We recommend implants for more support any time the patient does not have at least 10 teeth per arch, but if the patient has both mandibular canines and a full maxillary denture, we will make an appliance with appropriate informed consent.

Research shows clear associations between OSA and periodontal disease. The question of how much disease is too much remains up to the clinician and the patient to decide. Currently there is no definitive answer to this question. The prudent practitioner will evaluate the severity of the patient's OSA and compare that with any risk of treatment. Then the risks and benefits should be presented to the patient. Once the patient is adequately informed, the patient can accept this risk or decide on another form of treatment. Ultimately, patients are responsible for their own health care decisions.

Similar arguments exist for TMDs. Many patients with frequent microarousals due to an SRBD suffer from myalgia and myositis from bruxing and clenching. Over time, pressure can cause adaptive responses in the temporomandibular joint, including popping, clicking, and even crepitus. Still, the patient carries on with activities of daily living, moving their jaw. Adding a minimally protrusive, low-vertical opening MAD is not contraindicated in any but the most acute TMD situations. Resolving the SRBD and resulting microarousals is *treatment* for the TMD, not a causation of it. Considering the known medical risk of OSA, the risk of a sore jaw must be put into context for patients in your care.

References

1. American Dental Association. The Role of Dentistry in the Treatment of Sleep Related Breathing Disorders. https://www.ada.org/resources/ada-library/oral-health-topics/sleep-apnea-obstructive. Accessed 11 September 2024.
2. Lee-Chiong TL. Somnology 2: Learn Sleep Medicine in One Weekend. CreateSpace, 2011.
3. Ramar K, Dort LC, Katz SG, et al. Clinical practice guideline for the treatment of obstructive sleep apnea and snoring with oral appliance therapy: An update for 2015. J Clin Sleep Med 2015;11:773–827.
4. Levine M, Cantwell M, Postol K, Schwartz D. Dental sleep medicine standards for screening, treating, and management of sleep-related breathing disorders in adults using oral appliance therapy. J Dent Sleep Med 2022;9.
5. Gagnon Y, Mayer P, Morisson F, Rompre PH, Lavigne GJ. Aggravation of respiratory disturbances by the use of an occlusal splint in apneic patients: A pilot study. Int J Prosthodont 2004;17:447–453.
6. Kribbs NB, Pack AI, Kline LR, et al. Objective measurement of patterns of nasal CPAP use by patients with obstructive sleep apnea. Am Rev Respir Dis 1993;147:887–895.
7. Vanderveken OM, Dieltjens M, Wouters K, De Backer WA, Van de Heyning PH, Braem MJ. Objective measurement of compliance during oral appliance therapy for sleep-disordered breathing. Thorax 2013;68:91–96.
8. Phillips CL, Grunstein RR, Darendeliler MA, et al. Health outcomes of continuous positive airway pressure versus oral appliance treatment for obstructive sleep apnea: A randomized controlled trial. Am J Respir Crit Care Med 2013;187:879–887.
9. Edwards BA, Eckert DJ, McSharry DG, et al. Clinical predictors of the respiratory arousal threshold in patients with obstructive sleep apnea. Am J Respir Crit Care Med 2014;190:1293–1300.

Sleep is an investment in the energy you need to be effective tomorrow.

—Tom Roth

4

Integrating Dental Sleep Medicine into Your Practice

Improving a person's daily quality of life and elongating their health span are some of the rewards that stem from adding medical services to a dental practice and tackling the challenges of collaborating with medical colleagues. But business and professional growth demand change. If you want to be a better doctor and have a bigger impact on community health, your dental practice *must* change. And keep in mind that nothing changes without causing disruption. Choosing to add medical services such as dental sleep medicine (DSM) to your practice is one of the more disruptive opportunities you can embrace as a leader. This chapter helps you understand some of the necessary changes for developing a successful DSM practice, which will require office systems and staff responsibilities that are atypical in the dental field.

This chapter will not provide you with a template, script, or set of protocols to simply hand over to your team. We believe that the best system is the one created by you and your team that will help you thrive in the culture you have in your clinic. We provide some benchmarks, guidelines, and boundaries, but you and your team are in the best place to decide exactly how to implement them. As you design the necessary systems and workflows yourselves, you will be far more likely to put into practice what you know, what you learn along the way, and what you feel will lead to the best results. This will be hard. Embrace the certainty that you and your team will make mistakes but none of them will permanently harm anyone. Your office will make some money and also lose some along the way to a steadily positive cash flow from this new service.

BOX 4-1 SOAP notes

S	Subjective	What patients report about the issue for which they are seeing you
O	Objective	Data gathered through tests, examinations, and imaging
A	Assessment	Using the information to decide on a diagnosis
P	Plan	The chosen strategy to address the diagnosis

Documentation

DSM is not just about fitting acrylic devices for patients or adding a few more questions to your health history. Managing airway concerns always involves thinking about patient symptoms and how they relate to the complete medical history. We must look beyond the oral cavity and consider the whole person. How do health care providers record pertinent information with this perspective? In dentistry, we are used to keeping notes about the preventive, surgical, and restorative services we provide, and these notes can be verified by examination or imaging—we just take a radiograph to show a crown, filling, or smooth root surface. Non-surgeon physicians can rarely provide such evidence. Their documentation requirements differ from those of dentistry from the very beginning.

Notes are used to record the thoughts you have during a medical encounter. Dentists are often trained in the use of SOAP notes (Box 4-1). SOAP notes are not uncommon in a dental office during an initial visit or a comprehensive evaluation. If time is taken to get to know the patient, narrative sections about health concerns and history (the "subjective" part of the notes) can be entered into the record. A more limited intake process focuses on objective data and developing a treatment plan, with the narrative set aside. This results in electronic charts with a list of procedure codes to be scheduled without much supporting detail. As these tasks are accomplished, the codes are switched from "incomplete" to "complete," and billing support is performed. For dental billing, in which applying for benefits requires only submitting lists of completed, coded procedures, this is sufficient. Medical documentation to support billing is quite different.

In medicine, SOAP notes are also common, but often they are labeled differently, with some changes to the underlying structure. Medical visits are referred to as *evaluation and management* (E&M) *encounters*, and the level of coding (and the reimbursement amounts) are driven by the amount of detail recorded for each E&M visit. Government documents standardize medical notes.[1] While this level of detail is not (yet) required in dental offices, communication with our physician colleagues requires us to become aware of, if not familiar with, the format.

Labels for medical notes look like this:

- History: Chief complaint, history of the present illness, and past family and social history.
- Physical examination: There are specific ways of recording data—think of a multipoint checklist.
- Medical decision-making: Incorporating all the assembled data into a plan for care.

Keep in mind that the standards for medical note-taking were developed with full awareness that every field of medicine was to be included. Physicians have common training in the basics of physical examination and the review of systems. Every physician can listen to the heart, for example, but specialized physicians have a deeper knowledge of more specific parts of the body. The examination requirements of a cardiologist differ from those of a primary care physician (PCP). Likewise, dentists can assess and create records about the oral cavity and adjacent structures but cannot enter a note about the function of systems outside their area of training. What we must document is limited to our scope of practice. This chapter guides you in creating encounter notes that are appropriate to most dental training; if you've had a residency or other advanced medical training, your scope of practice is larger, and you may be able to provide more detailed notes.

Limited examination protocol

When a patient is referred to an oral surgeon for third molar extraction, the oral surgeon is not expected to do a full dental exam and diagnose, for example, incipient distal decay on a first premolar. The surgeon is not acting as the patient's primary care dentist. In the same way, when providing oral appliance therapy (OAT), dentists function as DSM specialists, and as the size of a DSM practice expands, it is common for providers to limit the amount of general dentistry that is performed. Many DSM providers do not employ hygienists, and some don't have a dental assistant. As a result, some DSM providers use a limited examination protocol.

In the limited examination protocol, the patient is not a dental patient of record but has been referred for OAT. In other words, this cannot be one of your own screened dental patients. New sleep patients are informed that as a DSM practitioner, you will not be acting as their primary care dentist and that you will be relying on their existing dentist to provide any examinations and diagnose any dental diseases or other conditions that need to be treated. The patient signs a release of liability and assumption of risk stating that the DSM practitioner is released from any and all liability associated with the patient's dental health and that the patient will maintain routine visits with their primary care dentist to ensure that their dental health is maintained.

Upon the patient signing the release, the DSM provider conducts an abbreviated examination to look for obvious problems. This protocol eliminates the need to take diagnostic radiographs, as well as the need for full-mouth periodontal probing. It is a protocol that one author (Ken Berley) uses frequently in various practices. This is because the reimbursement from medical insurance for providing a comprehensive dental exam and sleep intake exam for all new sleep patients is inadequate. Be aware, however, that if an OAT patient is a dental patient who was screened by your dental practice, this section does not apply. *You* are the patient's primary care dentist of record, and you are legally responsible for that patient's dental health. You cannot have the patient sign a release to mitigate your exposure.

Software

Dental software is designed to support ordinary dental office code-based documentation. Making a medical encounter note can be difficult in dental software because each one must be customized. Creating individual templates for recording common procedures and assigning these templates to an office-created code is a straightforward way to continue using dental office software. However, there are no standardized templates available, so it falls to each office to create new ones themselves, or perhaps copy from a colleague.

The difficulty comes when these notes must be transferred to a report form for sending to medical providers. Most individualized custom templates do not automatically transfer to a letter format, so the dental team is left repeatedly extracting and reformatting data to compose individual letters to physicians, or leaving off important information when standardized reports are used to save time. But studying medical encounter notes and sleep test reports received from physicians will reveal that these notes are unique to the patient and the encounter, and physicians will expect the same from the trained dental office. There are a few dedicated software options for DSM on the market to address this problem. Even though specialized software is not a necessity for providing excellent airway services, it will save you and your team a lot of the time and energy spent working around the limitations of standard dental office software. It is never easy to work with more than one software for the same patient base, but the value of a dedicated system comes in the ease of use, which translates into more frequent use and a more professional appearance to your notes. Additionally, innovative solutions are always being developed, and some medical software is now integrating with leading dental programs.

Medical-oriented computer programs are important because physicians are currently the gatekeepers to airway therapy, and they are looking for dentists who "know what they are doing." If you want to be part of the airway health team, having professional software is one step toward getting there. The investment will more than pay off by lowering barriers to creating new office systems, fostering professional acceptance, and increasing the number of referrals received as you build relationships with other providers. Another advantage to your team is the enhanced ability to think separately about the medical and dental services you provide.

Choosing the right software

Because the whole office team will be using any software that is chosen (perhaps the dentist least of all), this decision should be made by the people who will be the most hands-on with it. One method is to have a clinical staff member and an administrative staff member work together to investigate the available choices. They can search the market, trial the software, look online for references, talk to office users, and then come to the dentist with a suggestion on what they think will work best for the office. Taking part in the process will make them far more likely to learn and implement any new system.

There is no standard for how a medical database is constructed in a medical software or electronic health record (EHR). Thus, the industry lacks connectivity, and data cannot be easily shared between disparate programs. If the company that supports your program goes out of business, your data may not be able to be picked up by your next choice. Carefully consider the health of a software company before you invest the massive amount of time, energy, and capital required for the onboarding process. Many programs are cloud-based. Make sure you have access to and control of a backup of your data any time you wish. Ask about the file format to see if it will be useful if you must import it to another vendor's program. You will want to hear that the software is based on a common, commercially available platform. Current examples include Amazon's AWS and Microsoft's Azure. The most common software used in medicine is Epic. As of this writing, there is not a platform readily available to an individual dental office that integrates with Epic, but that could change at any time. Integrating with Epic should allow secure access to most patient chart data, greatly simplifying the record sharing necessary for collaborative care and medical billing.

Equipment Needs

Luckily, there is not a lot of new equipment needed to provide airway therapy.

Fax machines and scanners

You will need a fax machine (or an equivalent e-fax, as long as it is HIPAA compliant). Despite the ubiquity of electronic communications, medical record programs do not share a common format, and most medical offices do not permit outside access to their EHRs for posting messages or entering chart data, including via email. Security breaches at medical facilities cost these companies millions of dollars. Because most physicians work for full-service systems, the various providers have access to common software. When they must send notes to an "outside" doctor, they use conventional paper and electronic mail and fax. These are transmitted over phone lines rather than the internet, which provides security. It also means you must have a conventional phone line to your office solely for fax. While we can hope for a change, currently you will need a means of sending and receiving HIPAA-compliant faxes. If you must get a physical fax machine, ask the vendor if it is HIPAA compliant and can distribute incoming faxes directly into an electronic file for transfer into your electronic chart. These machines are not difficult to find, but your local big-box electronics store may not be familiar with medical office requirements.

USB card scanners are also very helpful for scanning medical insurance cards into your software, and they are easy to find online and in retail stores. Specialized small printers can produce labels for patient records sent to the lab and for the oral appliances before delivery. Machines capable of scanning full-size letters quickly are useful for adding any papers mailed to you from an outside source to the patient record.

Tools for taking vitals

You will need to record basic vitals data, including blood pressure, pulse, respiration rate, height, and weight. Do NOT rely on asking patients about their weight. Recording the patient's weight provides your team with a big opportunity to pass along your new commitment to overall patient health, including the airway. Because changes to weight can have a profound impact on airway performance, it is critical to be able to track it over time from baseline diagnosis through treatment and follow-up. You already have a blood pressure cuff, so it is just a matter of creating systems to use it and record what you find. Add pulse, respiration rate, and oximetry, and your vital signs record is complete.

The most unfamiliar vital to the office team might be oximetry, but an oximeter can provide patients with tangible imagery about their airway problems. Not

BOX 4-2 Explaining oxygen level and why it matters

Ask the patient to hold his or her breath to lower the oxygen level measured by the oximeter. Then compare the maximum change to what was noted on the home sleep apnea test (HSAT) or polysomnogram (PSG). Someone who can change their resting oxygen saturation (SaO_2) from 98% to 96% voluntarily but who sees an SaO_2 nadir of 84% from their sleep test might consider the suggested therapy with more seriousness.

everyone understands what we mean by "airway problems," but oxygen levels are easy to grasp (Box 4-2). Oximeters come with a variety of price points and accuracy. A medical-grade device is a good investment that should not entail a high cost. Pick one that looks good and that you have confidence will last. Oximeters used for overnight treatment assessment should be able to record for more than one night and come with software that is validated against hospital-grade oximeters. The higher-capability software that typically comes with the better units will allow you and your staff to spend less time troubleshooting software or repeating tests due to equipment malfunction. Chapter 5 covers the use of oximetry for screening patients with temporomandibular disorder (TMD), and in chapter 6, we look at the use of oximetry for assessing patient response.

Finally, an emerging test that may be considered a vital sign in our field is nasal function. Because we are concerned with respiratory function and nose breathing, an assessment of nasal function is appropriate at intake and during therapy. Equipment needs vary from nothing (asking the patient to breathe through their nose) to a mirror to check for fogging during exhalation to rhinomanometry (a test that precisely measures airflow through the nose; see chapter 16). Rhinomanometers are becoming more common in ear, nose, and throat (ENT) offices and will become more popular in dental offices as they focus more on nasal function as a means of optimizing DSM outcomes.

Imaging devices

Before fabricating a mandibular advancement device (MAD), practitioners need some means of evaluating the patient's dental health and periodontal bone support, as well as a way to screen for condylar health. CBCT is excellent for these purposes but not required for airway therapy. If you are considering purchasing a new office space, we suggest you plan for a CBCT machine. The chosen machine must have a large field of view so the entire upper airway can be included. The authors agree that a panoramic image is minimally sufficient for the fabrication of an oral appliance. If the software can generate 2D tomograms of the temporomandibular joints, you will be better able to determine joint health before OAT.

Telehealth equipment

The COVID-19 pandemic expanded medical and dental services offered via telehealth. For your office, you will need a private space to conference with your patients and an adequate camera and microphone. Many computers include this hardware, but external systems are not expensive. You will need to use a secure, medically compliant software program for patient conferences. Typical business-oriented programs, such as the one you logged into for your last webinar, are not yet sufficient for telehealth use. There are many telehealth programs available at no or low cost (possibly even embedded in your dental or medical software program). Once you begin using telehealth, you will find many ways of enhancing your patient services in low-cost, high-impact ways. Patients very much appreciate talking with their health professionals without the need to drive to the office, and regulations provide parity for billing in-office and telehealth services.

Consultation Services

Dentistry has a long history of consultants offering their services to help offices sort out new systems, provide training, and bring expertise to the team in many areas. Airway therapy is no different—there are consultant companies that can provide services and training for systems, diagnosis, billing, laboratory support, and follow-up. While the up-front costs may seem daunting, these services could save you a lot of time and offset the cost of consultancy. A careful check of what a consultant service offers and whom else they service may help you decide if they are right for your office. The added support can also help build team confidence and lead to better integration of airway services into your practice. Consider selecting two members from your team to investigate the different consultation companies and make a recommendation based on their findings. The dentist should then talk with several users of the company to complete the evaluation. Investment into a consulting company may range from a few thousand dollars to six figure deposits. Be careful what you sign up for, and choose wisely.

Preparing for Medical-Dental Collaboration

The best way to get to know your local physicians is to screen for at-risk patients in your practice, find someone you think would benefit from the expertise of a sleep physician or ENT specialist, and facilitate a referral (see chapter 3). As you do so, call the physician's office and ask if you can have a few minutes to discuss the patient's needs with the doctor, lead nurse, or physician's assistant. Whether you sit down with them face-to-face (preferred), use a HIPAA-compliant conferencing software, or discuss the patient over the phone, be sure to ask them how you can communicate best. Considerations include the following:

- How do they want to receive information? Letter? Fax? Phone call? What is their usual method of sharing treatment data with their referral sources? Do they have problems in this area that you can solve/approach differently?
- Can they accept emails with attachments, in case you want to send an image? Usually this is possible in a secure format, but physicians often are constrained by their security service.
- Would they prefer a custom letter, chart notes, or a form that they provide?
- How often would they like updates on therapy for shared patients?
- For sleep physicians, ask about their feelings regarding dentists ordering or providing home sleep apnea testing (HSAT). Some will want to perform all tests themselves; others will request that the MAD be titrated prior to the patient's return to the doctor's office. Being up-front about this sometimes touchy subject will go a long way toward building trust.

As you begin to work with physicians, study the reports you receive from them in detail, and make notes about preferences you see. Some physicians are more detailed than others and consistently comment on certain particulars of a patient's history. Others follow a different set of data points. Familiar patterns will begin to emerge that can help you to become more trustworthy in their minds. You use this same set of skills when you talk with your dental patients and treat them as individuals. Don't use form letters.

Information cards and brochures, sleep-specific business cards, and sample MADs for physicians to use in their offices are all tools that will make it easier for physicians to refer patients to you. Manufacturers sell sample devices, and you can create a custom plate or label to make sure physicians remember who provided these valuable items for their office. A tip: Give physicians only the device, not a pretty set of printed teeth with the device on it. It's hard for us dentists to think this way, but untrained physicians and patients can find it difficult to see just the MAD. Often, they view the entire thing (MAD plus typodont) as the device, and that looks big and intimidating. Surely not every patient or physician thinks this way, but eliminate the risk by giving them only a nicely presented selection of common MADs.

BOX 4-3 Minimum information required from the referring physician for medical insurance reasons

- Demographics with insurance
- Letter of medical necessity (LOMN)
- Prescription for a custom MAD—HCPC: E0486/ICD-10 G47.33
- Chart note—face-to-face interaction prior to diagnostic sleep study (documenting comorbidities and symptoms of OSA as medical reasoning for ordering the HSAT or PSG)
- Chart note—review of the diagnostic study that outlines the findings and treatment recommendations
- All studies (diagnostic HSAT/PSG, CPAP titration, oral appliance titration) signed and interpreted by a board-certified sleep physician

Insurance companies require specific information before paying for therapy. Fortunately, what is required is what physicians are used to signing off on for continuous positive airway pressure (CPAP) treatment. Still, the prescriber must send over details. Make it easy for them by providing them with the list of requirements—not what you need but what the insurance company insists on having before paying for what the physician is prescribing. At a minimum, make sure you request the information shown in Box 4-3.

All medical records are electronic, so any paper that you provide the medical office must be scanned into their computers. Traditional referral pads are often not useful for medical offices because it is easier for them to mention the referral in their notes and give the patient one of your cards and/or brochures. Adding notes to a referral pad will seem redundant and will not satisfy documentation requirements. Save your referral pads for your dental colleagues who do not want to add airway services to their practice.

Team Training

With the many challenges of adding airway services to your practice, success will come only with commitment to the new service from all members of the dental office team. The best way to learn something is to teach it, so anyone who has taken a sleep course has an obligation to share that information with the team. A series of team meetings in which the leader brings everyone along as they learn about airway health and the role of the dentist will encourage questions, promote brainstorming for problem solving, and allow new systems to be developed. Team huddles and debriefing sessions during the first months of providing airway treatment will highlight successes as well as the necessary updates to these nascent systems. Do not be afraid of mistakes or failures. These events simply point out opportunities for growth,

BOX 4-4 Training exercises to promote team growth

- At a team meeting, the leader plays the role of a patient new to the practice and asks each person a question about the airway-related parts of the intake forms. Practicing the answers and discussing how they should be presented will enable the team to become comfortable with explaining the "why" behind this new service.
- Divide the team into pairs and have each person take a turn playing an existing patient handed a new airway-related screening form. The objective of this exercise is to improve the verbal skills of the team members in presenting the form and answering questions about it.
- Improve communication skills using online resources, consultation services, and books. One book the authors have found helpful is *Communication Skills for Dental Health Care Providers* by Lance Brendan Young, Cynthia Rozek O'Toole, and Bianca Wolfe (Quintessence, 2015).
- At a team meeting, pass out copies of a detailed encounter with a patient and a sleep physician, one that includes a full workup, sleep test, and recommended treatment, and possibly even a positive airway pressure (PAP) trial and the results. Have your team go through the test with two colors of highlighters to identify the terms they know and the ones they are curious about. Talk about how these notes are different from your office notes. While they do not need to match, there are often ways to improve your notes. If the ideas come from your team, it is more likely that implementing changes will be successful. This exercise will reveal areas in which you can help your team gain a better understanding of sleep-related breathing disorders (SRBDs).

training, and course correction. The worst thing a dental team can do is allow untreated patients to stay on a downward health spiral, so every attempt to improve health is a step forward.

Cross-training is vital to the success of your DSM practice. Do not confine finance training to administrative staff or clinical tips to chairside assistants and hygienists. Letting people do what they are best at is a sign of great leadership, but having clinical staff members who are unable to answer basic questions about insurance or administrative team members who are unfamiliar with why dentists are involved in airway treatment in the first place will prevent patients from feeling that they have had the best encounter with your office. The market is responsive to the need for all team members to become trained, and online resources are widely available. Several professionals have created team-training consultancies to work online or in person to help patient flow in your office. Again, a clinical staff person and an administrative staff person should investigate training opportunities and come to the doctor with a suggestion for the most effective use of office resources. You must provide the facilities and time for training and then bring it to the rest of the group in a huddle or team meeting. When a dentist is passionate about mastering a new field of study, the team will follow (Box 4-4).

Along the way, someone on your team will emerge as a "sleep champion." This new service will become the most motivating part of their job. Although everyone is involved, the sleep champion will take on the tasks of organizing the rest of the team, keeping track of what systems need to be developed, assigning who is responsible for what, and generally being a cheerleader for airway therapy. You can think of the sleep champion as the project manager who is invaluable for your success. Often, this person is a chairside assistant or a hygienist who relishes the patient involvement, the deeper knowledge of the dental profession, and the rewards that follow successful airway therapy. The best way to find your sleep champion is to demonstrate adept leadership in the early phases of your airway services and watch carefully for the person who lights up when opportunities arise. Many dental hygienists lose the ability to practice their profession due to physical infirmities. Adding sleep services and/or myofunctional therapy skills can give them a way to stay engaged in dentistry in meaningful ways.

Marketing and Advertising Outside the Practice

Every dental practice harbors a certain number of CPAP failures within the patient base. The trick is to find these patients and introduce them to OAT. One author (Ken Berley) found 22 patients who were CPAP noncompliant simply by asking them during medical history taking. Because these patients were previously diagnosed and had a treating sleep physician of record, they were treated first. This provided the opportunity to connect with local sleep professionals while developing appropriate in-office systems and communication protocols.

Because many dentists are not trained in airway health therapy or choose not to provide these services, one fertile field for new patients is to become known in your dental society or study club as a go-to clinician to whom to refer at-risk patients. You can provide colleagues with screening tools, referral pads, and (quite critically) a pledge to refuse a transfer of general dental services. Communicate with your peers just like you do with your patients' physicians and your dental specialists. You can get tips from your own specialists about building relationships with general dentists; they do it every day. If your 2,000-patient dental practice has 600 patients who are at risk for airway problems, imagine treating many of them and just two or three of their friends. Add in similar numbers from a few colleagues' practices, and you will be plenty busy with airway therapy.

For other outside advertising, consider providing health and civic groups with short talks on airway health. Physician groups have grand rounds, and many community clubs are always looking for an interesting professional to give a program. The American Academy of Dental Sleep Medicine (AADSM) has a Member PR Toolkit, online branding, and a packet of research papers that you can use to assemble a compelling pitch for airway health awareness. Additionally, there are online resources, such as SleepApnea.org and SleepHealth.org, that you can use to provide information for your patients. Although many of these sites are CPAP-oriented, they can provide insight into what the public knows about our field. SleepHealth.org has a CPAP donation system in case you want to stage a "turn in your unused CPAP" public event.

Media advertising can be very expensive, and it is hard to gauge the return on investment. Dentists have used radio, TV, billboards, and even infomercials to get more people aware of airway health and their office. A few companies have emerged that focus on our niche market; tapping into their expertise may be more effective than listening to the marketing pitches of your local media outlets. The AADSM has a patient-facing marketing program to build support for DSM.

Marketing takes time and focused energy. It is likely that no one on your team has the capacity to devote time to these efforts. It might be a great choice for you to contract this work to a local marketing professional or hire an additional public relations person for your office who can work full-time developing materials, getting you in front of community groups, and meeting other doctors. Measure the investment you make in this person against your goals and improvements in airway services. Keep in mind that establishing yours as the go-to office is an investment that may take some time to pay off, but the results can carry on for years.

In Steve Carstensen's office, the team made a goal to attend the American Dental Association (ADA) meeting in Hawaii using sleep medicine as the way to fund the trip. An ambitious goal was set for appliance deliveries, and a sum of money for each case delivered above that goal was set aside for the trip. With $500 contributions, the team funded a $15,000, whole-office trip in only 6 months. Everyone on the team contributed—the administrative staff set up meet-and-greets with other doctors, we screened everyone, and the finance team set up systems for payment. It worked so well that we did it again a few years later for a trip to the ADA meeting in New Orleans on Halloween!

Recording the Medical Encounter

Breaking down a new system into its parts can help the team focus on step-by-step improvements and goals that will enable the best outcomes. The medical encounter can be thought of in five parts: check-in, intake, examination, sign-off, and checkout.[2] Your patients' medical visits to your office are completed by the same team members who facilitate the dental appointments, but the documentation is different. Creating excellent medical encounter systems can benefit your dental practice, and the effort to do so will pay off on many levels. The steps are described here. Considering the personal nature of medical information being shared in these encounters, a private space in the office must serve as the designated spot for the intake steps. Scheduling, staff resource allocation, and patient flow systems must take this into account.

Because airway therapy is a hybrid treatment involving the fields of both dentistry and medicine, there are more stringent requirements for documentation. Other health care providers need to know what work you have performed for shared patients. Using shared documentation style and terminology will enhance the sense of working together. Included in this book is a glossary of terms to help you "speak the same language" as your medical colleagues. You can even turn memorization of this glossary into a team-building game, with prizes for team members who master common terms.

Check-in

When someone visits a medical provider, the greeter usually makes a copy of the medical insurance card, front and back, for the patient's chart. A card scanner at the front desk makes this very easy. The insurance card will provide a number to verify benefits and how much to collect for office visit copays. If your dental practice is going to use medical insurance to cover visits for airway therapy, the insurance company policies will make no allowances for how you conduct your dental practice but instead will expect you to conform to their standards. Given that, the explanation of benefits for any encounter will list the copay amount as part of the overall reimbursement. While copays are not common in procedure-based dental benefit plans, they are part of nearly every medical plan, so make collecting the patient's copayments a routine part of your office check-in protocol. Check-in also includes letting the clinical staff know that the patient is ready for the next step, intake.

Intake

The initial encounter form used in your dental practice probably has questions related to the patient's chief complaint, health history, current medications, family history, and dental health and esthetic goals. The medical encounter has similar questions; however, they are likely arranged somewhat differently. Information that you or your staff should be gathering includes the following:

1. Verify the reason for the visit. Often, patients are confused by the medical process, curious as to why they were referred to a dentist for an airway issue, and unsure of what to expect compared to other dental office visits.
2. Make sure you record the patient's preferred pharmacy and the names of their other medical providers. Ideally, you should gather the names of any providers that the patient has seen within the last 10 years so you can provide those practitioners with a copy of your professional-looking intake examination. This is especially important for airway-oriented history, such as ENT consults/surgery. If your examination and intake is well done, frequently these physicians will become referral sources.
3. Record the patient's vital signs. This is an opportunity to distinguish this dental encounter from standard dental visits. Patients will view your office differently based on your protocols. This will be enforced by the fact that you are a dentist who monitors their height, weight, blood pressure, respiration rate, and blood oxygen levels. Your team members should explain why gathering this data is necessary, and this is a great time to make a value statement about your new airway awareness.
4. Record any allergies, current medications, and other medical problems. Patients will often disclose other problems in this setting that they have not spoken about to the dentist before, thinking they were not relevant to their oral health care. Much can be learned at this step.
5. Record the past medical, family, and social history. The goal is to document a complete history of the patient's known medical problems. You should explore the patient's appreciation for the seriousness of OSA and what therapies have been attempted. This can be a part of the medical history or consist of a separate discussion as part of the HPI (history of present illness). Additionally, you need to discuss other family members who have diagnosed or suspected airway-related disease. You should discuss SRBD therapies that have been attempted and determine the social conditions that are exacerbating the patient's OSA. In particular, document the patient's smoking status, sleep schedules and patterns, alcohol use, and exercise habits. Additionally, it is helpful to ask whether the patient has a regular bed partner, as you will need their feedback during the titration portion of your therapy.
6. Ask about surgical history related to airway. Have they been operated on for tonsils, adenoids, or other nasal or upper airway issues?
7. If your patient has completed an airway screener, such as the Epworth Sleepiness Scale (ESS) or STOP-BANG questionnaire, you can reference it here, or have them fill out another one if this is not a first-encounter visit.

8. Record the HPI. How do they define the condition for themselves, how long have they had it, what have they done to make it better, and what makes it worse? Asking these simple questions will go a long way in helping you to understand the condition the patient presents with and their attitude about their health. Spend the time needed to gather details. A valuable question to ask is "What else?" until nothing else comes to the patient's mind. Whoever does this portion of the intake should be the office's best listener-communicator. Enhancing listening skills is especially helpful for this role.
9. It is important to note in your intake that you have reviewed and incorporated the referring physician's notes into your record. The referring sleep physician will provide a complete ROS (review of systems). Dentists can add observations to this comprehensive physician-conducted ROS; however, it may be outside your scope of practice to attempt to perform a full review of systems.

This may seem like an exhausting list for intake, but it takes just a few minutes for a trained auxiliary to complete, and it provides valuable insights that will help you find the best way to treat the person, including key motivators that will help the patient initiate and maintain therapy.

Examination

The best and most valuable information is collected when the doctor joins the conversation for the examination. The first step of examination is the handoff from the clinical team, who summarize what they have learned to this point. The doctor can review this information on a screen while listening to a verbal report from the staff member. The conclusion of this handoff should always involve turning to the patient and asking simply, "What else would you like me to know?"

RECORDING THE CHIEF COMPLAINT

By law, the doctor must always ask and record the chief complaint, although often the patient writes this out first. It is critical for the dentist to ask and probe for the most important reasons the patient is seeking therapy. Ask about it in the following way:

- What in your life is worse because of problems related to breathing while you sleep?
- What would improve if this problem went away? How would your life be better?

Being able to reference the answers to this chief complaint throughout the treatment process will provide powerful motivators that the team can employ to help the patient see therapy as truly being in their best interest. Knowing your patient is one of the most critically important parts of dentistry and medicine, especially as it applies to treatments that require the patient's active participation. For example, if the history includes the rejection of nightguards, that should be explored in detail prior to making a custom-fabricated oral appliance.

There is another important patient history report that bears detailing here: If a patient reports claustrophobia as the reason for not tolerating CPAP masks, dentists are advised to simply make a note of that and move on with the interview. A sleep doctor who became a psychiatrist once told Steve Carstensen that these patients have a high likelihood of posttraumatic stress disorder (PTSD) from an abuse episode where their mouth and nose were held closed by a perpetrator to control them. There simply is no need to go into details with these patients, and the dentist is further advised to emphasize how easy it will be for the patient to breathe around the custom MAD. There are also anatomical reasons why claustrophobia may be a problem with CPAP masks, such as an epiglottis that is forced over the airway by pressure. The risk of triggering PTSD is high. However, patients who have rejected nightguards or have claustrophobia may be candidates for a trial appliance to help build their acceptance of OAT. Each patient is different. If it appears that the patient may reject OAT due to the apprehension of having something in his or her mouth, it may be time to mention a professional-level temporary device.

Finally, the doctor reviews and updates the HPI and ROS as recorded in intake, just to make sure the data is correct. The physical examination comes next.

PHYSICAL EXAMINATION

When it comes to the physical examination, there is very little extra data that needs to be collected beyond what most dentists do for a comprehensive evaluation, although familiarity with the anatomy and function of the airway is required.

You do not have to be a TMJ expert, but because MAD therapy moves the mandible forward as the means of addressing airway patency, it is important to have a degree of comfort with the ways people might respond to that (Box 4-5). In addition to the standard TMJ, muscle, and soft and hard tissue examination data, the range of motion of the mandible and tongue are evaluated. Ankyloglossia (tongue-tie) is best addressed before age 5, but often, quality of life in adults can be improved with proper therapy. You may be the first one to discuss possibilities for addressing this condition with your adult patient.

BOX 4-5 Gaining confidence to manage the TMJ

If it has been a while since you studied the complex anatomy, function, and neuromuscular control of the TMJ, or if you lack confidence when a patient complains of pain or discomfort related to movement of the mandible, it is time to refresh your knowledge and clinical skills. Seek out training if you discover shortfalls in your understanding or comfort level. Adding MADs to your practice will create complications. Like every other part of dentistry, skills can be obtained, practiced, and mastered to give you, your team, and your patients confidence moving forward with vital treatment.

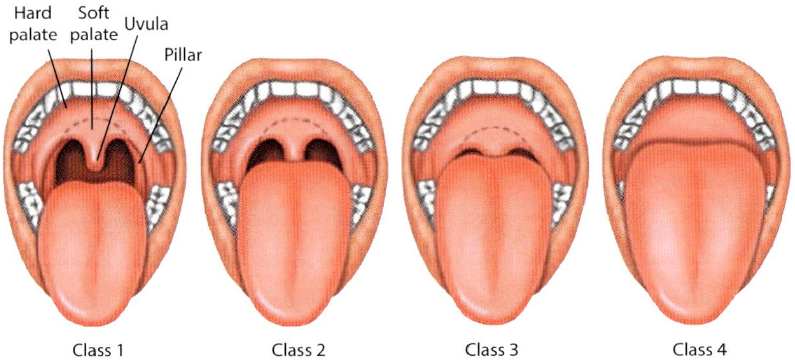

Fig 4-1 Mallampati scoring.

The oropharynx is evaluated using a Mallampati score[3] (Fig 4-1). This system, originally devised to help medical residents choose the correct size of intubation tube, is valuable for describing crowding in the oropharynx. The patient is instructed to sit upright, open as wide as possible, and protrude the tongue, with no sound.

- Mallampati 1: The posterior wall of the oropharynx is visible, with the tip of the uvula not contacting the tongue.
- Mallampati 2: The tip of the uvula contacts the dorsum of the tongue, but the entire soft palate is visible.
- Mallampati 3: The uvula is hidden behind the tongue, but the arches of the soft palate are visible, with a slight space above the tongue.
- Mallampati 4: There is no visualization of the oropharynx.

The Mallampati score is not indicative of any level of obstructed breathing, but people with scores of 3 or 4 are more likely to have a crowded oropharynx.[4] Mallampati scoring can be added to your hygienists' soft tissue examination protocol and reported to the doctor during preventive care visits.

Palatine tonsils are uncommon in adults. Typically, patients have either had them removed (as reported in the history), or they have naturally diminished in size with age. If the palatine tonsils are still visible, the patient should be asked about symptoms. These patients are often referred to an otolaryngologist, not for tonsillectomy but for a thorough assessment of the airway. Sometimes the recommendation is for removal of the palatine tonsils, but you never want your patient to think that surgery is the only choice. Children's tonsils are another matter entirely and are discussed later in this book (see chapter 12). Lingual tonsils and adenoids cannot be visualized during an oral examination but can be assessed with CBCT.

NASAL EXAMINATION

Another unusual place for the dentist to look is inside the nose. Also inquire about nasal breathing. The best way to evaluate the nose is to simply tip the patient's head back and lift the tip of the nose with a finger. Consider the nature of the nasal mucosa; it should be pink and healthy looking, just like the oral tissues. Redness, ulceration, crusting, or obvious inflammation is not uncommon and can lead to follow-up questions about allergies and nasal airway health. The dentist can see the shape and size of the inferior turbinates and whether the septum is deviated to one side. The black space around the turbinate is the only space there is to breathe through, so larger is better. Closing one of the patient's nostrils and then the other and asking if they can perceive a difference in breathing ability can provide more clues. Rhinomanometry is the most direct and precise way to quantify nasal function. Finding patients with significant nasal airway patency problems is very common in airway health examinations and requires forming a close relationship with an otolaryngologist who is aware of sleep breathing issues.

IMAGING

Most dentists have digital imaging capability. CBCT imaging, unlike panoramic radiography, provides accurate and undistorted images of the nasal passages and TMJs. Assessing the health of the periodontal bone support is part of the examination and is medically necessary. Unfortunately, because all imaging is performed on patients who are awake and there is no known method for translating that into what happens during sleep, it is not possible to predict effective mandibular position using any kind of imaging, though research is ongoing. Be cautious of making any kind of claim to provide a predictable treatment position. Because pictures on a screen can be powerful tools for visualizing the problem being addressed, they may be what motivates a patient to choose a path toward health. Make sure not to create unsupportable patient expectations.

Because the area imaged by CBCT is larger than most dentists have been trained to read, the authors recommend that all CBCT volumes be sent to maxillofacial radiologists for interpretation. Physicians are used to reading radiologists' reports and find this typical practice. Three brain tumors have been found in one author's practice using CBCT, identified by the radiologist. If you are considering purchase of a CBCT, we advise you to discuss with a few radiologists which machine provides volumes they find to be most accurate.

The latest CBCT machines are ultra-low–dose radiology devices. The benefits outweigh the increase in radiation. However, ALARA principles, standing for "as low as reasonably achievable," must be employed. Take images only when medically necessary. There is no benefit, for example, in taking an image in a jaw-protruded position to show the patient a larger airway during wakefulness because this is not predictive of airway responsiveness during sleep.

Assessment and planning

Dr L. D. Pankey called assessment and planning "applying your knowledge." In medical terminology, it is called "medical decision-making." The dentist takes all the information gathered, considers the personal nature of the patient, and creates a plan for addressing the diagnosed problem. Many of our airway health patients are already diagnosed with obstructed sleep breathing, and many at-risk patients are identified while conducting routine screening. These latter patients are then referred for testing and diagnosis. However, that is only a small part of the clinical picture. Dentists must also assess patients for their willingness to adhere to MAD therapy. While OAT compliance is much better than CPAP compliance, patients must be committed to the process. Managing OSA may involve nasal breathing techniques, positional therapy, weight loss, and exercise, along with some known side effects and other issues. Sometimes we must judge a patient who has been referred to us to be a poor candidate for our services. This level of decision-making is vital to airway health management, which in turn, is critical for the long-term health of patients. Dentists and their teams must be properly trained and aware of the role they play in their patients' overall well-being.

Once a patient accedes to a dentist's recommendations for custom OAT, it is up to the dentist to prescribe the best device. Staff can then take over and discuss finances and next steps, including scheduling requirements to begin therapy.

BOX 4-6 Financial considerations with MAD therapy

Financial management systems are disrupted by adding airway services because of the nature of medical benefit payments. Medical EOBs (explanations of benefits) do not follow the same pattern as dental benefit plans, with no different categories for adjustments. If the office engages with medical plans, calculations of production and collection can be difficult to perform. Team members used to dollar-figure goals and rewards can feel that there is too much chair time spent without payment for airway therapy. The leader must communicate the value by breaking down the time spent versus income generated and by helping the team see that it is financially viable. This may also be necessary to ensure that the team is clear that the fee for the device must support the necessary administrative and follow-up time devoted to airway therapy. Physicians, who are used to office encounters and ordering DME (durable medical equipment) services to be managed by a third party, often have a poor understanding of the significant time requirements of supporting OAT in the dental office. Patients may report comments by their sleep doctor about the cost of OAT. The dental team should be ready to support, in a positive, non-defensive way, the value of SRBD therapy with oral appliances in the dental office.

Sign-off

Sign-off is completed when the dentist has reviewed the check-in and the intake, performed the examination, and gathered sufficient data for completeness and accuracy. Letters can be created at this step to communicate with other providers what has happened during the encounter and what is requested next, if anything, to move the patient along the treatment path. Once satisfied with the details as recorded, the dentist signs off on the encounter. Some software packages allow only the doctor to "close the encounter," but if you are using a more standard dental software, it is important to place an attestation by the dentist at the end of the documentation that the data entered is accepted, coupled with initials or a signature.

Checkout

At checkout, the office staff discusses finances (Box 4-6) and insurance requirements with the patient, as well as the treatment sequence and next appointments. They can also see if the patient is comfortable with the huge amount of data just provided about their sleep and breathing. By devoting time and attention to this step, the patient will feel well cared-for, even if they acknowledge a bit of confusion. Patients often enjoy a phone call from the sleep champion a couple of days later for help sorting out their thoughts. Providing well-written materials or links to informative websites and videos is very helpful in preventing information overload, which can lead to inaction due to uncertainty over what to do next. Your practice's website can offer this information and include an action button that invites a call from the office.

Conclusion

Physicians involved with airway health include PCPs, otolaryngologists, board-certified sleep physicians, cardiologists, obstetricians/gynecologists, endocrinologists, neurologists, pulmonologists, and even oncologists. Your patients, depending on their health history, may have short or long lists of other providers. That care team now includes you. As our profession interacts with medical doctors concerning sleep breathing issues and we learn how to format our notes for professionalism and efficient, helpful communication, our standing in patient care will improve.

References

1. Evaluation and Management Services [publication ICN 006764]. US Department of Health and Human Services, 1997.
2. Athena Health website. https://www.athenahealth.com. Accessed 12 Feb 2024.
3. Kumar HV, Schroeder JW, Gang Z, Sheldon SH. Mallampati score and pediatric obstructive sleep apnea. J Clin Sleep Med 2014;10:985–990.
4. Bins S, Koster TD, de Heij AH, et al. No evidence for diagnostic value of Mallampati score in patients suspected of having obstructive sleep apnea syndrome. Otolaryngol Head Neck Surg 2011;145:199–203.

Sleep is the best and most natural painkiller in the world.

—Russell Foster

5

Treatment Decisions and Appliance Selection

Oral Appliance Therapy

When patients present to the dental office for oral appliance therapy (OAT), dentists must determine if they are good candidates for a mandibular advancement device (MAD). The decision for treatment lies with the medical provider who prescribes OAT, but dentists must use their expertise to decide if that prescription can be fulfilled. Whether a MAD can be fabricated for a given patient depends on the patient's dental, physical, and mental health. If a patient has severe periodontal disease or too few teeth to serve as anchorage for a MAD, the dentist must assess the risk of OAT and the likelihood of success and make a doctor-level decision about whether to proceed with treatment.

Some patients are incapable of placing, removing, or adjusting a MAD due to advanced arthritis or another issue. If none of the many oral devices available can be matched to a patient's physical abilities, that patient may be judged a poor candidate for OAT. Furthermore, because each patient must cooperate with therapy by wearing the MAD, cognitive decline or dementia may also be contraindications to therapy. For various reasons, some patients who otherwise qualify for OAT may refuse to consider wearing a device in their mouth. Every dental sleep medicine (DSM) provider must make a professional decision about whether OAT is a good match for treating a given patient's disease. If the dentist deems the patient to be a poor candidate for OAT, communicating that to the medical prescriber is critical. The physician may assume therapy has started when really they need to be thinking of what else they can do to help manage the patient's airway.

Setting expectations for OAT success depends on many variables. Every patient must be understood and treated as an individual. This may sound obvious, but every provider is subject to pattern recognition bias. In a cursory glance of a sleep report, focusing on only the Apnea-Hypopnea Index (AHI), oxygen desaturation index (ODI), or nadir SpO_2 can lead dentists to skip considering important details that may explain later shortcomings in therapy results. If the predictability of therapy can be improved up front, there will be better shared understanding between patients and providers and fewer negative encounters.

The medical history of every patient must be reviewed by the treating dentist, who searches for areas of concern. Many patients with obstructive sleep apnea (OSA) take sedatives, opioids, and/or central nervous system depressants to manage chronic pain and/or help them sleep. These medications frequently exacerbate OSA. Additionally, some patients take medications that affect sleep stages and quality. It is not uncommon for primary care physicians (PCPs) to prescribe selective serotonin reuptake inhibitors or antidepressants when patients present with a complaint of fatigue. Unfortunately, many of these medications reduce the total time spent in rapid eye movement (REM) sleep. Therefore, a thorough evaluation of every patient's health history and their medications is mandatory. Often, your software can be set to automatically download a patient's medication list. If so, that's a great place to start. Your team can also request a list of current prescriptions and commonly used supplements. Although you do not need to have a pharmacist's knowledge of these medications, familiarity with them is helpful. An excellent resource is Epocrates, which is free to download for desktop and mobile devices. Staying curious will help you find patterns, and soon, long lists of prescriptions reported by medically complex patients will not appear so daunting. If your review brings up concerns, keep in mind that challenging a prescribing physician with a "why did you..." question is far less productive than leading with a "please help me understand..."

OSA is also linked to dementia and cognitive decline. It is hypothesized that chronic intermittent oxygen desaturations result in the permanent loss of brain mass, particularly in the hypothalamus. As a result, it is not uncommon to encounter patients who have difficulty following instructions. If you suspect that your patient may have this challenge, in addition to providing all instructions in writing, you must obtain permission to discuss details with a reliable caregiver who can assist the patient with daily tasks. Dentists providing OAT are likely not the first medical professionals charged with managing chronic disease for these patients, so the patient and their caregivers are very likely to have a system that works for them already in place. Be welcoming to the caregiver and empathetic about the complexity of daily living for the patient.

OSA patients frequently present with temporomandibular disorders (TMDs) with no history of diagnosed sleep-related breathing disorders (SRBDs). When examining a patient for TMD issues, OSA or upper airway resistance syndrome must be a part of your differential diagnosis. When evaluating a possible airway insufficiency issue in a TMD patient, referral to a sleep physician is always the first choice. If you are fortunate enough to have a physical therapist in your area who understands the craniofacial respiratory complex, working with them could be very helpful (see chapter 15). Pulse oximetry screening may be appropriate. If your patient is a younger person with no significant subjective symptoms of SRBD, screening tools such as high-resolution overnight pulse oximetry with software that produces reports that include sleep quality can be invaluable for determining if the patient has an airway insufficiency problem associated with the TMD symptoms. Mild disturbances to airway function can induce sympathetic nervous system overdrive, resulting in a degradation of sleep quality and enhanced pain perception.

Examination

The physical examination of the patient includes checking and recording the following:

- BMI
- Blood pressure
- Neck circumference (in inches)
- Respiratory rate
- Upper airway
  - Soft palate
    - Elongated
    - Battered (bruised)
    - Inflamed
  - Uvula
    - Elongated
    - Battered (bruised)
    - Inflamed

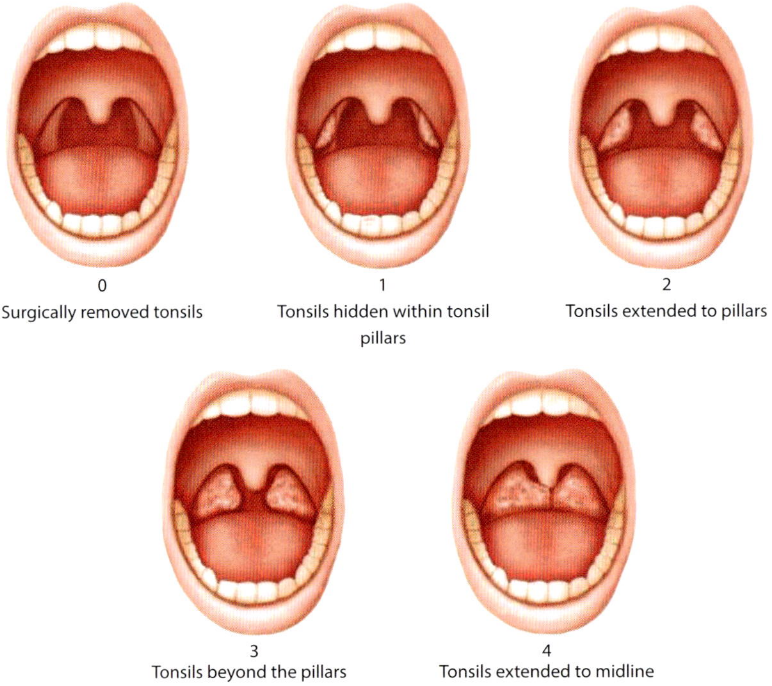

Fig 5-1 Grading of palatine tonsils.

- Palatine tonsils
  - Present
  - Absent
  - Obstructive
  - Purulent
  - Grade 1 to 4[1] (Fig 5-1)
- Tongue
  - Ankyloglossia (tongue-tie)
  - Enlarged
  - Scalloped
  - Inflamed (reddened)
  - Coated
- Mallampati score[2] (see Fig 4-1)

• Nose
- Inflamed
- Deviated septum

   - Turbinate enlargement
   - Nasal valve collapse with sniff
     - Right
     - Left
     - Both
   - Function: Can they pass a 2 minute nasal breathing test?
   - Need for referral to an otolaryngologist?
- Periodontal status (severe periodontal disease may be an absolute contra-indication to OAT)
   - Gingivitis
   - Periodontal disease (attachment loss) with the current periodontal chart made part of the record
   - Mobility
   - Hygiene insufficiencies
   - Consent discussion (must include the additional risk of exacerbating the patient's periodontal condition, plus tooth mobility, tooth movement, and tooth loss)
- Number, position, and health of the teeth in each quadrant and the number of teeth in each arch
   - There is no consensus on the minimum number of teeth necessary for OAT.
   - An edentulous maxillary arch can support a MAD in many cases.
   - An edentulous mandibular arch will not support a MAD without implants.
   - Most practitioners state that eight or more teeth per arch are needed to support OAT.
   - If the patient has less than eight teeth, a discussion and informed consent is required regarding the additional risk. One author (Ken Berley) has made a MAD on as few as two mandibular canines, but the patient signed a release of liability document.
- TMD symptoms (by palpation)[3]
   - Temporomandibular joint (TMJ) lateral capsule (right and left)
   - TMJ posterior capsule (right and left)
   - Anterior temporalis (right and left)
   - Middle temporalis (right and left)
   - Posterior temporalis (right and left)
   - Temporalis tendon (right and left)
   - Masseter body (right and left)
   - Masseter origin (right and left)
   - Masseter insertion (right and left)
   - Medial pterygoid (right and left)

   - Inferior lateral pterygoid (use provocation test)
   - Sternocleidomastoid body (right and left)
   - Sternocleidomastoid origin (right and left)
   - Sternocleidomastoid insertion (right and left)
   - Joint sounds (use a stethoscope or Doppler instrument)
     - Crepitus (right and left)
     - Early opening click (right and left)
     - Early closing click (right and left)
     - Late closing click (right and left)
     - Late opening click (right and left)
   - Range of motion
     - Anterior protrusion available from centric without pain (mm)
     - Maximum interincisal opening without pain (mm)
     - Right lateral excursion without pain (mm)
     - Left lateral excursion without pain (mm)
     - Deviation on opening (right or left) (mm)
     - Deflection on opening (right or left) (mm)
   - Informed consent: If TMD symptoms are present, the patient must be informed of risk. Start with less protrusion and advance the mandible slowly. Almost all TMD symptoms get better with time, but if you advance the mandible too far and too quickly, these patients will not like you and will often abandon therapy.
- Dental disease, decay, or infection
   - Oral examination
   - Radiographs (type and date)
   - If the patient has significant dental issues that need to be fixed but will not prevent you from making a MAD, you can have the patient sign an informed refusal and release.
   - You are not looking for perfect teeth, but they should be healthy.
- Crown/root ratio
- Amount of available voluntary non-painful protrusion
   - A range < 5 mm is not necessarily a contraindication for treatment.
   - Very slow advancement (< 1 mm/month) can result in additional flexibility.
- Bruxism
- Lack of sufficient axial contours that may cause retention issues
- Existence of periapical pathology
   - These patients must be treated or referred. If they refuse, they must sign an informed refusal and release of liability to be treated.

- Angle classification
  - Class I
  - Class II
  - Class III
  - Overbite (mm)
  - Overjet (mm)
  - Posterior crossbite (right, left, or both)
- Vaulted palate (mild, moderate, or severe)
- Mandibular crowding (anterior, posterior, or both)
- Maxillary crowding (anterior, posterior, or both)
- Interproximal open contacts
  - List any teeth with open contacts.

When the clinical exam reveals significant TMD symptoms or a lack of ability to protrude (< 5 mm), the patient should be informed that many practitioners consider this type of finding to be a total contraindication to MAD therapy. A conscientious and risk-averse practitioner who wishes to provide treatment for this patient should provide additional information to obtain a valid informed consent. The patient should be informed how the lack of voluntary protrusion will affect the titration of the appliance and potentially result in unsuccessful treatment. The patient should understand the need for slow advancement of the MAD over an extended period of time to achieve an adequate therapeutic protrusion. Additionally, the patient needs to understand that there may be an active elongation (stretching) of the sphenomandibular and stylomandibular ligaments, which can take months to accomplish. After adequate information is provided about the slower advancement and potentially compromised therapy, the patient's consent can be noted in the record.

Medical History

The patient's medical history should include the following:

- History of comorbid disease: Anxiety/depression, excessive daytime sleepiness (EDS), cardiovascular disease, hypertension, and insomnia all qualify a patient with an AHI between 5 and 15 for treatment.
  - Blood pressure (hypertension)
  - Stroke
  - Diabetes mellitus
  - Heart disease (stents, myocardial infarction, angina)
  - Chronic obstructive pulmonary disease
  - Dementia/Alzheimer's disease

    - Gastroesophageal reflux disease
- Diagnostic OSA evaluation
    - AHI
        - Total respiratory events
            - Obstructive events (% of total)
            - Hypopneas (% of total)
            - Centrals (% of total)
            - Central or complex apnea diagnosis
            - ODI (both 3% and 4% indices)
                - Nadir SpO_2
                - Time below 90% oxygen saturation
    - Sleep stage (%)
        - N1
        - N2
        - N3
        - REM
- Mental capacity/ability to follow instructions
- Significant arthritis
- Whether the patient has been successful with continuous positive airway pressure (CPAP)
    - Most patients with severe sleep apnea should try CPAP before MAD therapy.
        - If the sleep study shows significant central sleep apnea (CSA), it is a good idea to discuss options with the diagnosing physician if MAD therapy has not been specifically prescribed. CSA is a result of reduced or inadequate respiratory drive, which may not be improved by physically managing the patient's airway. Treatment options are limited, and many physicians will go ahead with MAD therapy even with high percentages of CSA events in the AHI.
    - Many insurance companies and Medicare require either a CPAP trial for any patient with severe sleep apnea before MAD therapy or a physician's note specifically stating why a trial is contraindicated.

Informed Consent

Once the decision has been made to proceed with OAT, a discussion needs to occur between the provider and the patient to inform the patient of the relevant facts about OAT and to obtain consent to begin treatment (see chapter 10 for details).

BOX 5-1 FDA-approved MADs

The FDA website includes a database search function for all snoring and OSA oral appliances that have received 510(k) clearance for commercial distribution: https://www.accessdata.fda.gov/scripts/cdrh/cfdocs/cfPMN/pmn.cfm.

Enter the product's LQZ or LRK code into the "Product Code" field, and click the search button. You can also enter the product's PLC code to find a list of appliances that measure patient adherence to therapy.

A Note on Brands

The goal of this chapter is to help you choose temporary appliances and MADs that will benefit your patients and provide successful early experiences. Rather than resort to labels that might be confusing (eg, "Device A"), we choose to provide brand names in this text. Neither author has any connection to the clinical sales of these devices (although both of us have been and continue to be hired to teach DSM at events sponsored by various manufacturers). Fortunately, many appliances have similar characteristics that allow for group discussion. It is amazing how many DSM practitioners use only one appliance. Do not fall into that trap! Your success rate will improve significantly as your knowledge of different appliances increases. Dentists who master three to five devices and who are adept at working with several more can meet the needs of nearly every patient. There are many FDA-approved devices on the market, and the trained and experienced dentist can select from a wide range of products for individual patients (Box 5-1). If we don't mention a specific device, it's not because we have any bias against it or are hinting at anything negative. If we wrote about every device available, the list would be too long to be useful and out of date before it was published.

An important consideration when choosing a device is its proven efficacy. The FDA approves MADs mostly by comparing them to similar devices already on the market. Some MADs have been rigorously tested for effectiveness, but most have not and have yet to make the list. Most MAD manufacturers have never had to submit randomized control studies to the FDA, and if you ask them for independent published reports backing their clinical claims, there will be none. That isn't to say that their devices cannot be useful, but if your intent is to provide evidence-based care, it is important to make informed decisions. Most studies that compare MADs find little difference between them in effectiveness, but sometimes patient preferences are starkly one-sided. We suggest that clinicians do their best to keep up with the large number of clinical reports being published every year to choose devices that are backed by solid science. Readers are encouraged to review the research behind TAP (Thornton Adjustable Positioner) appliances from Airway Labs and ProSomnus appliances for examples of MADs with well-documented efficacy.

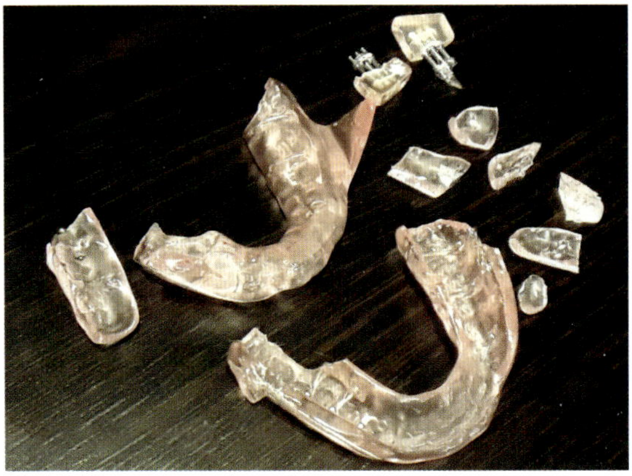

Fig 5-2 Unfortunately, MADs also make excellent chew toys.

BOX 5-2 Practice tip

If a patient sleeps with a dog in their bedroom, suggest that they contact their homeowner's insurance company to add a rider to the home policy for the MAD. These policies are simple and inexpensive and can save a patient lots of money if their new custom device proves irresistible to the family pet.

Temporary Appliances

All DSM providers are encouraged to stock temporary appliances in their offices. These devices are most frequently used when a patient's custom appliance fractures after a run-in with the family dog (Fig 5-2; Box 5-2). When an appliance is broken, a prudent clinician will provide a temporary appliance to be worn during the interim while the custom appliance is repaired or replaced. A temporary appliance may also be warranted when a patient presents for an initial examination and the polysomnogram (PSG) shows the patient to be dangerously hypoxic during REM sleep. OSA can be a deadly disease, and a temporary appliance could ensure that your patient safely returns to your clinic. If dangerous daytime sleepiness is a concern, every doctor on the care team has a responsibility to address it at every stage, including when successful OAT must be interrupted. You will notice on physician encounter notes that patients are directed not to drive or engage in other risky behaviors while sleepy. By providing a professional interim device, you could possibly help them with sleepiness while the custom oral appliance is being made.

Frequently, a question is raised regarding the use of a temporary appliance to predict the likely effectiveness of a custom-made MAD. Research has shown that some interim devices are as effective as custom laboratory-fabricated MADs, making this pathway a reasonable option for doctors and patients to consider. However, exercise caution when using temporary appliances as a trial device.

The danger of this type of trial is the false negative. The patient may wrongly believe that a custom-made MAD will not be successful if a temporary device fails due to poor retention, bulkiness, or poor fit, rather than a lack of effectiveness. This could cause a patient to abandon the therapy that would be best for them.

Although OAT is not typically recommended for patients with a diagnosis of CSA, experience has shown that some CSA patients respond well when the airway is opened with MAD therapy. This is particularly true for patients with complex sleep apnea that has been identified during CPAP titration. In this situation, the CPAP is blowing off too much CO_2, which results in respiratory depression. MAD therapy is sometimes a viable treatment option when the patient is unable to wear a CPAP device due to complex apnea. Because MAD use in this scenario does not have predictable therapeutic outcomes, a temporary trial appliance may be indicated with in-house testing. Testing can be accomplished using home sleep apnea testing (HSAT) after titrating subjective symptoms. One author (Ken Berley) routinely uses a myTAP (Airway Labs) temporary device for patients with CSA for a period of 1 month or more, performing an HSAT both before and after the myTAP trial to evaluate treatment efficacy. Once the temporary device is determined to improve the CSA, the permanent appliance is fabricated.

Over-the-counter temporary appliances

There are a number of over-the-counter temporary devices, and most are similar in design. Many use football mouthpiece–type materials with some type of hinge to hold the mandible in an advanced position. Poor retention and bulkiness are common problems associated with these devices, but they can be helpful in some circumstances. Typically, they are cheaper than semi-custom appliances and require no chair time for fitting. This is particularly helpful when a patient walks into your office with a broken appliance in the middle of a busy day. Having the ability to pull an appliance off the shelf that the patient can use during the time required to repair their MAD is valuable.

A good example of an over-the-counter appliance is the ZQuiet (Fig 5-3). This device comes with different amounts of protrusion, so patients must be evaluated to determine which ZQuiet should be dispensed. This temporary appliance is valuable to use when the patient is having a crown placed or when other extensive dental work is in progress. Because the appliance does not place significant pressure on any individual teeth, it is less likely to displace a temporary crown. Myofunctional Research Corporation also has a line of devices that serve double-duty as acute TMD therapy aids, and Steve Carstensen has found these to be very useful in practice (Fig 5-4).

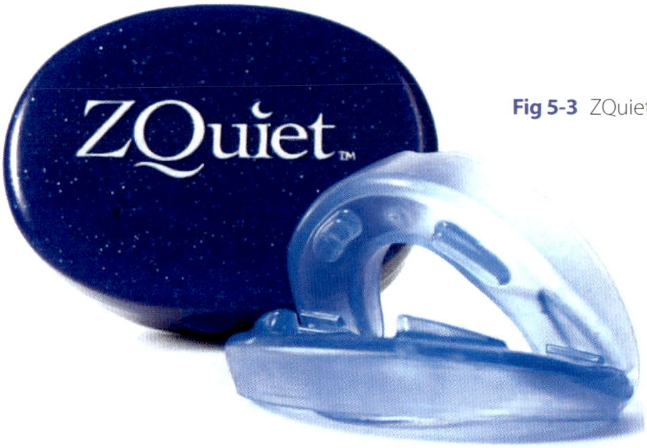

Fig 5-3 ZQuiet device.

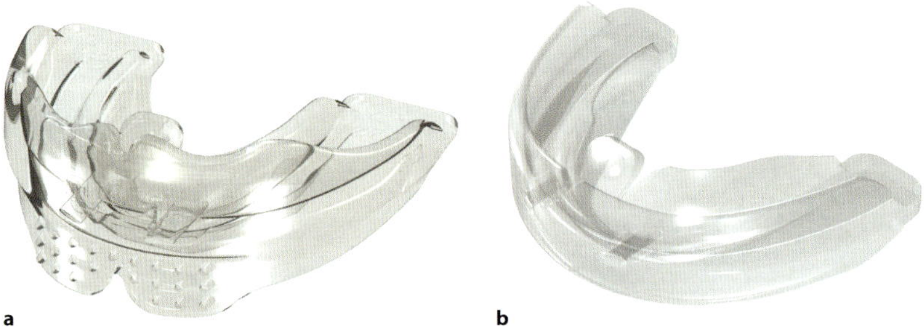

a b

Fig 5-4 *(a and b)* Examples of Myofunctional Research Corporation devices.

Semi-custom temporary appliances

All semi-custom appliances require some degree of fitting or adjustment before they can be used by a patient. Custom fitting in the dental office nearly always results in better retention but requires chair time and a team member. Some semi-custom appliances are just as bulky as over-the-counter options. The cost of the appliance and the required chair time must be considered when setting fees for this choice of therapy.

An example of a useful semi-custom—fit device is myTAP from Airway Labs. This is a thermoplastic appliance that can be molded to a patient's teeth (Fig 5-5). Heating the thermoplastic material softens it, which allows for a custom fit, and this step can be repeated as often as necessary should the patient be going through restorative dental changes. The appliance is also titratable,

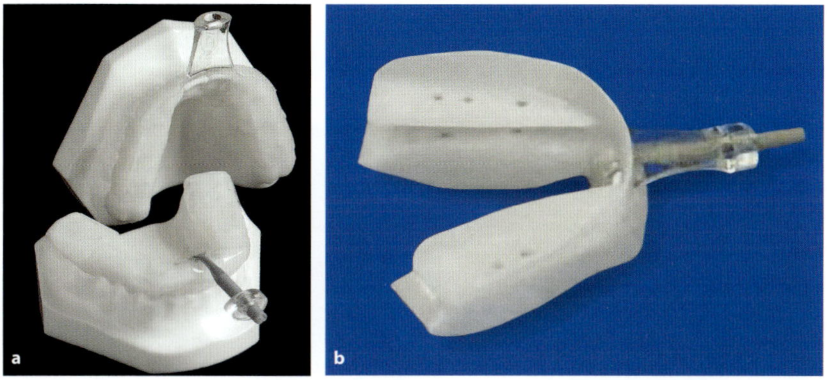
a b

Fig 5-5 *(a and b)* myTAP appliance.

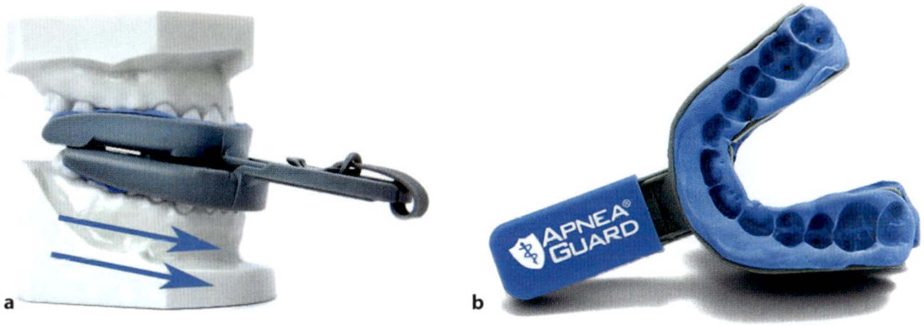

a b

Fig 5-6 *(a and b)* Apnea Guard appliance.

which research now shows can be used to predict the success of OAT. Titration is accomplished by turning the plastic nut on the front of the appliance. There is a millimeter ruler on the appliance that helps to determine the amount of protrusion. myTAP also comes with a mouth shield to promote nasal breathing and several soft spacers to vary the vertical opening while the mandible is being protruded. This provides an enhanced ability for the patient to evaluate whether OAT is for them prior to custom device fabrication. Using a myTAP device is challenging, however, if the teeth have little retentive shape.

Apnea Guard (Advanced Brain Monitoring) is another semi-custom temporary appliance that uses a heavy-body polyvinyl putty impression material to provide retention (Fig 5-6). It can be protruded, and the vertical dimension can be varied to some degree. Protrusion is done by sliding the lower tray out and locking it with a push pin that is inserted between the trays. There are millimeter measurements on the slide to assist in advancement. Unfortunately, the Apnea Guard feels bulky to some patients, and retention can be an issue for short, round teeth.

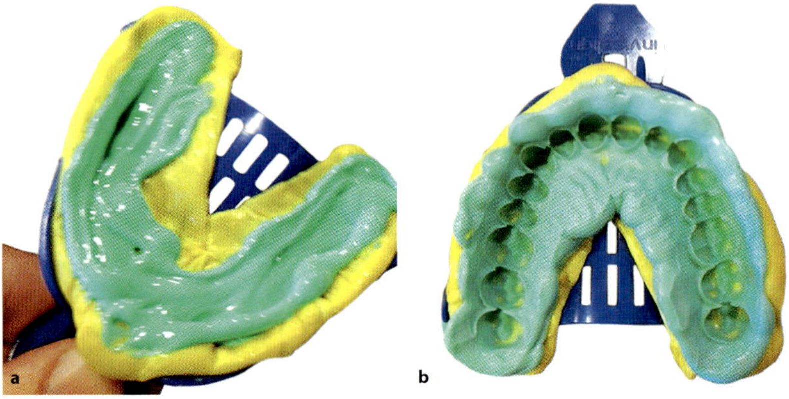

Fig 5-7 *(a and b)* Dual-system impression.

Clinical Techniques for MAD Fabrication

Impressions versus scanning

Both quality impressions and scanning are appropriate methods for MAD fabrication. Each technique has certain advantages and disadvantages, so use whichever one works best for you. Manufacturers are, however, steadily going digital. It may be some time before they refuse impressions or stone models, but there is no doubt that day is coming. If you are considering buying an intraoral scanner, be sure the supporting software makes it easy to capture whole arches and register a bite. Choose a software that automatically removes any registration material that is placed between the teeth, leaving the upper and lower teeth apart but connected on the screen. This is a common feature—just be sure that your choice includes it.

Scanning can be difficult when the patient is either obese or has little room between the maxillary second molars and the coronoid process. It may be quite challenging to scan the distofacial aspect of the maxillary second molar. If the patient has third molars, the task is virtually impossible. In some cases, a polyvinyl impression may be the best option. Picking a scanner that has a small tip and challenging your team members to master it can ensure that digital records are the first option for nearly every patient. In Steve Carstensen's practice, only three impressions have been taken in the past 9 years (as of this writing), and those were done because the scanner was inoperative on one day.

The best technique for taking a quality polyvinyl impression is a dual system composed of a heavy-body putty followed by a light-body wash (Fig 5-7). Commitment to the same quality required for a crown-and-bridge impression is the best route to ensuring a well-fitting custom oral device.

Bite registration

Dental sleep practitioners frequently disagree on protrusive bite registration techniques. As of this writing, there is no imaging system available that can predict a jaw position that will effectively support an open airway during sleep, especially during supine REM sleep. There are many ways to register the 3D bite but no consensus on the most effective technique. Some dentists swear by the use of acoustic pharyngometry, which involves using vocal exercises to identify a starting position for the jaw. However, most dentists who start patients between 25% and 75% protrusion get good results without significant TMD issues, so the authors recommend using the technique that is the simplest and least costly and requires the least time.[4] The initial protrusion depends on the severity of the patient's OSA and the results of the TMD examination. One author prefers 70% protrusion for a starting position, and the other author prefers 50% protrusion. The amount of initial protrusion must be comfortable for the patient. It is very important to test the starting position by holding the patient in that position for several minutes (10 minutes if time allows) to make sure that the position is comfortable. Studies about which vertical dimension is optimal are not helpful. Good results can be found with both minimal and quite large vertical dimensions. In accordance with patient preference, the minimum vertical dimension that allows for device fabrication is best, especially for females. When a crowded arch and obesity combine to give the tongue inadequate space, a greater vertical dimension allows for a more forward posture to diminish crowding in the oropharynx.

GEORGE GAUGE

The George Gauge (Great Lakes Dental Technologies) is a bite fork used to establish bite registration (Fig 5-8). To take a bite registration with the George Gauge at 70% protrusion, perform the following steps:

1. Place the George Gauge in the patient's mouth without the bite fork attachment.
2. Center the mandibular incisor notch over the anterior teeth.
3. Cinch up the mandibular incisor clamp to firmly grip these teeth, and tighten the lower turn screw to secure this position.
4. The upper bite forks are 2 mm and 5 mm thick. Choose the one that provides at least 3 or 4 mm of clearance between the back teeth, and slide it into the upper part of the George Gauge.

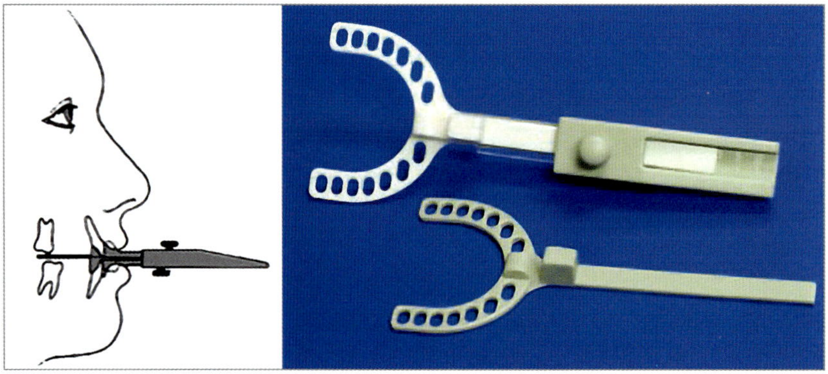

Fig 5-8 George Gauge bite fork.

BOX 5-3 Tips for using the George Gauge

- Repeat the measurement three times to ensure consistency.
- For most patients, two-thirds of centric to maximum protrusion is a valid formula. However, if there are TMD problems, it may be necessary to advance the mandible by gradually titrating forward.
- Once a position is obtained, ask the patient to hold that position for 3 (and up to 10) minutes and seek feedback. Adjust if necessary.

5. While the patient is holding the gauge securely by fitting their incisors into the notches, instruct him or her to slide the jaw forward as far as possible. Note the positive reading on the millimeter scale.
6. Ask the patient to move the jaw back as far as possible. Note the position on the negative end of the millimeter scale.
7. Add these two numbers without regard for the positive and negative signs. The total is the patient's protrusive range.
8. Multiply this sum by 0.7 (70%), and add this number to the negative number (retrusive position). The result is the number at which you should preset the George Gauge. Whichever starting position you choose, simply change the percentage number in this calculation, and the rest of the process is the same.

For example, if the patient can protrude to the +6 mark on the millimeter scale and can retrude to –4, their protrusive range is 10 mm. Take 70% of that range, which is 7 mm, and add it to the most retrusive position, which is –4. This gives you a setting of +3. Slide the marking end of the bite fork over the millimeter scale until its indicator rests over the +3 mark, and tighten the upper turn screw. Box 5-3 lists some tips for using the George Gauge.

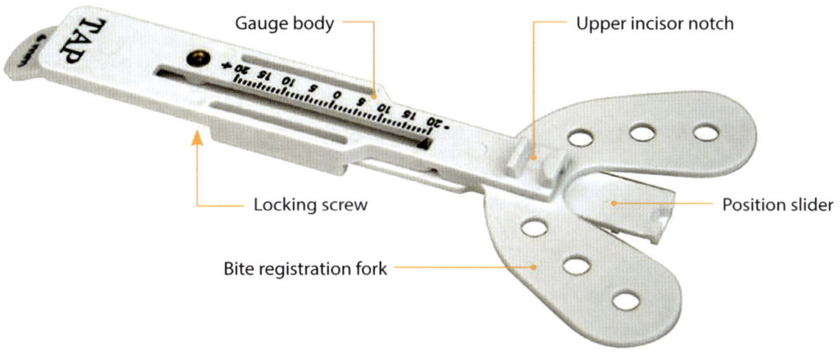

Fig 5-9 Assembled Pro Gauge.

Make sure to use enough recording material (eg, fast-setting vinyl polysiloxane [VPS]) on the bite fork. If you are scanning, you may need only two to four dots of VPS to stabilize the jaws while the intraoral scanner registers the arch position. If you are sending stone models to a lab, you must use enough VPS to keep the jaw position unambiguous for the lab artist. The procedure is as follows:

1. Apply bite material directly onto the mandibular teeth (going back to the most posterior tooth), and apply bite material to the top of the bite fork that is attached to the George Gauge.
2. Return the gauge to the mouth with the mandibular incisor notch centered over the midline, and instruct the patient to bite into the upper groove. Allow the registration material to fully set.
3. Unscrew the upper turn screw, and remove the bite fork.
4. Send the bite fork and impressions/casts to your dental laboratory, and keep the body of the George Gauge to reuse in the future.

PRO GAUGE

The Pro Gauge (Airway Labs; Fig 5-9) functions very similarly to the George Gauge but has positioning devices that allow for more vertical dimension than the George Gauge. It comes with 6-, 9-, and 12-mm interincisal positioning blocks. This capability is very valuable, depending on the appliance that is being fabricated. The Pro Gauge can easily accommodate patients with anterior open bites. This system also has an autoclavable measurement device and reusable plates.

BOX 5-4 Special instructions for when a 6-mm interincisal distance is too vertical for a starting position

1. Advance the lower part of the gauge 5 mm from the chosen starting position. For example, if you've chosen 0 mm, set the gauge at +5.
2. When positioning the loaded gauge into the mouth, instead of placing the lower notch over the mandibular teeth, position the end of the gauge against the facial surface of the incisors. The mandibular incisal edges will contact the plate.
3. The mandible is then rotated up as usual, with the maxillary teeth dropping into the upper notch. This provides a 4-mm interincisal distance.

Steve Carstensen's technique for using the Pro Gauge is as follows:

1. Have the patient close into maximum intercuspation (MIP), and observe the midlines.
2. Loosen the set screw on the lower side of the gauge.
3. The incisal notches in the gauge have blocks to place in contact with the facial surfaces. Align the lower midline in the center of the lower block, and close against the maxillary incisors. Note where the maxillary midline falls on the upper block. You can mark this if you wish.
4. With the teeth lightly holding the gauge, have the patient protrude and retrude the mandible two or three times, and record the maximum measurements at each position. There is no need for precision; just get it close.
5. Evaluate the posterior teeth to see if there is enough clearance for the device you wish to fabricate. If not, vary the interincisal distance by changing the slide. If the distance is excessive, see Box 5-4.
6. Remove the gauge, and set the bite at your preferred position by tightening the set screw.
7. Place the bite plate in the gauge, and apply the quick-setting registration material.
8. Place the loaded gauge back over the mandibular incisors, and instruct the patient to rotate the mandible up, dropping the maxillary incisors into the upper incisor notch. Ensure that the upper midline returns to the spot on the block you noted in step 3.
9. When the registration is set, remove the gauge, pop the bite plate out, and place it over the maxillary arch.
10. Verify that there is no rocking, and repeat the process for the mandibular arch.
11. Instruct the patient to close into the registration, and verify that the midlines have been kept in alignment.

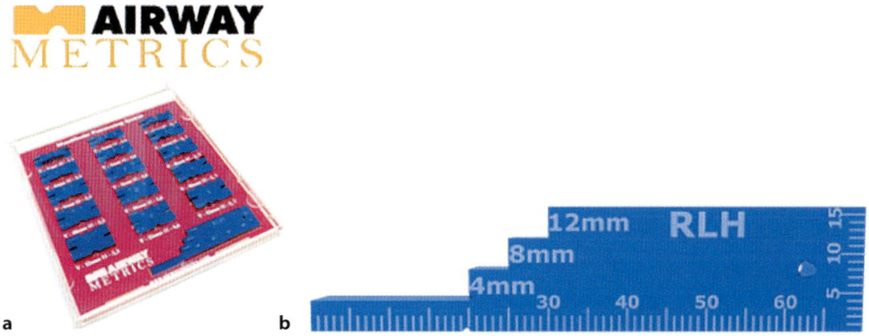

Fig 5-10 *(a)* Airway Metrics bite registration system. *(b)* Snore Screener.

AIRWAY METRICS

Airway Metrics (Kettenbach) bite registration system includes a series of preset plastic pieces with various amounts of vertical and horizontal protrusion (Fig 5-10a). It also comes with a Snore Screener that can be used to determine the best starting position based on the patient's ability to snore at each position (Fig 5-10b). If a patient cannot snore on command, logically, their ability to snore during sleep and occlude the airway will be diminished.

Ken Berley's technique for using the Snore Screener is as follows:

1. Place the Snore Screener in the patient's mouth, with the incisal tip positioned in front of the 4-mm ledge.
2. Ask the patient to bite into the plastic bar without protrusion and attempt to snore.
3. With the Snore Screener still in the 4-mm vertical position, ask the patient to protrude the mandible in 1- to 2-mm increments, and make note of the protrusive position at which the patient can no longer snore.
4. Reposition the Snore Screener to the 8-mm vertical position.
5. Ask the patient to protrude the mandible again and attempt to snore, and again, make note of the protrusive position at which the patient can no longer snore. If less protrusion is required to locate a position at which the patient cannot snore, the patient is a vertical patient.
6. Repeat the previous steps at the 12-mm vertical position.
7. The best vertical and horizontal positions are determined and then tried with the bite tabs.

The procedure for bite registration with the Airway Metrics system is as follows:

1. Insert the bite fork and handle into the slots on opposite ends of the selected mandibular positioning simulator so that the multiple notches are positioned on top and a single notch is on the bottom.
2. Position the maxillary central incisors into the notch that will allow for obtaining the desired mandibular position, and instruct the patient to close the mandibular incisors into the single lower notch.
3. Gently support the upper notch in position, and instruct the patient to open and close until the mandibular incisors smoothly fit into the lower notch (this usually takes two to four tries).
4. Place registration paste on the top and bottom of the fork, excluding the canine-to-canine area to preserve a clear visual of the anatomical center during closure.
5. Immediately upon closure, inject additional paste to cover the maxillary and mandibular areas that were left open for visualization. Connecting a second injector tip should not be required.

Photographs and casts

Photographs and casts should be used to document the original position of the bite and teeth before treatment. Tooth movement and jaw repositioning are the most common complications of OAT. Therefore, good records that show the patient's bite and tooth alignment prior to therapy are mandatory. For the most part, digital records have replaced stone models. If you send models to the lab for fabricating the MAD, request that they scan them and return the digital file to you. That way, you won't have to store boxes of stone models.

Photographic views should include the following:

- Full-face smile
- Lateral profile
- Anterior retracted in MIP
- Anterior retracted with teeth slightly apart
- Left retracted (MIP)
- Right retracted (MIP)
- Maxillary occlusal
- Mandibular occlusal

BOX 5-5 Medicare-restricted appliances

Go to https://www.palmettogba.com/pdac. Click on the option for DMECS, and enter "E0486" in the HCPCS Code box and click "Search." You will see a list of items with effective end dates. Items without end dates are approved for Medicare payments.

Definitive Oral Appliance Selection

Several factors must be considered when selecting the appropriate oral appliance for your patients. There is no flowchart, algorithm, or cheat sheet that can guide you to the "perfect" device. Each patient presents with unique characteristics that will require you to use your doctor skills to select the best device. Gaining clinical wisdom through thoughtful experience will provide you with the confidence to choose wisely.

Some details to consider when selecting a device include the following:

- Insurance and Medicare restrictions: Medicare and a significant number of insurance companies restrict the funding of appliances to those that have received a PDAC (Pricing, Data Analysis, and Coding) number (Box 5-5). Knowing restrictions in advance will improve the clinical encounter experience for patients. You don't want them to expect one device and then be delivered another.
- History of lateral bruxism and clenching
- Number and location of teeth
- Shape of the teeth (Do they provide enough retention for the design you choose?)
- Metal or material sensitivity or allergy
- Does the design allow for easy lip closure? If not, which additional therapy will you need to plan for?
- Ease of adjustment by the patient
- Can the vertical dimension (interarch distance) be modified during treatment if necessary?
- Can the appliance be modified to provide more protrusion if you run out of adjustment room?

Oral appliances can be further classified as one of the following types:

- Appliances that protrude the jaw by pushing
- Appliances that protrude the jaw by pulling
- Appliances that have an anterior attachment and interlock the arches
- Monoblock appliances that do not offer advancement or adjustment
- Appliances that have interlocking shapes that provide advancement

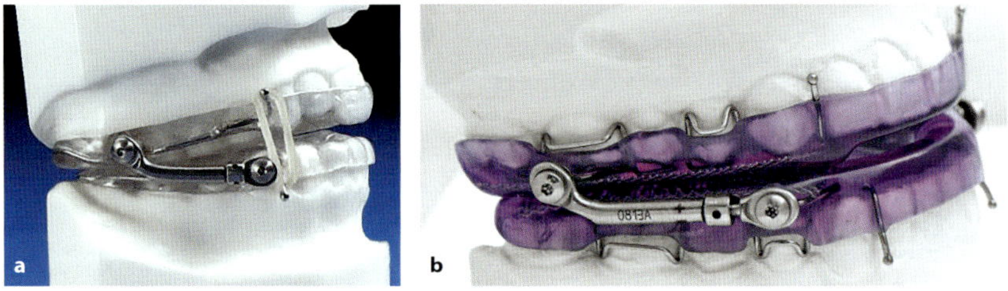

Fig 5-11 *(a and b)* Herbst appliance.

Appliances that push the jaw: Herbst appliance

The Herbst is a great example of an appliance that pushes the jaw to achieve protrusion (Fig 5-11). It can be used in patients with a limited number of teeth and in edentulous maxillary arches, and it is a workhorse for many practitioners. It is on the PDAC list and is made by every full-service DSM manufacturing lab. A Herbst device can be fabricated from many kinds of bases, including soft nylon, traditional methyl methacrylate, and milled acrylic, with or without adjustable ball clasps. Some manufacturers use proprietary acrylic-like materials, and others use printed nylon or even metal frameworks, like a partial denture. Dentists can choose whichever materials they and their patients are most comfortable with. Some devices can be customized with colors or logos to suit your patient's preferences (see Fig 5-11b).

Herbst appliances allow patients some lateral and vertical movement without disengaging the appliance. They can withstand some lateral bruxism and clenching, but if your patient has a history of extreme lateral movement, the bars can be stressed, bent, or broken. The bars come in different lengths, so they can be switched to a longer length if you run out of advancement. Some designs allow attachment points to be switched, which is a creative way of providing more advancement dimension. The bars are advanced in several different ways, including with keys, wrenches, and pins. Some advancement designs are easier to see than others. Patients with limited vision can still use a Herbst as long as the correct device is chosen. The office team should provide the patient detailed advancement instructions and coaching on how to use the appliance. Asking the patient to demonstrate their ability to advance the device at the time of delivery is a critical step for therapeutic success.

As with any device, the base for a Herbst can be bulky and take up tongue space. If your patient has prominent buccal maxillary tori, the upper posterior

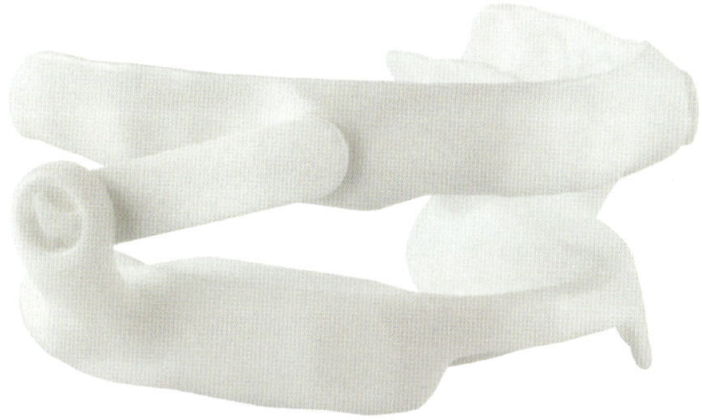

Fig 5-12 Panthera appliance.

mount may be difficult to locate. A wide maxilla may provide little space in the buccal corridor. During your examination, be aware of where the external hardware will be located. In the battle between a removable device and tender tissue, abandonment of therapy will win. Additionally, appliance adjustment may be difficult for some patients. Freedom of movement allows the mandibular arch to open and drop back, so all Herbst appliances must include anterior hooks or attachments for elastics to prevent the jaw from opening during sleep. However, not all manufacturers include these hooks as standard. You must specify them on the prescription form.

The Herbst is approved by all insurance companies and can be used on virtually any patient who is not sensitive or allergic to the nickel in the surgical stainless steel mechanism. This is a great appliance for your first few devices as you gain confidence. Some patients complain of the metallic feel and sound of the mechanism, but that is short-lived.

Appliances that pull the jaw: Panthera, EMA, and Avant appliances

PANTHERA DEVICES

Appliances that pull the mandible into a protruded position come in many varieties. Typically, these appliances have the maxillary attachment near the maxillary canine/first premolar and the mandibular attachment near the mandibular second molar. Thus, using them on a patient without mandibular posterior teeth can be challenging. Panthera has addressed this issue by designing the lower attachment on a wing that lifts it to the occlusal plane. This horizontal pull does not require the presence of mandibular molars to prevent dislodgment of the appliance (Fig 5-12).

Panthera D-SADs (digital sleep apnea devices) are produced by only one manufacturer, but you can order them direct or through many other labs. They are designed on computers with specialized software and built with

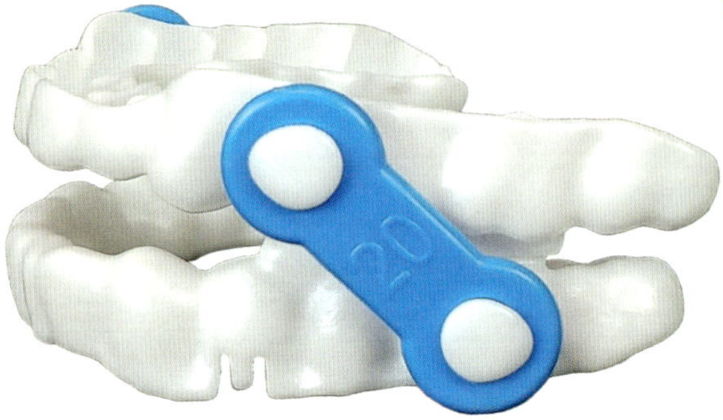

Fig 5-13 EMA appliance.

an extremely advanced additive manufacturing technique to produce some of the smoothest and strongest nylon oral appliances on the market. The material is easy to keep clean and feels comfortable for most patients next to their tongue. They are adjusted by substituting shorter arms bilaterally on the device. These devices seem to be long-lasting, requiring only a soaking once per week to supplement daily brushing.

Contraindications to Panthera are few. If the posterior teeth have very low retention, your patient may struggle. The most common problem occurs when the anterior border of the ramus lies close to the buccal aspect of the second molars. The wing mechanism holding the posterior end of the adjustment rod may impinge on the overlying soft tissue. A tip for using Panthera devices is to always choose the U-shaped device for the mandible between the canines. The flat plate design option allows for flexibility in the lower arch, which creates problems with device longevity and, in our practices, more tooth movement.

EMA DEVICES

The EMA (elastic mandibular advancement) appliance is another good representative of pulling appliances (Fig 5-13). EMA devices can be vacuum-formed, composed of acrylic, printed out of nylon, or milled from a puck. The bands placed on the sides indicate its identity. EMA devices can be made inexpensively, which may influence your selection depending on insurance reimbursement. However, you should be aware that most insurance companies require that the chosen appliance lasts for a minimum of 5 years, so make sure the EMA is made by a high-quality laboratory and from high-grade material.

EMA devices are advanced by changing the elastics, which come in varying degrees of firmness, to progressively shorter lengths. Unfortunately, the bands tend to stretch, which makes titration difficult, and EMA-generated forces may

Fig 5-14 Avant device.

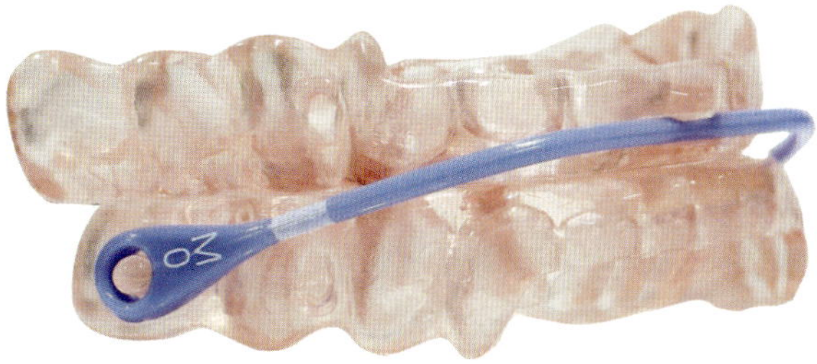

unseat the appliance if the mandibular molars have poor retention. Over time, these forces may cause the mandibular molars to erupt and tilt anteriorly. On the other hand, due to their potential to be very low cost, EMAs are a great appliance for patients who snore in the latter stages of pregnancy and who may not require any therapy when their body returns to normal postpartum.

AVANT DEVICES

Avant is a device from SomnoMed that is milled out of two different materials (Fig 5-14). One material is used to form a solid shell, and the other is used as a soft liner to cover the teeth. This combination makes the Avant comfortable and non-threatening for patients with extensive porcelain restorations. Avant shells have extensive opposing surfaces, so clenchers and bruxers generally find them quite acceptable. Adjustments are made with a strap that extends from the lower posterior area across the maxillary facial midline, where there is an anchor slot. The angle of force provided in this arrangement tends to close the mouth and promote nasal breathing. Avant does not require strong retention, and no metal is included in this device. Patients who struggle with lip incompetency, however, are poor matches for Avant because the maxillary attachment slot can interfere with lip drape. Some patients with extensive maxillary anterior restorations may be concerned about feeling pressure from the device on those teeth, which, although minor, is unavoidable with Avant.

Appliances with an anterior midline attachment: TAP devices

The dreamTAP appliance from Airway Labs is a comfortable device that pulls the mandible into a protruded position (Fig 5-15). Advancements can be made with the appliance in the mouth, which is particularly valuable when titrating a

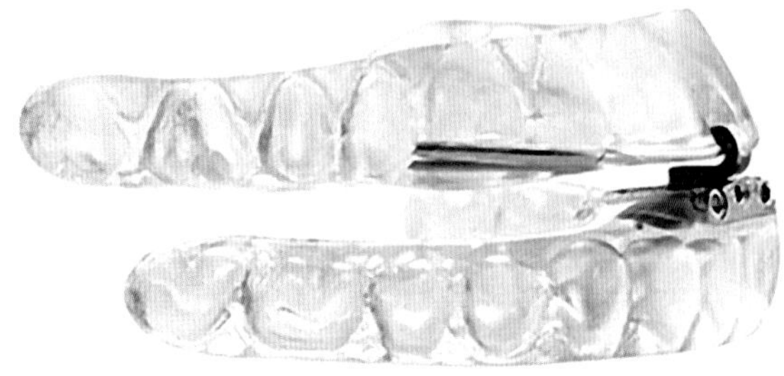

Fig 5-15 dreamTAP appliance.

patient in the sleep laboratory. The appliance is titrated by using a hex wrench to turn the hex nut on the front of the appliance counterclockwise. To keep track of the advancement, there is a millimeter ruler on the advancement bar on the mandibular arch. Because the arches are connected anteriorly, the maxillary and mandibular anterior teeth must be healthy and retentive. The appliance is typically comprised of a harder outside layer and a soft inside layer. The soft inside layer makes the dreamTAP easy to seat and comfortable to wear, and there are many other choices for TAP appliances, including a bonded thermoplastic layer that can be refitted using only warm water.

The dreamTAP has been designed with different metal hinges to allow for different vertical positions and increased protrusion. This appliance can pull the mandible farther forward than most other appliances, increasing the chances of treatment success. TAP devices are especially effective in supine-dependent OSA patients. dreamTAP and Airway Lab's other similar device, TAP3, can be directly attached to a CPAP mask for combination therapy, a feature that eliminates the need to use headgear to stabilize the mask. An accessory mouth shield can also be attached to the front of either of these TAP devices to seal the mouth for improved nose breathing, reduced saliva leakage, and fewer complaints of dry mouth.

Unfortunately, TAP3 and dreamTAP appliances can place significant pressure on the patient's anterior teeth, which must be healthy. You must discuss this expectation in your pretreatment conversations. Depending on many factors, including the patient's care of the device, TAP appliances sometimes turn yellow within a short time after placement, and the inner soft lining can delaminate before 5 years, requiring a reline or remake. Additionally, we have found that bruxers can cause the advancement mechanism to reverse with time, reducing protrusion. If the patient has a high maxillary incisal angle, path-of-insertion problems may contraindicate a TAP appliance. Therefore, this appliance is not ideal for any patient with periodontally involved or structurally

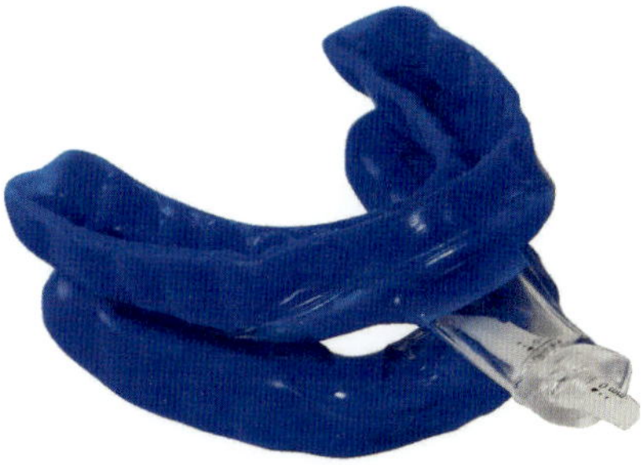

Fig 5-16 flexTAP appliance.

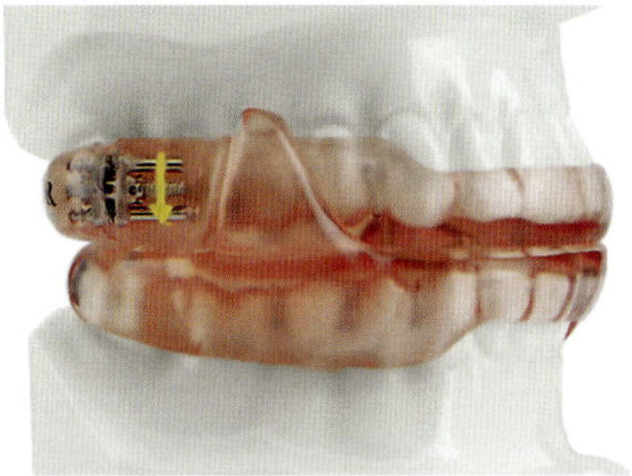

Fig 5-17 Dorsal fin appliance.

compromised anterior teeth. Furthermore, good retention is required because the maxillary and mandibular portions of the appliance are connected, so a patient with a limited number of posterior teeth may not be a good candidate for a TAP device.

Many of these concerns have now been addressed by a new TAP device—flexTAP (Fig 5-16). flexTAP devices are made from irradiated thermacryl, which can be modified with warm water but is stable for clinical use. The mechanism is designed to be more comfortable and place less strain on the TMJ complex. The arches are thinner to provide more room for the tongue, and the device comes standard with a mouth shield for better nose breathing. A major feature of the flexTAP is freedom of movement for the mandible. The jaw joints remain more comfortable as the mandible is allowed to seek a compatible position. Thus, the vertical dimension of OAT is set according to function and comfort, rather than at random by the dentist.

Dorsal fin appliances

Dorsal fin (posterior wing) appliances are indicated for patients who insist on the ability to open the mouth (Fig 5-17). The upper and lower components of the dorsal fins are not attached, which makes the appliance comfortable and leads to excellent patient acceptance. Dorsal fin appliances can be used with a limited number of teeth and minimal retention. They can be made of acrylic or dual laminate (many manufacturers) or be additively manufactured from nylon (eg, Panthera X3). The appliance is adjusted by moving a block adjacent to the fin with a finely threaded expansion screw or by replacing parts to position the jaw further forward.

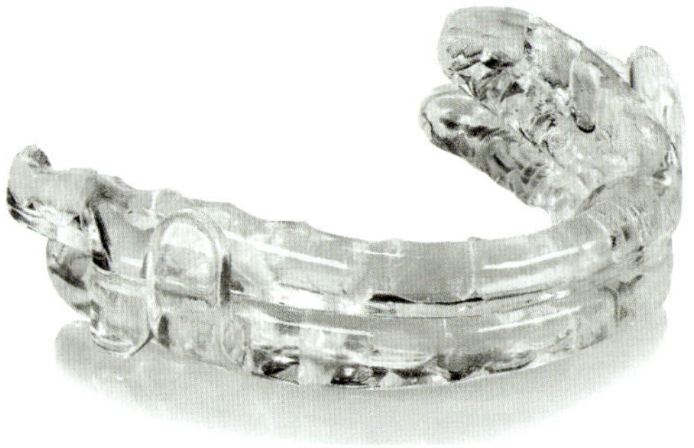

Fig 5-18 ProSomnus [IA] appliance.

Although many patients consider the ability to open the mouth a positive feature and not a problem, the mandible falls back when the mouth is open, which can result in increased respiratory events and snoring. Furthermore, an acrylic dorsal fin can fracture if the patient is a heavy lateral bruxer. Before deciding on this appliance, you should inspect for significant lateral wear on the canines or stripes on an existing nightguard that indicate lateral bruxism. Choosing a tougher material, such as nylon, may be the only way to stay with this design. The appliance should be fitted with anterior hooks or attachments for elastics to prevent the jaw from opening during sleep.

Interlocking shape appliances

PROSOMNUS DEVICES

The ProSomnus [IA] was the first CAD/CAM milled sleep apnea device available, offering precise and predictable results (Fig 5-18). It is a posterior fin-type appliance, but the fins are oriented 90 degrees to the plane of occlusion, which helps prevent the jaw from falling posteriorly during sleep. ProSomnus [IA] is milled from compressed methyl methacrylate pucks, though the advanced version (EVO) is milled from a proprietary material that is much tougher, with some flexibility that makes it more comfortable and less prone to breakage.

When ordering a ProSomnus [IA] or EVO, the desired protrusion must be specified and then several arches are included in the shipping box. Advancements are made similar to the way clear aligners are used to move teeth, by replacing either the upper or lower component with a new piece that is milled with a broader fin to result in more protrusion. These appliances fit very well and do not allow any significant tooth movement, so they are particularly indicated for patients who have recently completed orthodontic treatment. Making fine protrusive adjustments may involve selectively reshaping the wings, and additional advancement requires milling new arches with

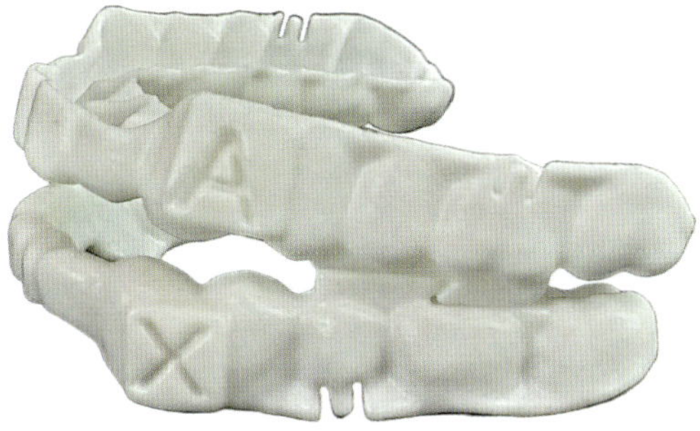

Fig 5-19 Elevate appliance.

differently positioned wings. This appliance has little to no material on the lingual aspect to maximize tongue room. Patient acceptance of these devices, especially the EVO variety, is quite high.

Because the ProSomnus [IA] achieves its retention by engaging the undercuts and embrasure spaces on the facial surfaces of the teeth, significant cross-arch buccal opposing surfaces are required for retention. Unfortunately, mandibular molars are often lingually tipped in patients with SRBDs, decreasing retention for this device. Additionally, changing the vertical dimension on this appliance may cause fin misalignment and fracture. Finally, this appliance may not be the best choice for a patient with lateral bruxism.

ELEVATE DEVICES

Elevate, a printed nylon MAD by Serena Sleep, has an innovative design with interlocking shapes that lie between the arches over the occlusal surfaces of the teeth (Fig 5-19). These shapes prevent the jaw from falling back, and further protrusion can be achieved with different upper and lower arches. The arches are not locked together, which affords lateral movement. The printed nylon is closely fitted to the teeth and serves as an excellent retainer, with very little tongue space impingement. This is one of the least bulky designs available and is excellent for patients with very tight buccal corridors lateral to the maxillary molars and those with scalloped tongues.

A disadvantage of Elevate devices is that the interlocking shapes can become disconnected, freeing the mandible to fall back. This can be avoided by using elastics. Because the arches are connected, the shape of the teeth must provide adequate retention, especially if elastics are going to be used.

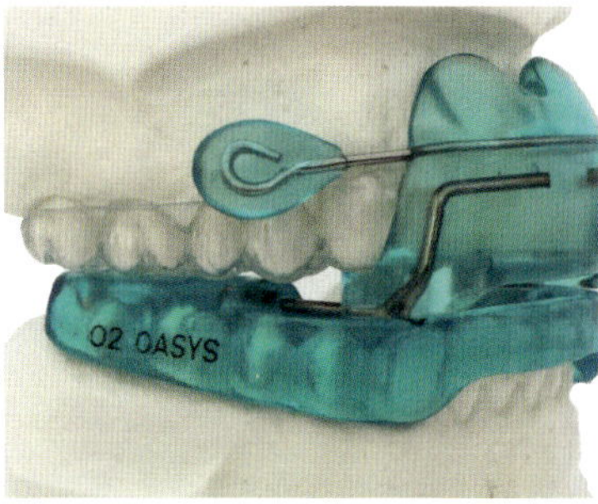

Fig 5-20 OASYS device.

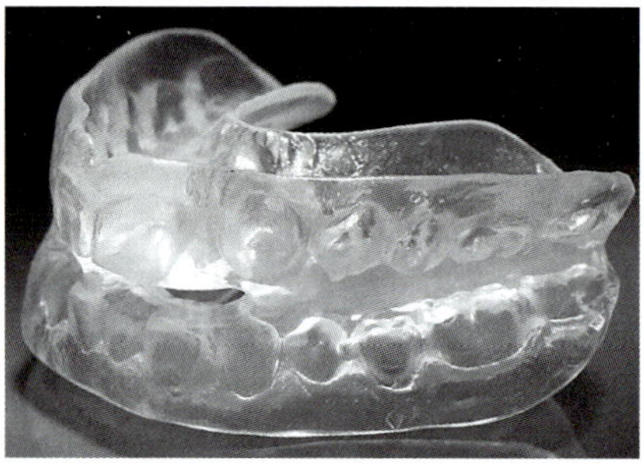

Fig 5-21 Traditional monoblock appliance.

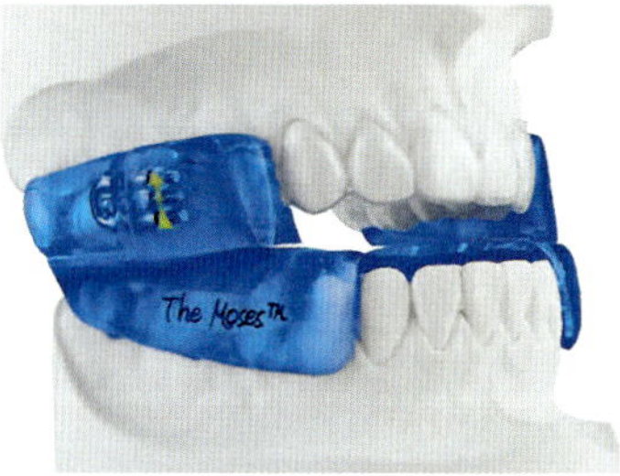

Fig 5-22 Moses appliance.

Combination therapy appliances

Some devices can be used to accomplish two changes at once. Often, these changes involve advancing the mandible and manipulating soft tissue such as the tongue or even the nose. One such device, the OASYS (Oral/Nasal Airway System, Oasys Sleep), has been shown to contribute to airway therapy significantly (Fig 5-20). Along with mandibular advancement, it has pads that can be adjusted to open the nasal valve and promote improved tongue position. This device can take the place of nasal dilators for those with high nasal airflow resistance.

Monoblock appliances

Historically, monoblock appliances were fabricated to hold the mandible in a set position and were nonadjustable (Fig 5-21). The name "monoblock" derived from the fact that there was not an upper component and a lower component. The drawback to this type of appliance was obvious. The successful treatment of OSA was made more difficult without the ability to advance the appliance. More recently, monoblocks have been redesigned to include a jack screw to allow for advancement. The Moses appliance is a good example of this (Fig 5-22). Patients

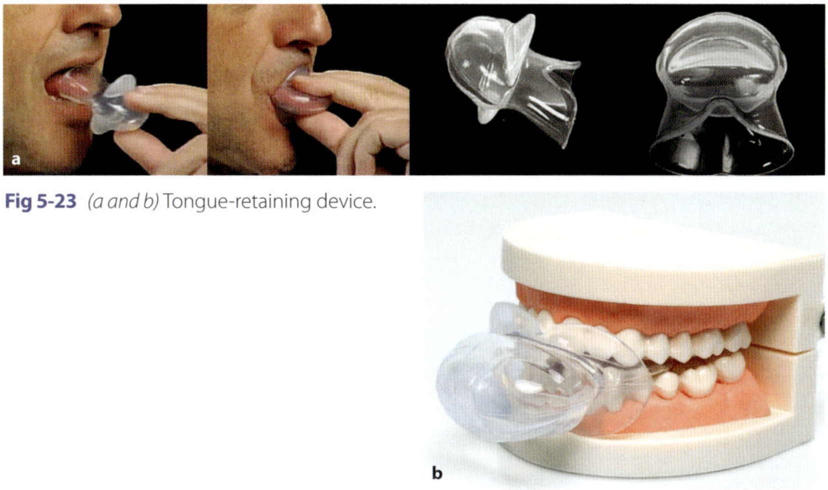

Fig 5-23 *(a and b)* Tongue-retaining device.

find the Moses a little bulky at first, but it is comfortable to wear and leaves plenty of tongue space. The appliance allows for fine adjustments with jack screws bilaterally and encourages anterior placement of the tongue.

The downsides of the Moses appliance include retention difficulties for the maxillary arch and the limited amounts of advancement that are achievable. Additionally, all monoblock appliances are contraindicated in patients with severe bruxism.

Tongue-retaining devices

Tongue-retaining devices (TRDs) act by suctioning the tongue into a bulb that sits outside the mouth (Fig 5-23). The lips and teeth prevent the tongue from falling back into the oropharynx during sleep. A TRD can be very effective if the patient can tolerate it. It is primarily indicated for edentulous patients, and some clinicians have reported success with TRDs when treating patients with Down syndrome. The AVEOtsd appliance uses progressive rings to titrate the amount of tongue protrusion for maximum medical improvement.

The negatives of TRDs include a sore tongue, drooling, and compliance issues. Most DSM providers use TRDs rarely or not at all.

References

1. Ng SK, Lee DL, Li AM, Wing YK, Tong MC. Reproducibility of clinical grading of tonsillar size. Arch Otolaryngol Head Neck Surg 2010;136:159–162.
2. Mallampati SR, Gatt SP, Gugino LD, et al. A clinical sign to predict difficult tracheal intubation: A prospective study. Can Anaesth Soc J 1985;32:429–434.
3. Smith MT, Wickwire EM, Grace EG, et al. Sleep disorders and their association with laboratory pain sensitivity in temporomandibular joint disorder. Sleep 2009;32:779–790.
4. Aarab G, Lobbezoo F, Hamburger HL, Naeije M. Effects of an oral appliance with different mandibular protrusion positions at a constant vertical dimension on obstructive sleep apnea. Clin Oral Investig 2010;14:339–345.

To achieve the impossible dream, try going to sleep.

—Joan Klempner

6

Delivery of a Custom MAD

Dentists are trained from early in school to fit devices to teeth. The challenge of oral appliance therapy (OAT) is mastering the new materials being offered for mandibular advancement devices (MADs). Fitting and adjusting variants of polymethyl methacrylate and nylon, as well as proprietary materials, requires specific skills. Fortunately, they are skills that any dentist or trained dental assistant can acquire easily.

Additionally, the delivery appointment consists of several detailed steps that must be understood by the patient for therapy to be successful. We suggest duplicating every instruction the patient hears in writing and/or in a video posted to your practice's website. We chose not to include the instructions our teams use not because we are protecting that information but because of how people learn. When you and your team settle on how information (such as MAD cleaning instructions) should be presented, it's best to write those instructions down as a handout. That way, when the patient reviews the document at home, they will recall the way your team explained things. This kind of review and recollection creates a more robust memory than reading words the brain has not heard before, especially if there are differences between the verbal and written explanations that might spark confusion.

The easiest way to develop handout materials is to discuss them as a team, then record or take notes for the first ten or so delivery appointments. Review these notes together, and create the documents based on what felt like the most effective way of saying things. Create a checklist for the team listing what must be done at each appointment in the treatment process, especially delivery. This exercise takes little time, and having everyone in the practice participate will ensure team mastery.

By FDA regulation, each MAD comes with an instruction book written by the manufacturer and approved by the FDA. Be sure to include this booklet with the materials that accompany delivery. Patients may not read the booklet, but in subsequent telehealth encounters, both parties can turn to the same pages for individualized coaching.

Quality Inspection

When the MAD arrives from the laboratory, the assistant must perform a quality inspection to make sure that the device is the one the doctor ordered, it fits the models, and there are no manufacturing defects. If the adjustment mechanism involves a key and a threaded shaft, ensure that the key fits the intended mechanism and that the shaft can be turned. If there are replacement parts for repositioning the mandible, be sure those parts are present and are the ones intended for that specific device. Inspect the MAD for rough spots, cracks, and interproximal fins that may make insertion more difficult. Record the serial number of the MAD, if present, in the patient's chart. The assistant then gathers the forms and educational material to be presented at delivery and sets them aside with the inspected device.

Intake and Try-In

When the patient is seated, a normal medical intake process is performed to update the medical history and any changes to prescriptions, and vital signs are recorded if significant time has passed since a prior recording. It's especially important to note the patient's weight at the beginning of therapy. After allowing for any top-of-mind questions the patient may have, the dentist reviews any additional information that came in since the patient's records appointment. If a CBCT scan was performed, the radiologist's report is discussed, and if there has been a consultation with an otolaryngologist, orthodontist, or other medical provider, those notes are brought out for discussion. Chart notes are made regarding the nature of these discussions, any questions the patient has, and any action items related to the new information. The radiologist's report is included with the patient packet, although it is not written in patient-friendly language.

It is important to keep in mind the patient's history of wearing oral appliances such as nightguards. The dentist should show and explain the orientation and features of the new MAD to patients, and for those with a history of oral appliances, allow them to insert the new MAD themselves. If a patient expresses any hesitation or reluctance, seat the device for them. Evaluate how

Fig 6-1 SomnoSeal device.

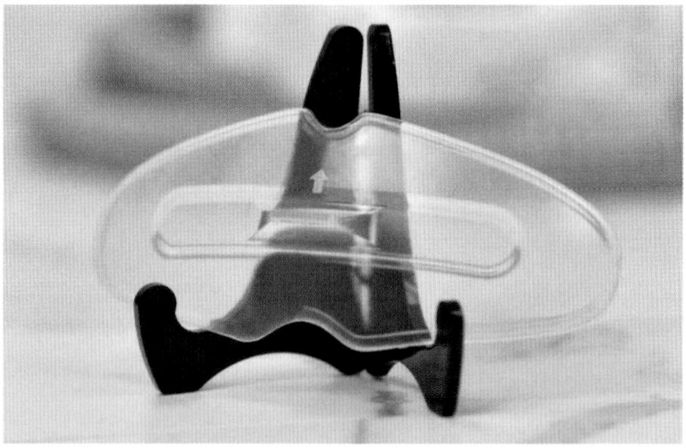

smoothly the device seems to go in, and check for the solid feel of a well-fitted device. There should be no rocking. A snug fit overall is acceptable, but being too tight on a tooth or the tissue is not. If the MAD has been chosen well and an excellent impression or scan and a good bite recording have been provided, the dentist should have few to no adjustments to make. If poor initial fits are common, the impression/scan technique should be revisited. The best person to seek counsel from is the lab technician who is responsible for working with the casts/data.

Take time to evaluate for lip closure. This is important because nasal breathing is one key to success. Because lip competency is one of the factors accounted for in appliance and jaw position decisions, it is uncommon for the patient to be unable to close their lips over the MAD, although a little strain is not unusual. Usually, the patient will learn to adapt, and soon the lips will seal on their own. Appliance design, such as a thick connector facial to the anterior teeth, can prevent the lips from draping over the front of the device. If the patient was a vertical grower, with a high mandibular plane angle and excessive maxillary gingival display, it's already difficult for them to keep their lips together, even without a device in place. Adding any more vertical dimension will make an open mouth nearly inevitable. This situation requires the aid of some sort of external agent, such as lip tape. Another strategy is to slip a silicone shape (eg, SomnoSeal; Fig 6-1) under the lips to block airflow no matter what position the lips are in. Patients returning with a dry mouth due to mouth breathing might have undisclosed nasal function problems (see chapter 14). If a patient has a known nasal airway restriction, this may be a good time to reinforce a proposed treatment strategy, such as nasal breathing exercises or referral to an ear, nose, and throat (ENT) specialist.

Next, the patient removes the MAD, with coaching from the dentist or assistant if needed. Patients will learn where to place their fingers and how to push the device off their teeth. Try to avoid doing this for them, but look for signs of trouble. If a patient is having difficulty inserting or removing the appliance, it is important to make the necessary adjustments for comfortable insertion and removal. Remember, there is a fine line between a tight appliance and a loose one. Improving retention can be difficult with some appliances, so be conservative when adjusting.

Patients with facially flared incisors are the most challenging cases for seating a MAD due to the lack of an easy path of insertion. The flared anterior teeth necessitate removal of the material on the distal aspect of the molars and/or the anterior facial flange (overlap) to allow the appliance to be properly seated. Remember, if the appliance is uncomfortable, compliance may be less than ideal. The more pressure there is on the facial of a flared incisal, the more torque will be felt in the periodontal ligament.

Patients should be cautioned that there is a normal accommodation period associated with OAT. One author (Ken Berley) informs all patients that it takes 21 days to develop a habit, so this appliance will take some getting used to. If they have problems falling asleep with the appliance, we recommend they take Advil PM (Pfizer) or another antihistamine with diphenhydramine (eg, Benadryl, Johnson & Johnson) to assist with sleep initiation for the first few nights. This medication is also useful if they experience excessive salivation with the new acrylic device. Be careful, however, because some people experience residual sleepiness the next day when using diphenhydramine in this way. You may also choose to prescribe a hypnotic medication or ask their sleep doctor to do so. This same strategy is frequently used during continuous positive airway pressure (CPAP) accommodation.

If the patient is going to have a tough time inserting the device because it is so foreign or because of a serious gag reflex, we suggest that they put it in during the evening while engaged in other activities, then take it out and put it in again. While they have it in place, they should breathe slowly and deeply through their nose, telling themselves that breathing is easier that way. This training of positive feelings around wearing the device while breathing through the nose goes a long way toward adherence to therapy. We also emphasize that they may not be able to wear it completely through the first, or first several, night(s). They may need to remove it partway through. Letting them know that this is a common behavior will help new OAT patients to avoid frustration and prevent them from prematurely dismissing their ability to use a MAD.

Fig 6-2 AM Aligner.

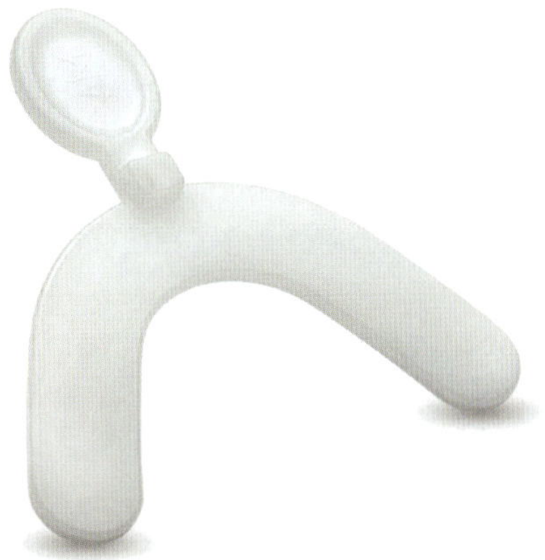

AM Aligners

The next step is making the AM Aligner. Chapter 7 covers the importance of this simple method for managing side effects. Dentists use many devices to help patients recover the maximal intercuspal position (MIP) of the mandible that they enjoyed prior to mandibular advancement therapy. Our favorite device is a simple index made from ThermAcryl (Airway Labs; Fig 6-2).

1. First, assess the patient's MIP, and look for a key contact on each side that you can use as a landmark. Hold a piece of shimstock (Almore International) in cotton pliers or Miller forceps and verify the contacts, then record them in the patient's chart as a benchmark.
2. Heat the AM Aligner in hot water until it turns clear (about 30 seconds).
3. Place it over the lower arch, and instruct the patient to bite together with the alignment block in the midline touching the maxillary incisors. Instruct the patient to bite firmly, then stay in that position while relaxing the muscles for comfort.
4. At about the 90-second mark, ask the patient to open so you can unstick the AM Aligner from the teeth. It is not set yet, so have them bite together, being careful to keep the tooth imprint/alignment the same.
5. After approximately 3 minutes, the AM Aligner is cool enough to carefully remove without distortion. You can accelerate this process by using air on the device to cool it.
6. Place the AM Aligner in cool water for 60 seconds to return it to opaque white. Seeing clear areas where the teeth were nearly in contact indicates that the condyles were in their most seated MIP position.
7. Hand the cool AM Aligner to the patient and instruct them to place it on the teeth and bite. Hand them a mirror so they can see how perfectly their teeth fit. Ask them to notice how solid the bite feels.

Cleaning the MAD

While the patient is waiting, teeth together, for the AM Aligner to firm up, go over how to clean the new MAD. We suggest that the patient remove the device in the morning and move the mandible around while brushing the teeth. This restores normal mobility to the muscles and temporomandibular joint (TMJ)–associated structures. Provide a soft denture brush with each MAD, and suggest the use of simple hand soap for washing to protect the device from more abrasive toothpastes. Using soap, a nonabrasive toothpaste, baking soda, or another gentle cleanser will preserve the surface of the MAD and prevent staining. We suggest soaking the device in denture cleaner as needed. Some patients' appliances accumulate more stains and tartar than others, so be ready to suggest the right strategy on an individual basis. Current devices that should not be soaked for longer than a few minutes include triple laminate bases on TAP devices from Airway Labs and the flexible liners found on some milled devices from SomnoMed and DynaFlex. This is because the laminates can become separated. Be familiar with the manufacturer's instructions, and reinforce them to the patient. One author (Steve Carstensen) suggests that patients soak these devices for only as long as they are in the shower. All appliances are stored dry. A list of the authors' favorite soaker/cleaners is found in the Recommended Materials section at the back of the book.

Using the AM Aligner

When the AM Aligner is ready, hand the patient a mirror and inform them how to use their new device. Once the jaw is moved around a bit, the index is placed over the teeth, and the patient bites gently against it. Because it is most likely that the mandible will be forward, the lingual part of the incisal edge of the maxillary teeth will contact the slope of the index. A little closing pressure, held to a count of four, will serve to drive the mandible distally. What is thought to be happening is that the inferior lateral pterygoid muscle shortens with mandibular protrusion. Using the AM Aligner stretches that muscle and allows the condyle to reposition into the glenoid fossa and the teeth to come back into contact. The patient should alternate squeezing and releasing against this index until the bite returns to normal. The time this takes varies between individuals. Before the patient leaves the delivery appointment, we verify MIP with the AM Aligner in place and ask the patient to describe how the AM Aligner is to be used. Any communication confusion can be cleared up here, before use of the protrusion device has a chance to affect the MIP.

Patient Considerations

Patients often ask, "How should I adjust my MAD, and how do I know it's working?" We do not advocate for any adjustments within the first week of use. That is the time for the patient to get used to wearing the device and identify any areas that need to be adjusted to improve comfort, as well as to adapt to using the AM Aligner. We expect patients to try to wear the device every night for the whole night. Some patients cannot complete a full night right away and prefer to remove the MAD partway through the first few nights, increasing the time they wear the MAD as they go on. We let them know that any pattern that works is okay, but we hope that they can achieve full-night wear quickly.

The patient then signs a form acknowledging receipt of the MAD. This form includes the name of the device, the quantity (usually 1), the serial number if known, and the date the patient took possession of the device. This documentation is specific to Medicare DMEPOS (Durable Medical Equipment, Prosthetics, Orthotics, and Supplies) requirements, but it is good practice even for non-Medicare patients. Patients are also invited to contact the office immediately if there is an acute problem with the device that prevents them from wearing it, such as a pressure point or a rough spot. This rarely happens, and normally our next visit is about a week later. It is only following the delivery appointment that any insurance claims for the MAD can be submitted.

A special caution is given to patients who have a dog that sleeps in the same room as them. Because the new MAD is foreign, it is not uncommon for patients to unconsciously remove the device during the night. A dog may find this new chew toy irresistible, and nothing good will come from that. Patients are cautioned to avoid sharing the bedroom with the dog until it becomes routine to continuously wear the MAD through the night. On a related note, a strategy suggested by a patient is to get a homeowner's insurance rider covering special medical devices. This patient's dog chewed up his new MAD, but he got it replaced at no out-of-pocket cost because he had added the rider for a $12 annual premium. Patients who travel might also want to consider this coverage.

Follow-Up After Delivery

Most patients are seen via telehealth for the follow-up appointment, but all are welcome to come in for an office visit should they prefer it or if there is any physical issue with the MAD that needs to be addressed in person. There is no copay or charge for this appointment, and it is mostly led by the assistant. The patient is invited to share any initial impressions, note any desired changes for comfort, and reflect on the use of the AM Aligner. If the appointment takes place in person, the bite is checked using shimstock on the index points identified earlier, and any corrections to the device or patient behavior are done prior to the doctor being called in. The dentist's role in this appointment is to address the emotional response of the patient to this new therapy—that is, to reinforce good early thoughts and assuage any trepidation about managing the airway. Reminding patients of their chief treatment goals is very useful in helping them through the early accommodation phase. The assistant coaches the patient on the self-titration process and ensures that they understand how to adjust the device on their own.

When to see the patient next varies according to individual needs. Most patients are seen again in 3 months, after they have had time to get used to the therapy, form use habits, and titrate their airway using subjective measurements. Occasionally, a patient needs to be seen in the interim, mostly for therapy reinforcement. Rarely do appliance fit adjustments need to be performed, but any perceived need by the patient is met by inviting them to contact the office at any time to ask questions. Certainly, we would rather see the patient early than be told at the 3-month mark that they have been unable to wear the device.

Patients are not given a protocol or adjustment timing scheme. We believe it is best if they are involved in their therapy to the maximum amount possible. One author (Steve Carstensen) provides detailed written instructions to the patient on how to advance their device, as well as training on the concept of titration until subjective symptoms are resolved. Staff members are always ready to consult on this issue, but most patients do their own protrusion as they feel necessary. It is important that they understand that titration may take some time as their airway responds to being open throughout the night, nasal breathing improves, and the various involved tissues gain flexibility. It is also important to tell them there is often no need to go to the maximum range of the device.

Smart phone apps can be quite useful for helping patients feel that they have some control over their treatment without additional cost. Dozens of apps are available, and many more are being developed. As of this writing, SnoreLab is the one we most often recommend. It is important that patients test themselves sleeping alone, though it is not uncommon for treated patients to use their app to convince their bed partner that they also have a sleep-related breathing disorder (SRBD).

Generally, the authors agree about practice philosophies; however, we take different approaches when it comes to titration protocols. In Dr Berley's office, the patients do NOT typically titrate their appliances, as they tend to titrate too aggressively, which can cause excessive soreness and inflammation of the teeth and TMJs. We try to supervise advancements, and when the patient's subjective symptoms are adequately improved, we use high-resolution pulse oximetry (HRPO) to determine if the patient is adequately titrated. If the HRPO indicates improvement of the patient's objective symptoms, the patient undergoes an overnight home sleep apnea test (HSAT) to bring the patient's Apnea-Hypopnea Index (AHI) below 10 before their final polysomnogram (PSG). The patient then returns to the sleep laboratory, where Dr Berley supervises the final titration of the device to normalize the patient's AHI and oxygen levels.

The American Dental Association (ADA) and American Academy of Dental Sleep Medicine (AADSM) have recently published policy statements and protocols that endorse the use of HSATs and pulse oximetry during the titration process. The use of these objective testing devices during titration allows for fine-tuning of the MAD before the patient returns to the sleep physician. With the advent of HSAT titration, OAT results have been greatly improved. However, it is prudent to discuss HSAT titration usage with your referring physicians to make sure they are open to this protocol.

Many patients ask about testing for obstructive sleep apnea (OSA) resolution. We advocate patience to allow for healing and the resolution of airway tissue inflammation and improvement in the nasal airway. Often, the timing of effectiveness testing falls near the 90-day mark (the second follow-up appointment). Patients generally see the diagnosing physician for this test, and if they are going in for testing near the second follow-up appointment, we delay our appointment until test results can be reviewed. It is important for the patient to understand that incomplete resolution of OSA at this first test is not a reason to abandon OAT but rather an indication to adjust the therapy or add additional strategies. Knowing the diagnosing sleep physician's typical philosophy about this early testing will help you set patient expectations. Some sleep physicians will counsel for return to positive airway pressure (PAP) as soon as OAT is shown to be incompletely effective, but most will refer the patient back to the dentist. We call the patient as soon as the results are sent over from the testing doctor's office, either to reinforce the good news or to offer an office visit to address concerns.

When Oral Appliance Therapy is Incompletely Effective

Testing may ultimately show that a patient's SRBD is not fully resolved with the use of a MAD alone. Patients are then faced with making a choice about how to move forward:

- Accept these results as maximum medical improvement.
- Abandon OAT and return to PAP.
- Adjust the jaw position further forward or add a vertical increase to provide more tongue space.
- Add additional therapy in combination with the MAD.
- Move to a more invasive therapy, such as surgery.

Accept these results as maximum medical improvement

Accepting the results as maximum medical improvement is rarely the preferred choice at this juncture, though it is not as uncommon later in the treatment sequence. It is not always possible to noninvasively fully resolve SRBDs, but sometimes, patients refuse to take the next step and decide that their treatment is "good enough." Nearly always, this means that subjective symptoms such as snoring and excessive daytime sleepiness (EDS) are much improved or resolved, even if objective testing reveals a persistent SRBD and/or intermittent hypoxia. The physician should advise the patient of his or her individual health risks at this level of disturbed physiology, and the dentist commits to ongoing management of MAD use. The informed patient then decides what to do next. We shorten our follow-up intervals to three times per year to monitor these patients, and we ask them about subjective resolution at each appointment. Overnight oximetry can be useful as an easy measurement of ongoing airway management. It is not uncommon for patients to think they cannot accept additional therapy early on, only to change their minds and ask for more information later. Preserving the relationship and referring to their initial treatment goals are important strategies.

Abandon OAT and return to PAP

Abandoning OAT altogether is a very uncommon response to early incomplete therapy, but some patients seem to need to prove to themselves that PAP was not so bad after all. Others struggle with using an oral device or conclude that the gagging or excessive saliva simply won't go away. If patients make the choice to return to PAP, the dentist's role is to congratulate them for their commitment to airway health and suggest that the MAD may be useful in the future, either to give full OAT another try or perhaps for intermittent use during travel. The dentist should offer full support for ongoing OAT use in the future and may need to remind the patient that this was one of the outcomes discussed during the informed consent process. Thus, there is no need to consider a refund for the abandoned oral appliance. While we in dentistry are used to our therapies succeeding, in medicine, unsuccessful outcomes are an unwelcome but known possibility.

Adjust the jaw position further forward

Adjusting the mandible further forward is by far the most common response to a sleep test that shows a persistent SRBD. The patient is counseled to continue to advance the jaw position, and a specific sign or symptom that can be tracked to indicate improvement is agreed upon. Common signs and symptoms include residual snoring (which is often reduced to a heavy breathing noise), frequent trips to the bathroom (> 1 per night), continued reports of apnea by a bed partner, or persistent daytime sleepiness. Notes are made in the chart, and a follow-up schedule is agreed upon. The patient confirms his or her understanding of how to make the adjustments, is reassured that it takes some people more time than others to gain the flexibility required to achieve an open airway, and commits to the effort required to continue OAT. The dental staff follows up with therapy-reinforcement phone calls at the times agreed upon by the patient. Making these calls too frequently will annoy the patient, so asking for their permission to call on a schedule will be more welcome support. There is no time frame for this ongoing effort—every night the patient uses the MAD is better than no therapy at all. When the signs or symptoms seem better, a repeat sleep test is indicated to check for additional resolution.

What about the vertical dimension of the appliance? The studies that have investigated this aspect have been contradictory. In our offices, we add vertical dimension when more protrusion does not seem possible and if the patient's oral structures were especially crowded before therapy. A patient with a high BMI and/or narrow, crowded arches and a tongue that spills over the occlusal surfaces is more likely to be helped by increasing the vertical dimension, but watch to make sure that they don't lose their ability to seal their lips around the front of the MAD.

Adding vertical dimension to acrylic devices is simple. The best method is to cut small pieces from sheet acrylic or polycarbonate available from a hobby store. These shims can be made in several thicknesses and are simply bonded to the posterior segments of the mandibular device with orthodontic acrylic. For TAP devices, the mechanism with the hook can be cut out of the embedding acrylic, a shim can be luted in place, and the hook can be re-bonded with orthodontic acrylic. Nylon devices cannot be reliably bonded to, and increasing the vertical dimension often requires reprinting one or both arches in a new orientation. Retesting with HSAT or oximetry will indicate if vertical changes are helpful and tolerated.

Additional therapy in combination with the MAD

There are many noninvasive choices for combination therapy for patients committed to full airway resolution. Positional therapy, nasal airway improvement, and combination therapy with PAP are the primary tools available to the dental office.

POSITIONAL THERAPY

Sleep testing often reveals a predominance of airway events during supine sleep. Patients will tell their providers that they do not sleep on their back, but testing shows that not to be entirely true, so therapy must be effective in all sleep positions. MAD (and sometimes PAP) therapy measurements can be improved in many patients by simply not allowing them supine sleep, either by blocking them from this position or by retraining their autonomic nervous system. Blocking devices include shirts with pockets sewn into the back or belts that are worn around the waist with foam or air-filled shapes that keep the person on their side (Fig 6-3). These products are well accepted by patients, inexpensive, and effective when used, but there is little long-term research about adherence to therapy. Specialized pillows designed to promote side sleeping are available, and in Steve Carstensen's experience, they are far more comfortable than the other choices. A newer approach is a sleep position trainer that uses gentle electronic or vibratory signals when the patient is supine (Night Shift, Advanced Brain Monitoring; Fig 6-4). These signals serve as negative reinforcement and turn off when the patient is no longer in a supine position.

Positional aids have been shown to improve SRBDs in patients who have more events while sleeping supine,[1] and after an initial training period, patients continue to show improvement in SRBDs even with intermittent use. Furthermore, no significant side effects have been noted with positional therapy. Patient acceptance and belief in the therapy are the biggest challenges, so dental staff must be adept at guiding the patient to achieve maximum success.

NASAL AIRWAY IMPROVEMENT

Assessing nasal breathing is part of a thorough examination. Patients with a history of restricted nasal airway are best seen by an otolaryngologist who is well-versed in SRBD management. Otolaryngologists are key allies in achieving

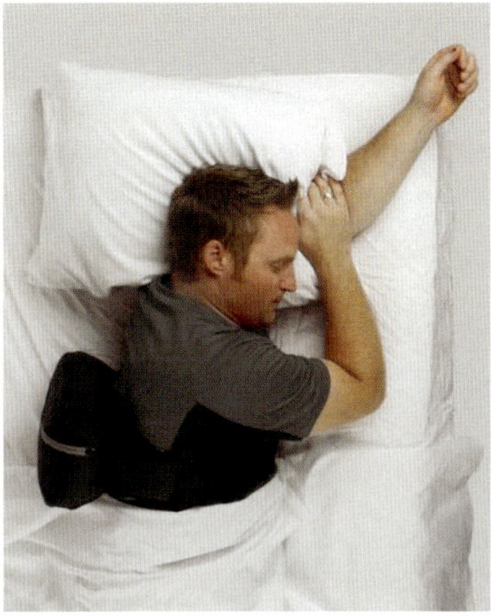

Fig 6-3 Belt-supported back pillow positional therapy.

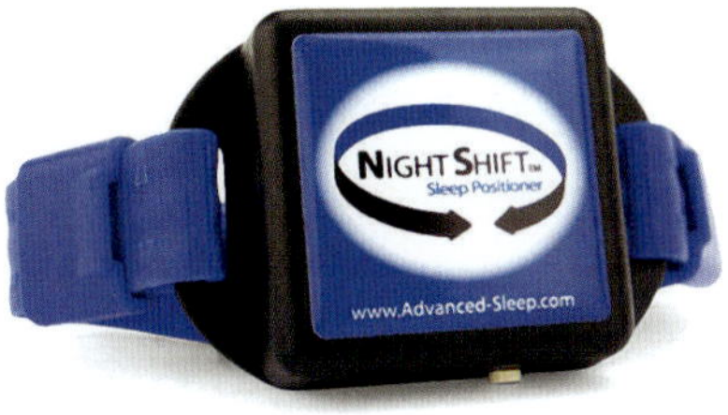

Fig 6-4 Night Shift positional trainer.

success with mandibular advancement therapy. Tissue restrictions, such as a deviated septum or enlarged turbinates, are frequently addressed by surgery. However, noninvasive therapies may be helpful for some patients. There are many reasons why nasal breathing is better for us physiologically than mouth breathing, but it is not important to go into those details with patients. They readily accept the concept that the nose is for breathing. Consistently improving nasal breathing can even result in the shrinkage of enlarged turbinates and other tissues, sometimes avoiding surgical approaches.[2]

One of the simplest noninvasive therapies is to have the patient decongest his or her nose at bedtime using a saline rinse or one of the various medications available. Many people have a low-level allergy to environmental conditions and can use over-the-counter corticosteroid sprays to minimize the allergic response and corresponding blockage. Patients with responses to over-the-counter solutions can be referred to an allergist or otolaryngologist. Saline rinses are also commonly used and are accepted by many patients. We suggest sprays and rinses that contain xylitol. This sugar alcohol changes the microbiome in the nose, which makes nasal clearing easier and reduces swelling of the nasal mucosa by drawing excess moisture from the tissues without drying them.

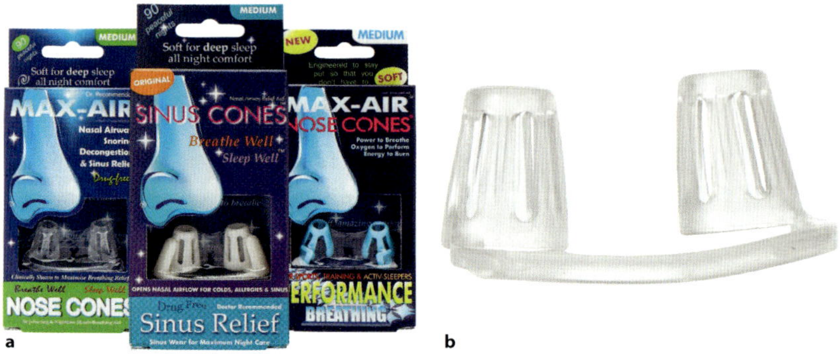

Fig 6-5 *(a and b)* Nasal cones to promote nasal breathing. (Courtesy of Sanostec.)

External nasal valve support devices, such as nasal cones (Fig 6-5), and adhesive strips for spreading the internal nasal valves are also on the market. Each of these approaches is simple for patients to use, and the effects are immediate and obvious. We have found a high acceptance rate for these simple devices, especially the external nasal valve support devices, because they are inexpensive, noninvasive, and there is no adhesive to irritate the skin. They come in various forms and materials, but they all insert in the nares to make it easier to breathe. Once patients accept the additional external device, many become happy users every night. There are also permanent ways to achieve this same outcome using minimal otolaryngologic surgery techniques to support external and internal nasal valves subject to collapse. ENT surgeons who understand how nasal function improves OAT are especially easy to collaborate with.

Many people who grew up with chronic stuffiness from allergies or other reasons have developed a mouth breathing habit and will continue to breathe through the mouth despite little restriction in the nasal airway. This habit can be overcome by making it more difficult to breathe through the mouth because of the design of the MAD chosen or by restricting the opening of the lips. Patients who have a mouth breathing habit will need to commit to change or they will feel claustrophobic if they cannot get enough air around the MAD. Most MADs have plenty of room for breathing, so restricting airflow requires sealing the lips. The most common way to do this is to use paper medical tape (Micropore Surgical Tape, 3M) to hold the lips together during sleep. Lip taping may seem radical to you and the patient at first, but it is often readily accepted, especially when the alternative is a visit to the otolaryngologist/surgeon. A short segment of paper tape is folded over at each end (for easy

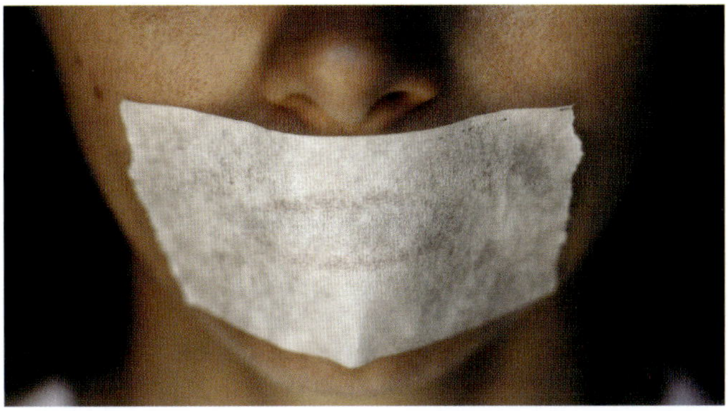

Fig 6-6 Lips sealed with paper tape.

removal) and placed horizontally or vertically across the closed lips (Fig 6-6). It is best for the patient to do this during the evening to get used to the new sensation of the nasal airway as the sole route of respiration. In our experience, it takes a committed patient and dental team reinforcement to achieve best results with this strategy, but when it works, lip taping can be a life-changer. It is worth the effort. We stock rolls of paper tape and hand them out; it is a small cost, but it removes the barrier to therapy that requires patients to buy the first roll of tape on their own.

Remember, all therapies require consent. There have not been any injuries reported secondary to lip taping, but if a patient has a medical emergency while wearing tape, that might result in a legal action. Dr Berley has drafted adult and child informed consent forms that can be obtained by request to kenberley@yahoo.com.

A new alternative to lip taping is SomnoSeal, a soft silicone oval that slips under the lips in front of the teeth/MAD. The sealed mouth requires the patient to breathe through the nose. One author (Steve Carstensen) finds this device invaluable for patient comfort and appliance success, with greater acceptance than lip taping.

COMBINATIONS WITH PAP

The combination of a PAP device with a MAD is another way to achieve success. Patients can use the MAD as a stabilization device to prevent the mandible from dropping back during sleep, which results in the PAP requiring less pressure to splint the oropharynx open. With less pressure, mask fit becomes better and there is less leakage, improving compliance. Coordination with the PAP-prescribing physician is important so the pressure settings on the flow

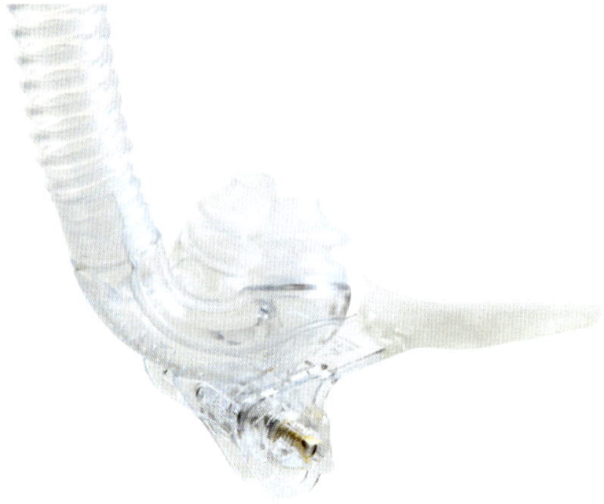

Fig 6-7 myTAP PAP interface.

generator can be adjusted. If the patient is already using an auto-adjusting PAP device, it is sufficient to simply notify the physician of the combination therapy approach.[3] A variant of PAP and MAD combination therapy is alternative use. Many of our patients use PAP at home, where it is minimally inconvenient, and use their MAD during travel or other times they want to skip the mask. If the MAD is proven to manage symptoms and the SRBD effectively, this approach is excellent; it provides patients with something they will accept every night. However, if they are going to use their MAD only occasionally throughout the year, they are at risk for requiring an accommodation period each time, so we counsel our patients to use the device several times a month to make sure that it is acceptable when it is time to rely on it fully.

One of the most frequent complaints patients have related to PAP use is poor mask fit and discomfort with the headgear and straps used to hold the mask in place. Manufacturers are constantly improving both issues, but dentists have a tool that the durable medical equipment companies do not—the ability to affix a PAP interface to the maxillary teeth. There are devices that are thermoplastic or can be attached to a custom acrylic device fitted to the maxillary teeth that extend between the lips and support nasal pillows that supply PAP pressure. A PAP interface that works in a similar manner is myTAP PAP (Fig 6-7). These devices are available from any CPAP supply store or from Airway Labs. The patient fits the upper tray and adjusts the nose pillows for comfort. Steve Carstensen keeps myTAP PAP masks in the office to offer to CPAP users.

Move to a more invasive therapy

Collapse of the airway during respiration is a mechanical response to pressure changes in an oropharynx made up of compliant tissues. Addressing this issue mechanically is helpful for many patients, making PAP and OAT valid management choices. Resolving SRBDs, on the other hand, requires structural change. Either the tissues must not move as much, or the pressure gradient of respiration must be less. Because it is impractical and unwise to decrease the action of the diaphragm or the volume of the lungs, the site of change is in the upper airway. Some breathing exercises have been proven to lower the AHI, presumably by enhancing muscle tone and making the area less collapsible.[4] Surgically enlarging the nasal airway can also allow air to flow more slowly at a higher pressure and produce less collapse.

If the nasal airway is restricted, it takes a higher airflow rate to fill the lungs in a normal respiratory cycle, and the resulting low pressure draws the walls of the oropharynx together. There are many types of surgery available for enlarging the nasal airway. Diagnosis often begins with a CBCT in the dental office and continues with nasal endoscopy and empirical treatment attempts, such as nasal steroids and nasal cone use. Because nasal airway surgery is not proven to fully resolve SRBDs a high percentage of the time, it is often adjunctive to other noninvasive and structural strategies. Any dentist managing the airway should get to know the otolaryngology physicians in the area for collaborative care at several levels.

The oropharynx may be constricted in two major ways. Structurally, the maxilla and mandible may be positioned too close to the spinal column to keep all the soft tissues far enough forward, or there may be excessive fat deposits surrounding the airway. Correcting the position of the maxilla and mandible in nongrowing patients is invasive and entails aggressive orthodontic and orthognathic techniques (ie, telegnathic surgery). If the maxillary and mandibular bones are brought forward, the soft tissues attached to those bones are also pulled forward, thereby enlarging the airway. If the transverse dimension of the maxilla is increased, the nasal airway resistance to flow is lessened, increasing pressure during respiration. If the mandibular teeth are uprighted to match the widened maxillary arch, the tongue has more space to rest forward, away from the back of the throat. Any airway therapy team will include an airway-focused orthodontist and an oral and maxillofacial surgeon who can evaluate and treat the structural component of airway restrictions.

Most patients will be dismissive of surgery when it is presented as a way to address their snoring and SRBDs, but many will return after using a MAD for some time to see if there is another way to resolve their airway issues. The younger the patient, the more nights they will have to use a removable device in their expected lifetime, and therefore the more benefit they might gain from a more invasive approach. Each patient deserves to be fully informed about treatment choices. In our experience, physicians often discuss nasal airway surgery with patients, but it is uncommon for them to present telegnathic options.

In growing patients prior to adolescence, telegnathic concepts are far less invasive and hold a different set of complexities. Those details are beyond the scope of this book, but again, an airway-oriented orthodontist can be an invaluable resource for addressing the airway before the jawbone positions are set. The use of functional appliances, proposed decades ago to help with orthodontic goals, are supported in the literature[5] as helpful strategies for telegnathic therapy in growing patients. Myofunctional therapy to correct tongue position and adjust swallowing habits allows the committed airway therapy team to address problems starting in very young children before they become a lifetime issue.

Lifestyle Changes

Weight loss is part of every sleep physician's conversation with the appropriate patients. However, although there are many case reports of successful management of SRBDs with weight loss, the population-based success rate for weight loss is abysmal for adults in the United States, and therefore this strategy is not a viable option to address SRBDs in a meaningful way. On the other hand, overweight or obese individuals will improve their health with any weight loss, and perhaps airway trouble is the motivation that person needs to make the necessary lifestyle changes. Thus, the airway team should continue to support weight loss for the appropriate patients.

One helpful fact to share with patients is that an SRBD, when there is significant adipose tissue, creates an imbalance between some key hormones involved with caloric intake and glucose processing. Resolving the SRBD can help restore those hormones to homeostasis, which will decrease carbohydrate craving and increase the effect of exercise on the metabolism. We tell overweight patients that getting their airway open will not cause them to lose weight, but it will make their other efforts more effective. Very often, a good night's sleep provides the patient with enough energy to start an exercise program. Connecting your airway therapy practice with local weight loss clinics can be an effective marketing strategy. Improved sleep often results in improved mood for both the SRBD-afflicted person and the bed partner.

With better attitudes comes a greater likelihood that partners will participate in healthy activities together, compounding success.

Additional strategies for maintaining a patent airway are being developed, and there may be more choices for clinicians and patients to consider soon. Implantable hypoglossal nerve stimulation devices (Inspire, Inspire Medical Systems) detect airway closure and trigger the genioglossus muscle to move the base of the tongue forward, out of the oropharynx. You may want to discuss this strategy with your otolaryngologist to see if you should be referring certain patients.

References

1. Beyers J, Dieltjens M, Kastoer C, et al. Evaluation of a trial period with a sleep position trainer in patients with positional sleep apnea. J Clin Sleep Med 2018;14:575–583.
2. Scadding G. Non-surgical treatment of adenoidal hypertrophy: The role of treating IgE-mediated inflammation. Pediatr Allergy Immunol 2010;21:1095–1060.
3. Morgenthaler TI, Kapen S, Lee-Chiong T, et al. Practice parameters for the medical therapy of obstructive sleep apnea. Sleep 2006;29:1031–1035.
4. Rueda JR, Mugueta-Aguinaga I, Vilaró J, Rueda-Etxebarria M. Myofunctional therapy (oropharyngeal exercises) for obstructive sleep apnoea. Cochrane Database Syst Rev 2020;11:CD013449.
5. Bernardes R, Ferreira LMDB, Machado AJ Jr, Jones MH. Effectiveness of functional orthopedic appliances as an alternative treatment among children and adolescents with obstructive sleep apnea: Systematic review and meta-analysis. Sleep Med 2023;105:88–102.

Sleep is not a luxury. It's a necessity. The quality of your sleep directly affects the quality of your waking life.

—Dr Michael Breus

7

Complications of Oral Appliance Therapy

The body is an adaptable system, yet it is also subject to homeostasis—a tendency for physiology to stay within a narrow zone of parameters that define health. Challenges kept within customary limits and an undefinable "comfort zone" are easily handled by the body. For example, people can exercise and become overheated (an acute response) but quickly return to normal with no permanent effects. Such disruptions are termed allostatic challenges if they do not result in changes to homeostasis. If we repeat the exercise enough, our bodies can adapt to the challenge and change, with increased flexibility, stronger muscles, and greater respiratory capacity. Homeostatic norms are reset, and the body functions within the "new normal" parameters. This process is called adaptation.

Use of a mandibular advancement device (MAD) to maintain airway patency is a challenge to the tissues associated with the mandible. The early nights of use create an acute response as the body senses disruption in homeostasis. Our patients vary in their comfort zones and their ability to adapt to the stresses associated with MAD therapy. Some patients have little trouble during the accommodation phase with a new MAD, whereas others have more. After the early phase, acute painful complaints are less common, and the dentist's attention turns to the adaptive response.

Understanding Anatomy

To address the "why" behind the various complaints patients present regarding the use of MADs, it is important that you have a thorough understanding of the anatomy. Dentists and dental hygienists learn the relevant anatomy and functions during professional training, but because most dental services do not create more than allostatic challenges, the dentist/hygienist can practice without drawing on that knowledge very often. Most practicing dentists believe that *(1)* temporomandibular joint (TMJ) troubles are best left to the few dentists with particular expertise in this subset of patients and *(2)* treating patients with acute or chronic temporomandibular disorders (TMDs) is difficult and unrewarding. Combine that with a lack of consensus about how to treat TMDs, and it is no wonder why many dentists have little interest in becoming adept at managing acute and chronic orofacial pain problems.

It is not necessary to become your town's TMD expert to successfully manage MAD use in your practice, but if you are uncomfortable with your familiarity of TMDs, seek out refresher training. Courses and books are widely available, and it does not take intensive study to be able to confidently manage most patient complaints. Again, dentists *must* be able to thoroughly evaluate the patient's TMJ status prior to ordering a MAD. A history of TMD does not contraindicate MAD therapy, but that history should be explored prior to initiating oral appliance therapy (OAT). This also has a great deal to do with the patient's attitude about wearing such a device and how they should prepare themselves for the allostatic challenge likely to come. Other medical professionals with less expertise in the area might have uninformed opinions about TMD and MAD use. Check to see if your patient has been told that there is a contraindication to OAT because of TMD history, or that MAD use always results in TMD.

Range of Motion Exercises

The mandible, of course, has 3D limits to its movement, determined by the various soft tissues. When the mandible is postured forward during sleep, the tissues of the orofacial complex are stretched, resulting in an allostatic challenge. The tissue elasticity of the TMJ and the associated muscles of mastication means that effort will be required to return the mandible to its resting posture. This imposed stretch is an acute challenge to the temporomandibular tissues. The MAD prevents a return to a resting position and actively stretches the TMJ complex while in use, often for 6 to 8 hours. Inflammation occurs when a challenge exceeds the allostatic capacity of any tissue. Most patients will experience an inflammatory response during the first few days or even

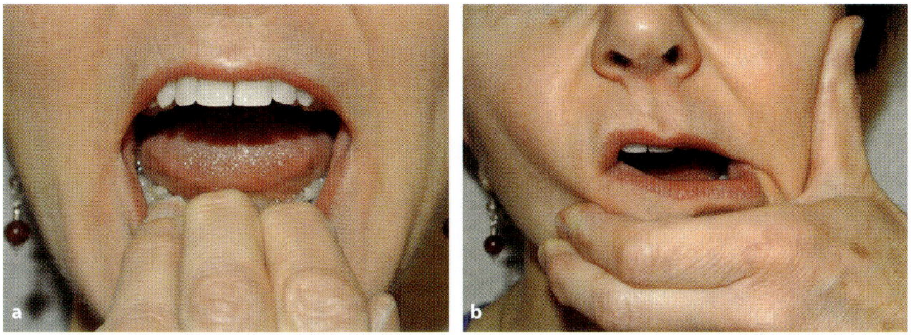

Fig 7-1 *(a and b)* Stretches to improve ROM.

weeks of using a MAD until the tissues have time to adapt. We explain this consequence to our patients using the analogy of starting a new exercise: The involved muscles will be a little bit sore at first but will quickly allow the new movement without protest.

A history of muscle pain and limited range of motion (ROM) increase the chances for early discomfort. Asking these patients to perform ROM stretches before beginning OAT will help them in the early phase (Fig 7-1). Demonstrate these exercises and have the patient show you how they will do them. It's important for them to understand that they must use other muscles (a hand, for example) to achieve increased ROM. They can't just use the muscles of the mandible. Often, when asked to "show us what you do," patients will move their jaw in exaggerated ways, open, left, and right. You must help them understand that they need to relax those jaw muscles as much as they can and use extrinsic muscle power to manipulate them. Stretches include holding the mandible in one hand and moving it left and right, trying to increase the lateral limits of movement. By pulling down on the mandible with fingers on the incisal edges, the patient can stretch the mouth open to increase vertical ROM. Pushing the mandible forward with fingers behind the ramus on both sides is another beneficial stretch. We ask our patients to do these stretches in threes: Stretch to a count of three, and do it three times, three times a day. Patients who perform these recommended stretches seem to have less trouble getting used to wearing their MADs.

Inflammatory Responses

The most common inflammatory response is myositis that produces myalgia (ie, pain in a muscle). Although many patients point to the masseter muscles as the site of the pain, there have been no studies that differentiate the pain response among the many muscles that move the mandible. There is no reason to be specific, as the therapy to help your patients through an acute myositis is the same no matter the location of the myalgia: moist heat, massage, stretching, and perhaps a nonsteroidal anti-inflammatory drug (NSAID). When these palliative efforts are accompanied by assurances about the short-term nature of the problem and the virtue of patience, the problem becomes less troublesome to patients. It is very helpful to guide your patients to recall another instance of body pain associated with an allostatic challenge, like when they mildly twisted an ankle or jammed a finger. When they remember how quickly that pain resolved, they will gain a positive feeling about the MAD discomfort.

Another common problem is capsulitis. As the name implies, the inflammation occurs around the condyle. There are many areas and tissues that can become inflamed, and like with the muscles, there has been no scientific inquiry into which tissue is most likely to be the culprit. Capsulitis can be differentiated from myalgia by asking the patient to bite on a tongue depressor or similar device. When the device is positioned between the incisors, the activation of closing muscles will apply seating force to the condyles, and the patient will quickly be able to identify the site of the pain. When the device is placed bilaterally over the molars (usually it takes a few layers of depressors over the posterior teeth), biting will produce pain in inflamed muscles but will spare enough pressure in the condyles to show the difference. The patient can isolate even further by biting on each side to see which is worse, but that rarely affects therapy recommendations.

Treatment of capsulitis takes time and NSAIDs, as stretching is ineffective. Assure the patient, prescribe a low-challenge diet, and recommend an appropriate NSAID regimen. Applying a cold pack to the area several times a day can also be very helpful. If you have access to a cold laser, a device common in physical therapy, this is where we have found it to be most useful. Many dentists supply condyle-relief appliances, such as daytime splints that support posterior tooth contact. The Aqualizer is one appliance that the authors have found useful (Fig 7-2).

For both myalgia and capsulitis, an increasing number of patients are reporting good results with CBD oils and ointments. There is no standardization of these agents so far, so there is no way to make a recommendation based on anything but anecdotal evidence. Because the use of CBD products seems benign so far, there appears to be little reason to dismiss a patient's idea to give them a try. Follow up with the patient, and you might find a product that can be recommended to other patients in pain.

It is important for capsulitis patients to exercise the affected area to return their bite to maximal intercuspal position (MIP) while the capsulitis heals to

Fig 7-2 Aqualizer splint for TMJ relief.

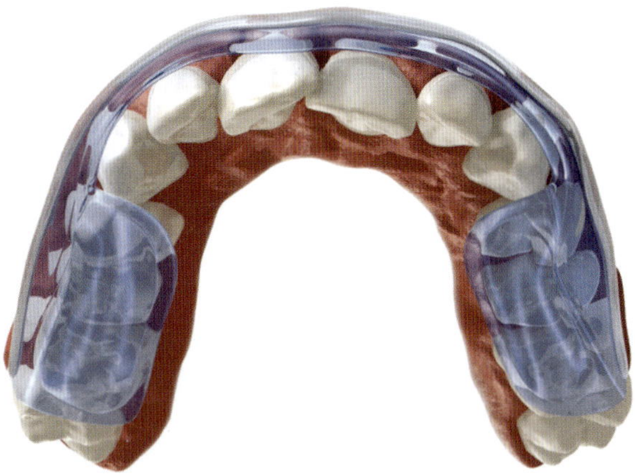

ensure that the condyles can return to the same orientation they had prior to the injury. This can be uncomfortable during the early acute phases of capsulitis, so patient assurance is very important. The most painful capsulitis presentations can be treated with a course of steroids, such as a methylprednisolone dose pack.

For some patients, there seems to be a direct causal link between how aggressively they use their morning repositioner and the severity of the capsulitis. The retrodiscal tissues contain vessels that fill with blood and lymph during MAD use. This fluid must be removed from the retrodiscal area for the bite to return to normal occlusion, which is one of the functions of a morning repositioner. The more aggressively a patient performs these morning exercises, the more likely they are to experience inflammation associated with the joints. In one author's office (Ken Berley's), the first treatment for any TMJ symptoms is palliative (eg, anti-inflammatory medications), with further instructions given regarding diet and evening use of the morning repositioner. Using the morning repositioner right before going to bed seems to relieve this problem. During the day, normal eating and swallowing help to return the mandible to its original position. We instruct the patient to eat a relatively soft breakfast followed by a normal lunch and dinner. Then before bed, after brushing his or her teeth, the patient uses the morning repositioner to make sure the bite is back to normal. Adding this technique to our practice has helped eliminate TMJ issues for many patients.

History of TMD

Many patients initially present with a history of TMJ dysfunction, such as clicking. It is important to thoroughly draw out this history, as it provides proof that the patient's TMJ had adapted anatomy prior to MAD use. There is no reason to order magnetic resonance imaging for every patient with a significant TMJ history, but establishing that they had some prior episodes will make it easier for you to help them through any problems they may develop.

Both authors have had a very small number of patients return within days of delivering the MAD without pain but with a posterior open bite. Dr Berley attributes this phenomenon to bilateral disc recapturing due to mandibular protrusion. When the patient has a preexisting nonreducing disc displacement that then recaptures, the result can be a posterior open bite. Physiologically, the joints are in a healthier (more favorable) position when functioning on the disc; however, we are then faced with the decision of whether to "dislocate the joints" to facilitate posterior occlusion. Typically, the posterior open bite is about 2 mm, which compares favorably with the thickness of the TMJ disc. We have noticed this occurring most commonly in patients who have a Class II, division 2 deep overbite type of malocclusion. To date, no patient has told us that they've discontinued therapy due to a posterior open bite. Patients routinely state that they do not even notice that their back teeth are not touching. Try to enforce the positive aspects of the therapy and how much better the patient is feeling with their chief complaint addressed.

In these instances, it can only be assumed that there has been a shift of tissues within the joint that did not cause inflammation but did change the position of the condyle within the fossa. If you have accurate pre-therapy TMJ images from a CBCT, you can discuss taking a follow-up to compare. Steve Carstensen rarely does this because the repositioning explains itself, and no matter what is found in the CBCT volume, therapy will continue. However, in the few instances where two volumes were obtained not too far apart, the pretreatment joint showed diminished space between the condyle and the fossa surface compared to the second image. That's exactly what we would suspect with this clinical presentation. Having an excellent history, a thorough understanding of the anatomy, and proper informed consent helps maintain a good relationship with these patients.

Another class of patients to take careful notice of are those whose condyles are posteriorly postured within the glenoid fossa while in MIP, as noted in the CBCT scan (Fig 7-3). Because normal muscle function pulls the condyle against the anterior wall of the fossa, this adapted position to the back has

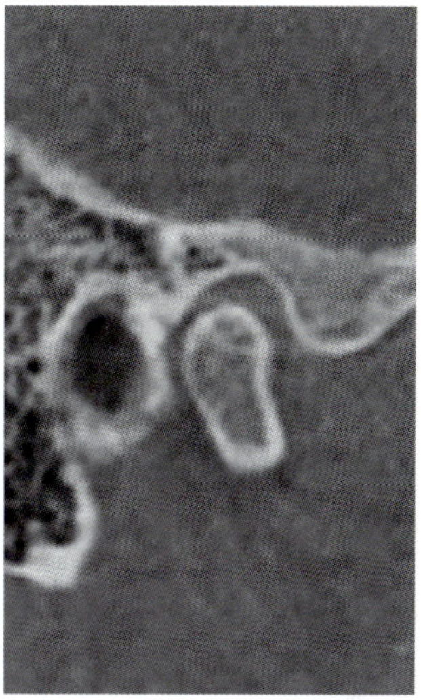

Fig 7-3 Posterior condyle position.

been followed by a higher incidence of condyle position shift in the early use of a MAD. We caution patients very carefully and emphasize the use of the AM Aligner.

Is there an appliance design that is more likely to cause early acute problems? There is nothing in the literature that supports this claim, and in our clinical experience, response is determined far more by the patient than by the device that holds the jaw forward. Choosing a device with an infinite adjustment rather than discrete steps allows patients to feel more in control of their jaw position. One patient found herself able to adjust her MAD forward only by quarter turns of the adjustment screw (0.025 mm) at a time, while others jump in millimeters between positions. Sadly, the only way for you to predict this is to employ clinical wisdom gained from previous experience with your patient or others like them. Sometimes, clinical judgment is insufficient, and you will have to replace a device early with one of a different design. Those unfortunate episodes are rare.

Patients who present with TMJ complaints should be checked for midline discrepancies or other protrusion issues in the MAD. Frequently, it is found that the jaw was protruded or deflected to one side or the other during the bite-taking process due to crowded incisors not fitting the registration device very well. If the patient is attempting to accommodate for tooth overlap, a shift in the protrusion may be the result. To determine if a shift has occurred, have the patient protrude the jaw and mark the mandibular midline. Then have the patient place his or her appliance in the mouth and see if you can detect an unnatural shift. If so, adjust the appliance to correct any shift from the patient's natural protrusion. If severe TMJ issues develop, you should discuss the possibility of discontinuing appliance use until symptoms resolve. However, if the patient has very severe obstructive sleep apnea (OSA), caution is advised, and depending on comorbid disease, daytime sleepiness, and other risk factors, interim CPAP use may be necessary. Emphasizing the transient nature of this recommendation may help them bridge this gap during TMJ healing. When OAT is resumed, it is best if the appliance is retruded (moved distally) to the initial setting or less, if possible, and then gradually protruded after a new accommodation period.

If patients are very reluctant to proceed with custom MAD use because of a history of TMD, they may elect to use a professional-grade temporary MAD to test their ability to manage a protruded posture. Use sound clinical judgment, and have detailed conversations about this. Everyone is expected to have transient allostatic challenges, and worried patients may jump too early to the conclusion that OAT is just not for them. Others, and in our clinic most, will find that a protruded position is quite safe for them, and they will gain confidence in the custom MAD solution. The patient who expects therapy to not work for them is often right. Remember, even when using a temporary appliance, informed consent is mandatory. One author (Ken Berley) has seen a significant posterior open bite develop with short-term temporary appliance usage. Therefore, a well-drafted consent and regular clinical oversight for temporary appliance usage is advised. Keep in mind the risk and office time required for managing even a temporary MAD when considering your fee for this service. Because the use of these devices is never covered by medical insurance, one business model that works is to include the temporary device in a global fee for TMD service, with a cash pay.

Other Acute Problems

Other acute problems are less troublesome than myalgia or capsulitis. If there are problems with appliance fit, the patient will be able to point to the sore tooth or pressure spot on the soft tissue, which will simply require adjustment of the MAD for resolution. Such requests are easily fulfilled. Use of pressure-disclosing paste inside the device or tissue-marking ink for a pressure spot will enable quick resolution of fit issues. With today's high quality manufacturing processes, if you consistently have fit issues, look first to your impression or scan technique. Optimizing them with feedback from the lab artists creating your oral devices will help your team develop. When devices fit the first time around, everyone feels better, and practice efficiency improves. Another detail to observe is when one manufacturer's devices seem to be troublesome at delivery, but others are not. Steve Carstensen has experienced these patterns and the manufacturer's representative was able to pass these observations along to the lab, where flaws in the process were discovered. Ultimately, patients benefit when everything moves smoothly from start to finish.

Excessive salivation commonly accompanies new MAD use. Like initial muscle soreness, this nearly always fades in time. However, if excessive salivation becomes problematic, diphenhydramine 50 mg taken 30 minutes before bed is typically very effective in reducing the saliva and helping the patient sleep. Some methyl methacrylate devices have an acrylic taste and smell at the time of delivery due to off-gassing. If the acrylic taste is an issue, soaking the appliance in water for a day should resolve the problem. The results are better if the water can be replaced several times during the day. Nylon, heat-pressed, and milled MAD bases have no such problems, so they may be better for patients who express sensitivity to acrylic odors or taste.

The Morning After

When your patient removes the MAD after a blissful night's sleep with an open airway, they may feel refreshed, but it is unlikely their teeth will fit together the same way as the night before. This is an acceptable situation. We compare it to sitting in one spot for a while, like on an airplane. It may take a minute to get the jaw moving like normal, so we instruct our patients to remove their device, brush their teeth, and simply move their jaw. If their morning routine includes a shower, warming their face under the running water and massaging the facial muscles will improve mobility. They can try to bite their molars together. Responses range from an immediate ability to touch the teeth together all the way to a real struggle to do so, with most patients able to achieve their normal bite with a little bit of work.

But how can we know if patients are successful achieving their original bite? While it seems obvious to occlusion-aware dentists, many people have little sense of tooth contact. Focus on helping patients achieve their normal MIP by giving them easy-to-follow instructions and tools. The most common ways patients can reposition include waiting on a natural reset, using a rubbery tab, employing a device that is custom-made in your office, or placing a laboratory-made repositioner over the mandibular arch (see chapter 6).

Waiting it out is successful for many patients, but this method is dependent on the patient being aware enough of the bite to not only perceive the full MIP but also to think about it at some point during their day to realize that things are, indeed, the same as before. It is not really in patients' or our best interest to make them think about their bite all day. Sometimes patients will ask about chewing gum to help accelerate the bite recapture. This can work well if the patient chews intentionally to feel the teeth contact on both sides, but this is not the nearly automatic pattern most of us use when chewing gum. Of course, the gum should be sugar-free, preferably with xylitol.

Repositioning the condyles using something between the incisors, generically termed a Lucia jig (Fig 7-4), is common in many disciplines in dentistry. This jig can be custom-made from acrylic and adapted to fit using a premade

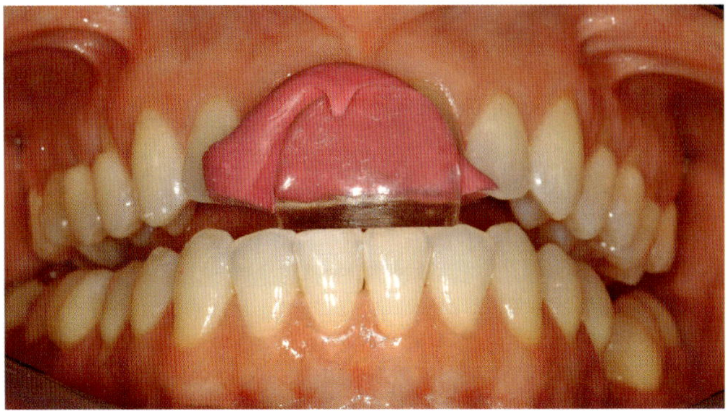

Fig 7-4 Lucia jig.

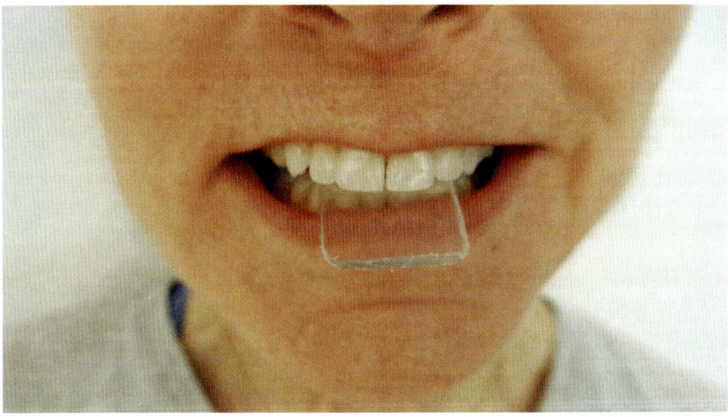

Fig 7-5 Leaf gauge.

shell. A leaf gauge (Fig 7-5) or even a cut piece of thick bite guard material can also be used. While holding this jig between the incisors, activating closing muscles will predictably position the condyles within the glenoid fossa. The disadvantage of this technique is that the patient has no proprioception of molar contact or visual confirmation of MIP.

Custom fabrication of a bite support in the laboratory, which is a common add-on to MAD fabrication, gives the dentist a ready-fit and easy-to-use strategy to help his or her patients. These devices cover partial or full arches and typically have an anterior or posterior support molded in (Fig 7-6). While it is easy to hand them to patients, and the fit is not critical, these devices sometimes add to the lab expense and perform the same function as a Lucia jig. The patient remains unable to feel or see the posterior tooth contact without removing the device.

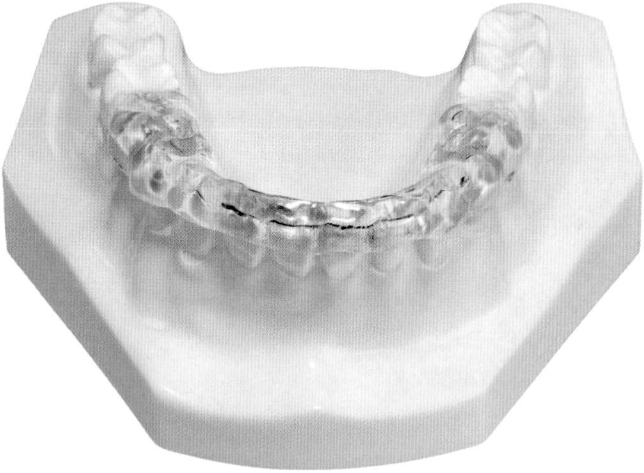

Fig 7-6 Custom-fabricated bite repositioner.

Creating an AM Aligner, as detailed in chapter 6, is the best way to help patients achieve their normal MIP. They can see when their incisal edges fit precisely into the thermoplastic material, and they can feel their posterior teeth fit back into the molded material. This hands-free technique, with both visual and tactile feedback, is more easily adopted into the patient's morning routine. With the low cost of material and ease of fabrication, the dental office can supply the patient with several AM Aligners or replace lost ones without much cost, adding value to the therapy and maintaining the dentist's ability to provide MAD therapy without forgoing a fine occlusion.

At each evaluation and management visit, the patient is asked about TMJ comfort and muscle function. The contacts first found with shimstock are checked to see if they still touch. Although most patients report only transient problems, some will present with longer-term discomfort and new pain locations, and many will lose that initial tooth contact.

It is important to titrate the jaw position to achieve optimal airflow (see chapter 8). By locating the least-protruded effective position, the allostatic challenges are minimized, leading to as few adaptive changes as required. Sometimes the need for protrusion to achieve an open airway leads to a perpetuating allostatic challenge. The difference between adaptive changes and a perpetuating allostatic challenge is the ability of the body to reduce perception of the problem to subclinical levels. Perpetuating challenges lead to sensitization, and that leads to allodynia.

Allodynia is a central sensitization where pain is felt following normally nonpainful stimuli, often from repetitive motion. More commonly associated with migraine, fibromyalgia, or trigeminal neuralgia, allodynia can also result from jaw repositioning. If your patient develops pain like this, check right away for whether their airway is being sufficiently treated; if not, continue to advance the MAD until they can breathe easily. This can pose a communication challenge—they think pushing their jaw forward is causing the pain, and you are going to tell them to move it further. If they are breathing well, you can try medications such as NSAIDs, methylprednisolone, or even gabapentin to break the pain cycle. Many patients will take themselves off OAT until the pain subsides. Most times, these complaints do not return once the initial presentation is addressed, and OAT resumes uneventfully. No literature exists to support the authors' many clinical observations that the central sensitization becomes an adaptive response over time if the airway is open and sleep is uninterrupted by intermittent hypoxia. As the response decreases pain, the therapy becomes routine, and the chance for a repeat painful episode decreases. Even if it returns, the patient's experience provides confidence in continuing therapy. A supportive conversation from a trained team member reinforces the value of therapy during any of these negative intervals.

These issues emphasize the importance of being knowledgeable about TMD and the 3D function of the involved tissues. Patients often overreact to dysfunction in this area, but if met by calm confidence in their provider's office, the episode becomes a learning experience, like many other small injuries in their life. If, however, their dentist (or worse, another dentist not involved with the therapy) reinforces an "all MADs cause this" attitude, patient confidence in the therapy may be diminished. One reason to carefully gather all the names of your patient's health care team and make a commitment to communication is to allay their concerns with open invitations for dialogue.

Dental Problems from MAD Use

Preventive care during airway therapy should be tailored to the patient's risk factors. No study in the literature suggests an increased risk of caries or periodontal disease due to MAD use, but all patients should be coached on proper preventive efforts. People with slightly mobile teeth or persistent periodontal inflammation may benefit from the splinting effect of the MAD and the limiting or redistribution of forces on weak teeth at night. Resolution of sleep-related breathing disorders will reduce systemic inflammation, which may aid local preventive therapy.

Fig 7-7 Posterior open bite due to MAD usage.

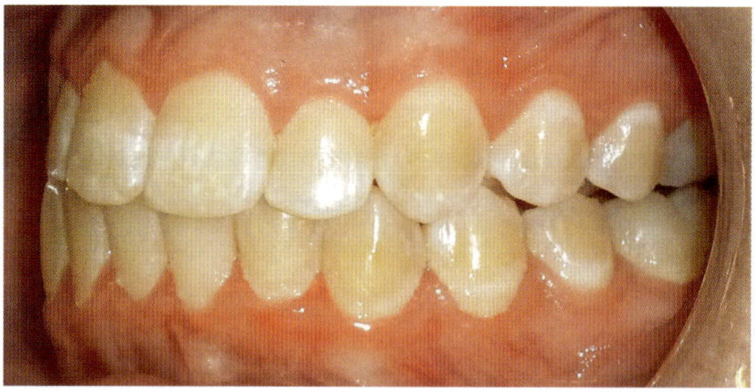

Xerostomia from mouth breathing has been covered previously, and an emphasis on nasal breathing is a consistent goal in airway therapy. Maintaining saliva on the teeth is part of overall health. If your patient consistently has a dry mouth and is not capable of full-night nasal breathing, the use of saliva substitutes, especially those containing xylitol, may help.

Tooth movement caused by MAD use is well documented in several short- and long-term studies. Because the anchorage for the forward posture consists of teeth supported by periodontal ligaments with pluripotent cells that can form osteoclasts and osteoblasts when subjected to pressure, tooth movement cannot be considered a 100% avoidable consequence of this therapy. Orthodontic forces move teeth under carefully controlled situations the exact same way MADs can move teeth, albeit most airway treatment devices lack the precision of brackets, wires, and clear aligners.

Typically, movement involves posterior tipping of the maxillary anterior teeth and anterior flaring of the mandibular anterior teeth. Additionally, the mandible will slowly reposition forward, which will frequently cause a posterior open bite (Fig 7-7). Most patients are unaware of these changes and only become aware when they go back to their primary care dentist for routine preventive visits. The reason behind this unawareness seems straightforward: If a new restoration is "high," the resulting pressure is immediately felt in the periodontal ligament. However, if a new change is *out* of occlusion, there's no signal to send, and the person remains unaware. Even an arch with only one contact and the rest of the teeth out of occlusion can remain undetected.

Every patient must be counseled regarding the probability of tooth movement. Like many other aspects of medicine, this risk must be carefully and clearly discussed with patients so they can make the medical choice that is most comfortable for them. Reminding patients of the reason they sought treatment in the first place often helps mitigate the emotional response to this tooth movement. No one ever died from tooth movement. This will help the patient focus on the seriousness of OSA and realize that tooth movement is a minor complication and not a barrier to this treatment choice.

MADs are made from different materials with different means of fabrication. It makes sense that the most rigid devices with the intaglio surfaces most tightly adapted to the tooth surfaces will result in less tooth movement, and there are emerging studies that document this clinical finding. The softer, less highly adapted materials provide less control over tooth position. Adding in consideration of the forces on the teeth from protrusion and nighttime masticatory muscle activity, it is easy to see how teeth can move over time. In fact, it may be unreasonable to expect no change in tooth position. Patients who have completed orthodontics as an adult seem to have more minor tooth movement than those whose treatment was in adolescence. If the adult has solid retainers, such as with clear aligner therapy, we encourage them to wear them during the day part-time. Some MADs can be fabricated to work with clear aligner trays, so that may be a comforting choice for concerned patients. The keys to success are having the informed consent conversation prior to any MAD therapy and applying your knowledge to the individual patient in a precise and personal manner.

Laboratory Considerations

If the dentist finds that many devices are fracturing or wearing out or that patients are having trouble with the advancement mechanisms, the best thing to do is to consider whether the right laboratory is making the devices. In the authors' experience, MADs typically last 3 to 6 years with few problems because we supply our high-quality labs with top-quality data. If the lead assistant contacts several labs, interviews the people he or she might work with, and chooses based on quality, the office can provide devices they will be proud to offer. One differentiating step is to have the assistant ask the lab artist what can be done at the dental office to improve outcomes. Improvement in impression/scan quality or precision in the 3D bite will go a long way toward simplifying MAD therapy.

It is important for patients to understand that they are being given a device intended to address a serious medical problem that they will use for 7 to 8 hours every night for several years. Guiding your patient to understand that this is a simple device put under rigorous service will help them set appropriate expectations for its clinically useful life span.

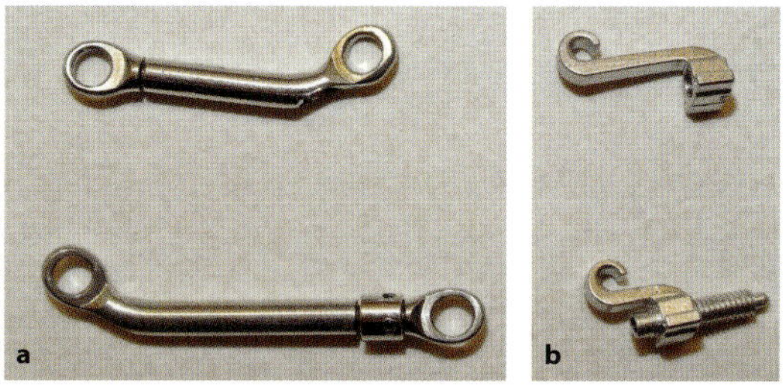

Fig 7-8 Replacement or substitution parts for a Herbst appliance *(a)* and a TAP appliance *(b)*.

Every practice wants to keep the cost of doing business to a minimum. However, basing treatment decisions solely on lab fees can be shortsighted because labs have different business models. Because only FDA-licensed labs can produce MADs, quality standards must be maintained to retain certification. You should keep in mind that there is service that accompanies the product, and many times the value of the service is overwhelming justification for a higher lab fee. If one lab produces devices that take less chair time to deliver and fewer adjustment visits, your cost of providing therapy will be less with that lab or device design.

Each MAD design has its own adjustment mechanism. Most are quite straightforward and serve for the life of the device without becoming the failure point. Adjusters that become impossible to turn can often be freed with ultrasonic cleaning or, in extreme cases, a return to the lab for replacement. The dentist is often capable of freeing a stuck mechanism with a little ingenuity in the office. Although most patients will not exceed the adjustment range built into their device, occasionally the jaw must be advanced further. Some devices have parts that can be substituted, such as a different hook or arm mechanism. For example, you can replace the arms on Herbst appliances and change out the advancement arms on TAP appliances (Fig 7-8). If the appliance has an acrylic base, you can reposition the hinges using ordinary acrylic skills common to dentists. Some labs give you the option of designing the appliance with additional advancement incorporated into the appliance. One manufacturer's Herbst appliance comes with an extra posterior bar attachment that can be engaged once the Herbst bar reaches its maximum protrusion (Fig 7-9).

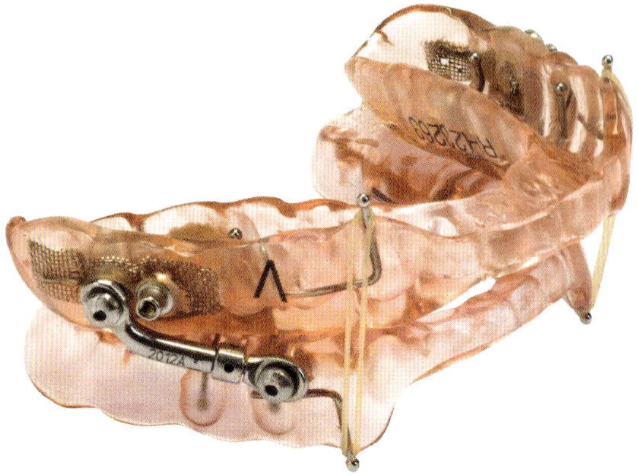

Fig 7-9 DynaFlex Herbst appliance with an extra posterior bar attachment.

The use of acrylic shims is also helpful. Dentists should consider adjustment needs and have the confidence to choose a path to achieve that range of adjustment with the skills they already have. Contacting the lab will most likely result in a return of the device to the lab with a fee to make the change. Any such return is costly, and the patient cannot be left without treatment. Providing a temporary MAD increases costs. On the other hand, modifying the MAD in the office often voids the manufacturer's warranty. By necessity, any dentist providing sleep devices will become adept at developing unique strategies to solve individual clinical problems. We consider this opportunity for creative problem solving to be one of the positive aspects of dental sleep medicine—one that is not generally available in restorative and preventive care.

High perceived benefit is the first, and perhaps the most important, step on the road to increased treatment acceptance and utilization.

—Meir Kryger

8

Evaluating Therapy and Ongoing Care

Patients request sleep diagnostic and treatment services because they have symptoms they want to eliminate, such as snoring and excessive daytime sleepiness, or they are determined to improve their health in manageable ways. They cannot change their genes, but they can control some gene expression and improve their health span. In our offices, we always use two coexisting definitions of success based on *(1)* what problems the patient wants solved and *(2)* what numbers the medical professionals want to see normalized. Eliminating snoring as a social issue and maintaining SpO_2 above 90% are two common examples.

Each sleep physician that you work with may have a different definition of a successful oral appliance therapy (OAT) case. Some sleep physicians adamantly demand that OAT resolve the patient's subjective symptoms and completely control the patient's apnea. Sadly, the authors have seen symptom-free and medically sound patients with an Apnea-Hypopnea Index (AHI) of 7 after mandibular advancement device (MAD) titration placed back on continuous positive airway pressure (CPAP). Obviously, this approach is counterproductive, as most patients are using a MAD to avoid CPAP. It certainly can be challenging to work with sleep physicians who insist that all your cases result in an AHI < 5. Discuss with them why they think this threshold is so important.

The science of defining treatment success is constantly evolving. If you engage with your referring physicians regarding the length of time each therapy is typically used, most practitioners will realize that OAT is a reasonable

TABLE 8-1 Comparison of OAT and CPAP effectiveness* according to Hoekema[3]

Patient group	OAT	CPAP
Total population (N = 103)	76.5% (39/51)	82.7% (43/52)
Nonsevere OSA (N = 50)	84.0% (21/25)	80.0% (20/25)
Severe OSA (N = 53)	69.2% (18/26)	85.2% (23/27)

*AHI < 5 or decreased AHI of at least 50% from baseline to less than 20 in a patient who had no symptoms while using therapy.

alternative to CPAP. Surveys reveal that most OAT patients use oral appliances significantly longer per night than CPAP[1]; therefore, it can be argued that the length of use of oral appliances counters the higher levels of efficacy of CPAP. In chapter 3, we introduced the concept of mean disease alleviation, which is a mathematical computation of total apneic event elimination based on the efficacy of the therapy and the length of use. Using mean disease alleviation, it is easy to argue that OAT is as effective or more effective than CPAP for most patients.[2] Because OAT is generally less effective at normalizing AHI than CPAP on an hour-by-hour comparison, dental professionals sometimes redefine success in terms that are more favorable to OAT. The definition of OAT success that is frequently used by dentists is a reduction in AHI of at least 50%, with improvement in subjective symptoms. Any time you read an article on OAT success compared to CPAP, always check the definition of OAT success used by the researchers.

In dental sleep medicine (DSM), we frequently cite the Hoekema study,[3] which shows a nice comparison of successful OAT and CPAP patients (Table 8-1). However, when viewing these results, you will notice that "successful" cases could have a residual AHI as high as 19, as long as they showed symptom improvement and a 50% reduction in AHI. The American Board of Dental Sleep Medicine (ABDSM) uses a final AHI of 10 or less, with symptom improvement, as the measure for success for ABDSM case submissions.

Dentists are at a disadvantage when declaring or determining that any OAT case is successful, because ultimately success is defined by the supervising or referring sleep physician. Always remember, however, that sleep physicians certify that CPAP therapy is successful if the patient uses CPAP therapy at least 4 hours per night for 70% of nights. Neither PAP nor OAT is the perfect solution to obstructive sleep apnea (OSA). Astute clinicians provide the best treatment by planning for the individual patient, considering their preferences and choices.

BOX 8-1 Factors that influence MMI

- Dental health limitations, including the number of teeth, the periodontal condition, etc
- Temporomandibular joint health, including painful joints/muscles and limited range of motion or protrusion
- Appliance choice, tongue space, lingual appliance thickness, and the ability to change the vertical and horizontal advancement
- Starting position choice (vertical and horizontal positioning)
- Co-therapies employed, including positional therapy, weight loss, bariatric surgery, and exercise
- In-office titration technique and subjective symptoms, such as home sleep apnea testing (HSAT) and pulse oximetry
- Final sleep study titration technique (eg, dentist in laboratory, registered polysomnographic technologist in laboratory, HSAT)
- Referral for maxillomandibular advancement surgery, uvulopalatopharyngoplasty, or tracheostomy

Maximum Medical Improvement

Maximum medical improvement (MMI) is the ultimate endpoint of OAT. Virtually all patients will experience improved health with OAT, but not all will reach a normal AHI (AHI < 5). Therefore, when patients reach their MMI with OAT, their OSA may still not be adequately controlled. All dentists who treat OSA should be aware of techniques to improve OAT outcomes (Box 8-1).

Dentist-Facilitated Appliance Titration for Increased MAD Efficacy

Sleep physicians typically determine OAT success or failure based on a single-night follow-up sleep study. Dentist-facilitated appliance titration can be accomplished based on either improved subjective symptoms or improved objective data, such as oximetry. However, it is important for the MAD to be titrated as closely as possible to an effective position before sending the patient back to the sleep physician. If the OAT tests ineffective, your patient will likely be placed back on CPAP, and your referrals may suffer. Therefore, practitioners should make every effort to ensure that their patients are effectively titrated *before* being seen by the sleep physician.

Dentist-facilitated titration protocols can take several forms. In some cases, your patient may be perfectly capable of titrating their appliance with appropriate instructions, or that process may need to be performed by your office staff. The goal of dentist-facilitated titration is to advance the appliance to a point where the patient's subjective symptoms are at a minimum and the objective data show disease control, without creating side effects that may prompt the patient to discontinue therapy. Some patients require little advancement, whereas others require significant advancement, even beyond the point they were able to protrude at the initial seating of their MAD. During the titration process, patients must be seen on a regular basis to evaluate any side effects and monitor subjective symptoms. With titration, progressive improvement of subjective symptoms should be noted. Patients should report improved quality and quantity of sleep. Comparing the patient's "after" symptoms with the list of "before" symptoms that were detailed upon the patient's first visit is important. Studies label pre-experiment evaluations "T0" (time zero) at the beginning of the treatment and subsequent data points "T1, T2, T3," etc. This construct could be useful in correlating symptoms with jaw position changes.

Several factors can affect the success of titration, including medications, BMI, the positional component of OSA, dental classification, tongue size, arch width, lymphoid tissue size, size and length of the uvula, and alcohol consumption.

Goals of oral appliance titration

There are three goals of oral appliance titration:

1. The patient wears the appliance all night, every night.
2. The appliance is titrated adequately for all or most of the patient's subjective symptoms to disappear.
3. The MAD is titrated adequately for all or most of the patient's objective sleep data to recover to normal levels.

THE PATIENT WEARS THE APPLIANCE ALL NIGHT, EVERY NIGHT

If you are new to DSM, you might think that it is easy to get patients to wear their appliances during sleep all the time, but sadly, this is not the case. The list of excuses that we have heard from patients explaining why oral appliances remain on the counter is quite long. Reasons for not wearing an appliance may be associated with its size or comfort. Some problems revolve around social issues: "My girlfriend has been staying at my house, and I don't want her to know that I have to use a thing." In each of these situations, encourage the patient to commit to wearing the appliance. Reminding them of the reasons they sought treatment in the first place is a great place to start, so make sure that data is readily available at every follow-up appointment. Having a patient-centric response is imperative. Telling a patient that it is better to wear the appliance than to have a stroke or heart attack may work well to motivate patients with that concern but will sound trite to a young adult with no thoughts of cardiovascular complications.

In any case, MADs must be comfortable to wear. Obviously, some appliances are naturally more comfortable than others due to the materials used during fabrication. The MADs that seem to be the most uncomfortable when initially seated are those fabricated from traditional, powder and liquid polymethyl methacrylate (PMMA). When acrylic is processed, longitudinal shrinkage occurs toward the center of the appliance, causing pressure on the anterior teeth and tightening the acrylic on the distal portion of the posterior teeth. Typically, adjustments to a PMMA-processed appliance will be on the distofacial aspect of the maxillary posterior teeth and the facial aspect of the anterior teeth. The mandibular arch is adjusted on the distolingual aspect of the mandibular molars and the facial aspect of the mandibular anterior teeth. Additionally, the embrasure spaces may be excessively tight if an inadequate amount of block-out was used by the laboratory artist. More flexible liners or whole devices created out of softer materials may be acceptable for patients with a history of nightguard rejection, for example.

MADs should be fabricated with 1 mm or more of retrusion available from the starting position in case the patient cannot tolerate even the minimal protrusion you chose. When the appliance is initially seated, it is ideal that the patient be allowed to wear the appliance in the dental chair for 10 minutes or longer to ensure reasonable comfort. Make sure you address any soreness issues before the patient is released. It is much easier to fix a simple problem during the seating appointment than to allow the patient to get so sore that he or she refuses to wear the MAD. Most devices today do not cause tooth or tissue pain, but keep in mind that the periodontal ligament is very sensitive and the perception of discomfort varies greatly between individuals. Because inflammation takes a few days to become established, it is not uncommon to get a call from a patient a week or so after delivery of a MAD in which they state that the device is too uncomfortable to wear. Don't encourage the patient's worry or offer to change device; just invite them in for a fit adjustment and some needed reassurances about the therapy process.

THE APPLIANCE IS TITRATED ADEQUATELY FOR ALL OR MOST OF THE PATIENT'S SUBJECTIVE SYMPTOMS TO DISAPPEAR

During your initial intake examination, you should document the patient's subjective symptoms. The most used marker is the Epworth Sleepiness Scale, but patients will report what they feel are the most important problems sleep-disordered breathing is causing for them. With successful titration, patients should report improvement in their list of subjective symptoms. Documentation of these improvements is helpful to reinforce therapy in the times ahead. You may find that many patients have had significant symptoms for many years and are unable to determine when they feel normal. Any slight improvement for these patients can be life-changing. However, once the patient thinks the subjective symptoms are gone, testing is required.

Many patients use consumer sleep technology (CST) to supplement their perceptions of symptom improvement. Fitbits, Apple Watches, the SnoreLab app, and Oura Rings are a few examples of popular devices, but there are many more, with others being developed. Clinicians should explore how much trust the patient places in these CSTs and work with them to interpret results carefully. It does little good to dismiss data from CST if your patient has chosen it as their means of understanding treatment outcomes. People tend to understand that the data is a guide and not diagnostic, and it has value to improve self-care without precluding professional assessment. People who are engaged in their own health are the most successful at managing chronic disease. On the other hand, some people can become obsessed with CST numbers and wonder why their snoring score is not 0, or why it is 7 on some nights and 9 on others. During your new patient intake, a few pointed questions about how they use CST data to guide decisions can provide you with valuable insight into later behavior. Cautioning patients not to obsess over clinically insignificant data requires the dental team to focus on empathetic communication that includes proper education.

THE MAD IS TITRATED ADEQUATELY FOR ALL OR MOST OF THE PATIENT'S OBJECTIVE SLEEP DATA TO RECOVER TO NORMAL LEVELS

The only way for dentists to know if the patient's objective sleep data are at normal levels is to use some type of testing. Technology is available that rivals in-lab polysomnography (PSG) for gathering biodata, and software algorithms that interpret physiologic responses are sophisticated. Artificial intelligence will soon be the norm for interpretating vast amounts of biodata, and the process for evaluating sleep quality will become easier and provide more insights. Determining whether additional titration is needed and whether positional therapy would be beneficial depends on good data collection.

Dentist-Facilitated HSAT and Pulse Oximetry for Titration

DSM practitioners disagree on MAD titration techniques and the use of testing during titration. It is the opinion of the authors that some level of testing is necessary to ensure reasonable results with OAT.

Before you invest in home sleep apnea testing (HSAT) or pulse oximetry equipment, you need to be aware that, as of this writing, most state dental boards have not ruled on whether a dentist can order an HSAT. Thus far, owning and using HSAT equipment is illegal for dentists only in New Jersey (though the New Jersey State Board of Dentistry is not currently enforcing this position). All readers should be aware of the applicable regulations in their state and make their treatment decisions accordingly. At this time, the American Dental Association (ADA) and the American Academy of Dental Sleep Medicine (AADSM) have both endorsed the use of home testing during patient titration to facilitate therapeutic results.

The patient's subjective symptoms should show significant improvement almost immediately after seating the MAD and improve further with titration. Once the patient's OSA symptoms are improved, an HSAT/pulse oximetry study should be considered to see if further advancements are needed to reach MMI. If the patient is sent to a sleep laboratory with significant residual apnea, he or she may not be capable of advancing adequately to achieve normal results. By performing oximetry studies to aid in titration, the patient will generally find the physician-directed treatment efficacy study a confirmation of adequate treatment rather than serving as a "let's see how we're doing test"—which would be viewed as a waste of resources.

The following example demonstrates this technique. A patient's initial AHI was 24.6. The patient spent only a few minutes on his back during his diagnostic PSG, so his supine AHI was only 4 (Box 8-2). The patient was delivered a Herbst appliance, which was advanced until the subjective symptoms were eliminated. The patient was then sent home with an HSAT (Nox T3, Nox Medical). The results of the first titration study showed an overall AHI of 11.5, a supine AHI of 34.8, and a minimum SaO_2 of 86% (Fig 8-1). As a result of this titration study, the patient was advanced 2 mm over a 2-month period and placed on a Night Shift (Advanced Brain Monitoring) to prevent supine sleep. The patient was then tested again. The results showed an overall AHI of 4.6, a supine AHI of 0, and a minimum SaO_2 of 86% (Fig 8-2). As a result of this study, the patient was appointed for a final PSG with titration in the sleep lab.

BOX 8-2 Pretreatment parameters of a patient with significant OSA

Respiratory parameters

- 41 total apneas (38 obstructive apneas, 3 central apneas, and 0 mixed apneas)
- 11 hypopneas
- Overall AHI = 24.6/hr
- REM AHI = 32.4/hr
- Non-REM AHI = 23.2/hr
- Supine AHI = 4/hr
- Longest event = 72 seconds
- Snoring noted

Oximetry and cardiac data

- Mean SaO_2 = 92%
- Minimum SaO_2 during total sleep time = 85%
- Minimum SaO_2 during REM sleep = 85%
- Minimum SaO_2 during non-REM sleep = 87%
- Percentage of sleep time below 89% = 9.4%
- Maximum heart rate = 70 bpm
- Minimum heart rate = 56 bpm
- Mean heart rate = 61 bpm

Respiration summary

	A+H	OA	MA+CA	Hyp	Desat	Snores	Cardia	Movements	Paradoxical
Total events	74	44	9	21	29	14	0	50	0
Total duration (min)	29.3	15.8	2.6	10.8	12.8	2.7	0	12.5	0
Total duration (%)	7.6	4.1	0.7	2.8	3.3	0.7	0.0	3.2	0.0
Index (#/hr)	11.5	6.8	1.4	3.3	4.5		0.0		
Longest event (s)	90.4	86.0	24.0	90.4	48.0	23.1	0	92.9	0
Average event duration (s)	23.7	21.6	17.6	30.8	26.5	11.8	0	18.0	0

Position summary

Position	AH-Index	A+H	OA	MA+CA	Hyp	Desat	ODI	Average SaO_2 (%)	Snores	Paradoxical
Supine	34.8	48	30	7	11	19	13.8	91.1	1.1%	0.0%
Prone		0	0	0	0	0				
Left	19.5	4	3	0	1	1	4.9	94.2	3.5%	0.0%
Right	4.5	22	11	2	9	9	1.9	92.7	0.5%	0.0%

Oximetry	
Average SaO_2 (%)	92.4
Baseline SaO_2 (%)	92.4
Minimum SaO_2 (%)	86.0
Desaturations	29
Average low desat (%)	90.1
Desaturations < 90%	10
Desaturations < 85%	0
SaO_2 below 90% (%)	5.7
SaO_2 below 85% (%)	0.0

Pulse	
Average pulse rate (bpm)	55.8
Highest pulse rate (bpm)	71.0
Duration above 100 bpm (%)	0.0
Duration below 40 bpm (%)	0.0

Signal quality		
Oximeter	100%	Good
Nasal cannula	100%	Good
RIP belts	100%	Good

Position	(min)	(%)
Supine	82.6	21.1
Prone	0	0.0
Left	12.3	3.2
Right	291.1	74.6
Upright	3.9	74.6

Activity	
Time in bed (hours)	6.4
Sleep efficiency (%)	95.8%

Fig 8-1 Respiration summary after initial titration.

Respiration summary

	A+H	OA	MA+CA	Hyp	Desat	Snores	Cardia	Movements	Paradoxical
Total events	14	11	0	3	5	1	0	38	0
Total duration (min)	5.0	4.0	0	1.0	2.7	0.2	0	14.5	0
Total duration (%)	2.7	2.2	0.0	0.5	1.5	0.1	0.0	8.0	0.0
Index (#/hr)	4.6	3.6	0.0	1.0	1.6		0.0		
Longest event (s)	60.0	60.0	0	28.5	81.0	13.9	0	424.2	0
Average event duration (s)	21.3	21.7	0	19.8	32.3	13.9	0	42.0	0

Position summary

Position	AH-Index	A+H	OA	MA+CA	Hyp	Desat	ODI	Average SaO_2 (%)	Snores	Paradoxical
Supine	0.0	0	0	0	0	0	0.0	93.0	0.0%	0.0%
Prone		0	0	0	0	0				
Left		0	0	0	0	0				
Right	4.6	14	11	0	3	5	1.6	92.6	0.1%	0.0%

Oximetry	
Average SaO_2 (%)	92.5
Baseline SaO_2 (%)	92.6
Minimum SaO_2 (%)	88.0
Desaturations	5
Average low desat (%)	89.6
Desaturations < 90%	3
Desaturations < 85%	0
SaO_2 below 90% (%)	0.7
SaO_2 below 85% (%)	0.0

Pulse	
Average pulse rate (bpm)	57.7
Highest pulse rate (bpm)	72.0
Duration above 100 bpm (%)	0.0
Duration below 40 bpm (%)	0.0

Signal quality		
Oximeter	99%	Good
Nasal cannula	98%	Good
RIP belts	100%	Good

Position	(min)	(%)
Supine	0.1	0.0
Prone	0	0.0
Left	0.5	0.3
Right	182.0	92.6
Upright	13.8	7.0

Activity	
Time in bed (hours)	3.0
Sleep efficiency (%)	85.3%

Fig 8-2 Respiration summary after second titration.

In-Lab Titration

In-lab titration is difficult to discuss because the titration protocols used in the authors' practices are very different. Ken Berley is from northwest Arkansas, and most of his patients are closely followed by their referring sleep physicians. In Arkansas, PSGs are routine, and HSATs are rarely ordered. Ken has sleep lab privileges and oversees the final titration of all patients. Steve Carstensen is from Seattle, where his patients are not closely followed by their sleep physicians, and frequently his patients do not even return to their physicians after the resolution of subjective symptoms. In Seattle, PSGs are rarely performed, unless the patient is very sick or if HSAT results do not correlate with the patient's clinical presentation. Therefore, Steve does not adjust his patient's appliances during a final titration sleep study.

Ken Berley firmly believes that an in-lab PSG is far superior for final titration because it allows either a well-trained sleep technologist or the treating dentist to titrate the MAD for maximum efficacy. However, some dentists may have difficulty achieving hospital privileges, and insurance companies may resist final titration PSGs. Consider the protocols in your area of practice. You will need to work with your local sleep labs, sleep physicians, and insurance companies to determine the best approach to titration in your community. You will come to discover the diagnostic approaches of the physicians in your geographic vicinity. Design your practice protocols to comply with local requirements. Based on the dictates of the medical insurance companies in your part of the world, sleep physicians will use either PSGs or HSATs to diagnose OSA and confirm the efficacy of your therapy.

If the treating sleep physician orders an HSAT to determine the efficacy of the appliance, adjustments are not possible. If the referring sleep physician orders a final PSG, the treating dentist should attempt to arrange for the MAD to be titrated during that test. Think of this as a titration study and not necessarily as an efficacy study. Prepare your patient for the test and make sure there are no issues with the fit of the device.

Titration by the lab technologist

Titration can be performed by well-educated lab technologists. Visit the lab with models of the appliances that the lab will regularly titrate, and offer a workshop on MAD titration. Provide a handout to the sleep lab for each appliance that you regularly use. Make sure the name and picture of the appliance is on the handout. The handout should include detailed instructions on how to advance the appliance and how many turns, quarter turns, or half turns are necessary to advance the appliance by 1 mm. Make sure you include which direction to turn the gears for advancement. Provide any wrenches necessary for the adjustments. If the MAD advances by replacing side straps, the patient should bring them to the test, but it is wise to provide the lab with a supply as well. Make sure the lab is aware that they cannot adjust MADs as frequently as they make adjustments for CPAP titration because the patient must be awakened for adjustments. During those interruptions, the technologist should try to stimulate the patient no more than necessary. No turning on bright lights in the patient's room! Make sure the lab has rubber bands for the anterior hooks and understands the necessity of having the patient's mouth closed. Include your phone number, and assure the lab technologist that you will answer a call at any time during the night if your help is needed.

It is important to inform technologists that you need them to use BiPAP titration software for your patients. Your studies need to be named "Mandibular Advancement Device Titration Study." They will need to place the current appliance's vertical dimension, which you supply from the appliance fabrication notes, as the top number in the BiPAP titration software. The bottom number is the current horizontal protrusion at the beginning of the sleep study. At the beginning of the study, this bottom number includes any initial advancement plus any advancement that was made during dentist-facilitated titration. The horizontal number is the number that changes during the in-lab sleep study. Each time the appliance is titrated during the study, numbers start over, so you will get an AHI and oxygen saturation nadir for each level of protrusion.

In the physician's report shown in Fig 8-3, you will see that there was 10 mm of vertical dimension built into the appliance, and the appliance was advanced 3 mm during the lab titration. At the final titration position, the patient spent 51 minutes of sleep at 6 mm of advancement, with 20.5 minutes in NREM (non–rapid eye movement) sleep and 30.5 minutes in REM sleep. The minimum SaO_2 level at that titration was 91%. The AHI at the final position was 1.2. These results are possible only with titration.

Titration by the dentist

You can also perform in-lab titration personally. This approach has many advantages. During your time in the sleep lab, you will learn a lot. The sleep technologists will enjoy teaching a doctor about sleep, and you can teach the technologists about the appliances that you are using and how DSM works. Ultimately, these technologists can become a great referral source for your office. You do not necessarily have to stay all night, but if you really want to see how your patient is doing, you should stay until you see the last REM session

MAD level	TST (min)	Wake (min)	NREM (min)	REM (min)	Supine REM (min)	Sleep efficiency (%)	Apn	Hyp	AHI	Min SaO_2	Average SaO_2	Max SaO_2
Off	0.0	0.5	0.0	0.0		0.0%	-	-	-	-	-	-
10 3	12.0	4.0	12.0	0.0		75.0%	-	-	-	91.0	92.5	94.0
10 5	263.0	126.0	237.5	25.5		67.6%	1	14	3.4	88.0	93.0	99.0
10 6	51.0	11.0	20.5	30.5		82.3%	-	1	1.2	91.0	93.5	97.0

LIMB ACTIVITY: The Limb Movement index was 0.2 per hour while the PLM index was 0.0 per hour. No movements in REM were suggestive of REM behavior disorder. No bruxism was noted. No seizure activity seen.

EEG SUMMARY: Limited EEG demonstrated no epileptiform activity.

DIAGNOSIS:

1. Moderate obstructive sleep apnea.
2. Excellent titration of MAD.

RECOMMENDATIONS:

1. The MAD appears to be set appropriately with normalization of the AHI in its final position.
2. Exercise and weight loss to normal BMI.
3. Do not drive or operate machinery if sleepy.
4. RTC 4–6 weeks.

Fig 8-3 Physician's report from the sleep study.

of the night, which occurs right before the patient wakes up in the morning. Going to the sleep lab with your patients will impress the sleep professionals you are working with.

Titration by the patient

If your patient has shown the ability to advance their appliance, you can have your patient titrate the device during this sleep study. In this scenario, when the technologist feels that the appliance needs to be advanced, the patient is awakened, often with the overhead lights being turned on. The drawback of this scenario is that the patient becomes fully alert. When patients are stimulated to this degree, it may be very difficult for them to get back to sleep. Additionally, they must understand exactly how to advance the appliance and be able to see well enough to make the changes.

No titration

Some dentists simply refer the patient back to the sleep lab for an overall PSG during which the appliance is not titrated; however, research and the personal experience of the authors confirms that you will not get the best results if the appliance is not titrated. Plus, if you do not have personal contact with the lab technologists, they will not become a referral source. Additionally, they will not know what to do when the patient has a problem during the study.

Dentist-Facilitated Final Sleep Study

Again, the authors are challenged over the need for a final sleep study. In Seattle, many patients do not return to their sleep physician and do not get a final sleep study after the improvement of subjective symptoms, despite entreaties from the treating dentist. Both authors strongly believe that all patients should have a final sleep study. If one is not performed by the patient's physician, it is imperative that the treating dentist facilitate a final study. Ken Berley always stresses the need for all patients to be followed by their sleep physician. If the patient refuses to return to their physician, the treating dentist can use one of the HSAT services to secure a final study. This choice may be influenced by insurance limitations.

All practitioners should be aware that there is an element of risk associated with failure to get a final sleep study. All patients should be informed of the need for a final sleep study and either be referred to their sleep physician or have the study facilitated for them by the treating dentist. Failure to get a final sleep study has resulted in malpractice actions in some cases. However, as of this writing, there have not been any jury awards. If the patient refuses to undergo a final sleep study, practitioners should have the patient sign a release of liability.

Physician/Dentist Monitoring

Once diagnosed with OSA, patients will always need to be monitored. OSA generally worsens with age. The loss of bone density in adults, especially women, decreases hard tissue support for the soft tissue lining the airway. Less support and lower muscle tone caused by aging means a more collapsible airway and worse breathing. (The good news? Less bruxism!) Increased weight and menopause also exacerbate OSA. We are always changing and getting older, so regular monitoring is a must. It is ideal for DSM practitioners to recall their patients on a 6-month basis for the first year and then yearly after that, with an open invitation if symptoms change.

At each recall appointment, several factors must be evaluated (Fig 8-4). The treating dentist must determine whether the patient's OSA is being adequately controlled. When interviewing patients, be aware of the level of alertness they exhibit and their ability to follow the conversation and answer questions appropriately. Based on an assessment of the patient, the treating dentist should develop a plan for further treatment or evaluation.

Vital signs, intake, and subjective symptoms*:
1. Patient age:
2. Blood pressure:
3. Weight:
4. Body mass index:
5. Changes to health history since last appointment:
6. Changes to medications since last appointment:
7. Positive or negative weight change since last appointment: Yes or No
a. Weight gain ________
b. Weight loss _________
8. Time of MAD use in hours:
9. What percentage of the patient's sleep time is MAD used:
10. Patient dreaming: Yes or No
11. Appliance stays in place all night: Yes or No
12. Uses morning repositioner or exerciser every day: Yes or No
13. Patient able to get his/her bite back to normal each day: Yes or No
14. Patient needs a nap during the day: Yes or No
15. Patient frequently falls asleep when watching TV: Yes or No
16. Patient is snoring: Yes or No
17. Appliance hurts patient's teeth: Yes or No
18. Appliance makes patient's jaw hurt: Yes or No
19. Patient takes medication for jaw/tooth pain: Yes or No
a. Medication name ____________
b. Amount of medication ____________
20. Patient takes any sleep aid: Yes or No
a. Medication name ______________
b. Amount of medication ______________
21. Patient is satisfied with oral appliance results: Yes or No
22. Rate the patient's experience with oral appliance therapy: Poor, Acceptable, Good, Fantastic
Objective symptoms:
1. TMD signs or symptoms
a. Maximum opening ___
b. Maximum protrusion_____
c. Left/right excursion _____
d. Muscle tenderness
i. Temporalis: anterior, middle, and posterior
ii. Temporalis tendon
iii. Masseter: origin and insertion
iv. Medial pterygoid
v. Lateral pterygoid
2. Tooth mobility
3. Tooth interproximal contact: anterior and posterior
4. Posterior and anterior occlusion
5. Mandibular protrusion
6. Tooth sensitivity
7. Appliance condition

Fig 8-4 Factors to evaluate at each recall appointment. *Subjective symptoms should be compared with those reported at the original intake visit.

A typical plan may involve the following:

1. Have the patient return to the clinic in 6 months or 1 year for reevaluation.
2. Perform objective testing, such as pulse oximetry, to evaluate for adequate management of the airway.
3. Refer the patient to the sleep physician for further evaluation.
4. Review positional therapy, weight loss, exercise, and sleep hygiene.

American Academy of Sleep Medicine guidelines direct sleep physicians to place patients on a yearly recall schedule to evaluate therapy effectiveness. The treating dentist and referring sleep physician should keep each other informed of any changes that might signal the return of symptoms that could place the patient at risk and require additional treatment.

References

1. Vanderveken OM, Dieltjens M, Wouters K, De Backer WA, Van de Heyning PH, Braem MJ. Objective measurement of compliance during oral appliance therapy for sleep-disordered breathing. Thorax 2013;68:91–96.
2. Uniken Venema JAM, Doff MHJ, Joffe-Sokolova D, et al. Long-term obstructive sleep apnea therapy: A 10-year follow-up of mandibular advancement device and continuous positive airway pressure. J Clin Sleep Med 2020;16:353–359.
3. Hoekema A. Oral-Appliance Therapy Obstructive Sleep Apnea-Hypopnea Syndrome: A Clinical Study on Therapeutic Outcome [thesis]. University of Groningen, 2007.

In our 24/7 society, the idea of getting a full night's sleep can sound quaint. But it is increasingly clear that a full night's sleep is vital to our health, and that of our children.

—*Shari Roan*

9

The New Reality

Dr Lindsey Pankey Sr held that the key to a successful dental practice is to balance four critical areas of focus: know yourself, know your patient, know your work, and apply your knowledge[1] (Fig 9-1). Now over 50 years since it was founded, The Pankey Institute for Advanced Dental Education, founded and named for Dr Pankey by those he mentored, is stronger than ever, testifying to the timelessness of this wisdom.

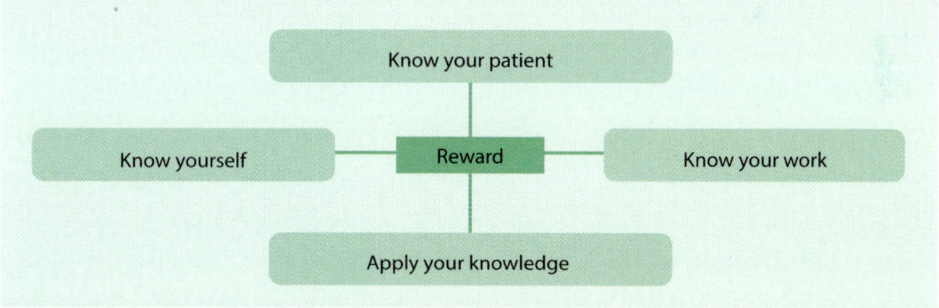

Fig 9-1 Pankey's cross of dentistry.

Knowing Yourself

Adding sleep services to any dental practice, large or small, busy or with capacity to fill, is disruptive and requires much work to assimilate. The dentist-leader must be ready to address the challenges that will arise and marshal the resources necessary to communicate and achieve the vision. Remember, there is no value judgment on any dentist's vision for their practice—no right, no wrong, no best, no unworthy. Once basic ethical and legal thresholds are met, there are as many ways of serving patients as there are professionals with intent to make a difference in their communities.

The process of clarifying what you want to achieve in your career, in the long and short term, is the critical first step to take that will serve as a guide for organizing your work. If you are unsure whether the addition of sleep services is going to fit with your preferred future, it will be difficult to overcome the challenges that will pop up. The authors maintain that every dentist must be able to write down, words on paper, with clarity and detail, what he or she needs from the practice to feel fulfilled. It is insufficient to "think about it" or to "know"—there is power in seeing the words in front of you. If you have not done this key step, why not? If your vision is clear, this will be an easy exercise, although you will probably discover something new as you go. If your vision is not clear, you may put this exercise off in fear that you are not really doing what you want to be doing with your practice. The first step in overcoming fear is to name it.

When opportunities come along, like providing sleep services, this written vision will serve as a guide and filter for the decisions that must be made. From time to time, this document should be revisited to see if what you have since learned has changed what you want to accomplish. Likely, core values will not change much, but opportunities for growth may add possibilities unforeseen at previous stages. There are many paths for fulfilling the "know yourself" portion of Dr Pankey's teaching, from introspective guidance to fully facilitated retreats.

Knowing Your Patient

The more traditional work begins here, where the connection between the doctor and the patient can be transactional or relational. Transactional encounters are simple: Clinical findings are presented, decisions are made, procedures are accomplished, and money changes hands. These transactions are common in a dental practice and serve many needs. But some patients seek more than simple solutions, especially patients who want to know more about the "why" behind their disease and how it affects their future. These patients will want to share more with their health care provider about their current story than can be contained in a transactional encounter. There is history to be shared, desires to be recorded, and a future to be described. Open-ended questions and excellent communication skills, as well as dedicated systems for recording this vital information, are hallmarks of dental practices committed to knowing their patients. Setting aside the time, preparing a trained team member (who should not be the dentist, in the interests of practice efficiency), and creating a private space within the practice for these conversations are all necessary steps.

Time spent on this phase of patient engagement with your practice will distinguish your team from all others and pay dividends because the dental team can offer clinical advice that is well matched to patient wishes. Optimum communication skills are at the heart of knowing your patient, and investing in improvements in this area for every team member is highly recommended. It is sometimes difficult to schedule the right amount of time for the initial visit; team members taking an initial phone call can be trained to recognize different needs of prospective patients. Some will require a longer, and others a shorter, initial visit. These are skills most experienced health care administrative team members quickly acquire; those responsible for scheduling will protect their schedule by allocating the right amount of time, with the right team member, if the office culture allows such flexibility.

Knowing Your Work

Some of the easiest and some of the most challenging aspects of sleep services fall in this category of knowing your work. The dentist's primary strategy is providing custom devices to be worn in the mouth. Fitting, delivery, and management of these devices is the process most comfortable for any dentist; we are trained in dental school to fit acrylic to teeth for several reasons. The fact that there is a mandibular-protrusion feature to these devices is only a modification. Naturally, the details of each chosen mandibular advancement device (MAD) must be mastered.

One suggestion is to have your lead sleep assistant do a study for each of the devices you will regularly use; there should be three to six types on that list. The assistant researches the choices available for each device, such as materials, laboratory support, the means and increment of adjustment, care instructions, and common indications and contraindications. He or she can identify lab choices and fees for each device as well. During a team meeting,

BOX 9-1 Practice tip

Every day you think about treating SRBDs, find a journal article or a chapter in a textbook and learn something new. This discipline will go a long way toward increasing your comfort in embracing the links between medicine and dentistry.

these data are presented so everyone benefits from the research. The sleep assistant can role-play the questions and answers that patients will provide in the safe environment of the dental team.

When it comes to creating office systems to take care of all the business in the dental office, the best people to design and implement those systems are the people who will run them. Providing visionary leadership and making final decisions is the role of the dentist, but it is the team who should research new software or billing systems, different scheduling schemes, and how patients should flow through the office. If your team is given support and encouragement to create systems that support the service values of the office culture and create efficiencies, they will not only come up with more and better ideas than the dentist can alone, but their investment will pay off with enthusiastic implementation.

Sleep-related breathing disorders (SRBDs) have implications beyond the position of the mandible and even the opening of the airway. Many adult patients have accumulated chronic noninfectious diseases related to the disruption in health that accompanies poor breathing at night. While science is still emerging to link with certainty airway problems and the myriad other health concerns, these patients are often seeing multiple medical providers, taking several medications, and living with unstable health. The more dentists can learn about the interrelationships between disruptions to homeostasis that come with airway problems and chronic disease, the more confidence they will have in taking a proper medical history or following their patient as they deal with ongoing medical challenges. Because of the whole-body effects of SRBDs, it is not enough for the dentist to provide only airway support and not collaborate with the other medical providers. The dentist must learn how to communicate with those doctors and how to coordinate care. Combining oral appliance therapy (OAT) with positive airway pressure devices is a common solution, but without knowledge of what this implies, the patient will be underserved. Research into the physiologic effects of SRBDs and the treatments available is ongoing, with hundreds of papers published yearly (Box 9-1). All professionals benefit from increasing their knowledge in related fields, and if you enjoy physiology, there is no more unifying process than respiration. If the dentist falls into the pattern of being concerned only with opening the airway, other symptoms might go unnoticed, and the patient might be underdiagnosed due to lack of a timely referral.

Applying Your Knowledge

Applying your knowledge is the step that brings the entire concept of medical decision-making together. It involves combining the office culture with the patient data collected by the team, the clinical wisdom of the dentist, and the choices endorsed by the patient. Often, it takes some time to gather and review physicians' notes, possibly follow a patient through a trial device, apply interim testing, and wait for patient decisions to be able to come to the best treatment plan. There is no hurry in this process—it is far better to arrive at a treatment strategy fully endorsed by the patient than to rush through to some preordained conclusion. Management of chronic disease benefits from an unhurried, while not unnecessarily delayed, process. Following the patient as he or she accommodates to MAD therapy and benefits from improved respiration is part of applying the clinical wisdom so necessary in health care.

Systems must be in place to stay connected with the patient and ask the right questions about symptoms, impacts on health, and side effects of whichever treatment is current for the patient. Dental offices with well-established recall systems are already set up to help manage chronic disease. Because patients with medical conditions have different needs and nondental data that must be recorded, it is best to keep evaluation and management of the medical diagnosis separate from ongoing dental periodic examinations. The same patient might have three appointments in one continuing care visit: one with the dental hygienist, one with the dentist for a periodic examination, and one with the sleep champion plus the dentist for SRBD management. The dental visit might be paid for by a dental benefit plan, while the checkup related to the medical diagnosis is covered by medical insurance. You cannot charge both coverages for the same services, but if you are documenting dental health in one chart and medical evaluation and management in another and the data is not duplicated, you can properly code and bill for both services.

Dr Pankey's four-part construct is still being taught and used every day by uncountable numbers of dentists. It is applied to patient-doctor-team encounters around the globe and provides dedicated professionals the means to engage in relationship-based treatment for individual people seeking better health. By employing this structure, the dental team can create a culture that cares more about what works for individual patients and every member of the patient's provider team.

Conclusion

There are many good reasons to introduce sleep services to your practice, and each dentist must know why treating patients with sleep-disordered breathing is important. If you do not know why you are doing this, the "hassle factor" will overcome your motivation. A dental sleep medicine (DSM) practice is difficult to launch, and you need a clear reason for doing so. Both authors have met dentists with physical limitations who were unwilling to give up patient care. Other dentists are approaching retirement age but are not ready financially. It takes a determined team to navigate the DSM maze. Those dentists who are successful know why they are making the effort.

Once you know why you are doing this, setting goals for your practice to accomplish is the next step. There are many philosophies around goal setting. Should they be easy to ensure early success to gain momentum? Should they be challenging, requiring a "stretch" of new and existing skills to provide a true sense of accomplishment? The leader chooses the right mix for themself and their team. Goals should include educational benchmarks as well as marketing and clinical goals. Ken Berley started with education, screening patients, finding continous positive airway pressure (CPAP) failures, and crafting letters to sleep physicians. Steve Carstensen began with a patient's need ("Can you fix my sleep appliance?") and encouragement from a mentor, which led to one successful treatment and a need to satisfy a new curiosity of "What is this all about?"

Once your goals are set, make sure you can measure your success. Keep track of the screened patients whom you have referred to a sleep physician. Follow their treatment successes and failures. When you first start referring, it is not unusual for most of your patients to end up on CPAP. Monitor their treatment and be ready to provide OAT if CPAP fails. Additionally, find the CPAP failures in your practice. When you treat these patients, make sure that you communicate with the local physicians and keep them informed. Count the number of physicians that your office has contacted and their responses. Try to talk to physicians personally and establish working relationships with these practitioners. It is quite productive to assign one person to track every aspect of sleep services in a database and provide frequent reports to the team. If your current clinical or administrative team members don't have capacity for extra tasks, investing in a part-time employee for this function will pay off in smoother operations, clearer opportunities for improvement, and more reliable relationships with other health care providers.

Each step of this process modifies your "why." You may wish to contact primary care physicians (PCPs) because they do not know what to do when patients refuse to wear CPAP. You can help those PCPs by providing a valuable service for their patients. That becomes your why. The goal then is to personally speak with at least one PCP per week, who then decides to refer their CPAP failures. The process is continuous.

Look for your "why," set your goals, and measure the results. And you will be successful.

Reference

1. Pankey LD, Davis WJ. A Philosophy of the Practice of Dentistry. Medical College Press, 1985.

No organic law can ever be framed with a provision specifically applicable to every question which may occur in practical administration. No foresight can anticipate, nor any document of reasonable length contain, express provisions for all possible questions.

—Abraham Lincoln, *First Inaugural Address (March 4, 1861)*

10

Legal Issues Related to the Practice of Dental Sleep Medicine

Ken Berley

Much has changed since the first edition of this book was published. The practice of dental sleep medicine (DSM) has gained a measure of acceptance with many physicians, and patients are much more aware that there is a viable alternative to continuous positive airway pressure (CPAP). With new leadership in the American Academy of Dental Sleep Medicine (AADSM), the use of home sleep apnea testing (HSAT) by dental professionals has been expanded greatly, resulting in an explosion in the numbers of patients being treated. As a profession, DSM is moving rapidly, with the law lagging far behind. As a defense attorney, I am preprogrammed to be cautious. It is much easier to prevent a legal problem than to try to get out of trouble. This chapter is included so you can be aware of the controversies that currently exist in DSM and the most ethical practice techniques.

The AADSM and American Dental Association (ADA) are currently in a tug-of-war with sleep physicians (American Academy of Sleep Medicine [AASM] and American Medical Association [AMA]) over the appropriate scope of practice for dentists. Both the ADA and AMA have published policy statements on sleep-related breathing disorders (SRBDs). Unfortunately, these policy statements are in direct conflict with one another. While the struggle is ongoing, state dental boards have continued to embrace the expanding role of dentists in the screening, diagnosis, and treatment of SRBDs. Dental board complaints based on the use of HSATs by dentists are uncommon as of this writing. This does not mean that the fight is over, but the good news is that most referring physicians just want their patients to be successfully treated and do not care about the politics.

As the turf war continues, I am asked almost daily by a dental client why a dentist cannot diagnose obstructive sleep apnea (OSA) and snoring. Many of my legal clients want to be able to treat patients who complain of chronic snoring without referring them to a sleep physician. Many dentists believe that an in-lab sleep study is unnecessarily costly and generally results in the patient being placed on CPAP and not given the option of oral appliance therapy (OAT). In response to this growing demand for simpler testing, a cottage industry has emerged. HSAT companies are now selling testing equipment and encouraging dentists to test their screened patients for SRBDs.

In this scenario, the screening dentist evaluates the need for a sleep test, then orders an HSAT to determine the existence and severity of the patient's SRBD. Even though it is recommended that a sleep physician always evaluate a sleep test, there seems to be a growing propensity for dentists to provide treatment without any physician oversight. However, providing treatment without physician participation and oversight opens up the treating dentist to significant legal exposure. Therefore, I would caution all DSM practitioners on the in-office use of HSAT for the diagnosis of OSA. Many dentists screen and administer a sleep test to their patients to achieve an OSA diagnosis, with the test then scored and diagnosed by a sleep physician who has not personally examined the patient, even though protocol still requires a face-to-face examination by a physician. This treating physician is then available to assess the general health of each patient and provide care for the numerous comorbid conditions that can accompany OSA.

All protocols currently place the treatment of sleep-disordered breathing under the control of physicians, even though oral tissues are responsible for the nocturnal airway resistance. This is difficult for some dentists to understand because we provide treatment for the conditions of the oral cavity. I am asked frequently, "Why do I need a physician to help me provide dental treatment?" The truthful answer is because doing so minimizes your legal risk. With a sleep physician overseeing the treatment of each patient, your liability is minimal, even if your patient were to have a bad outcome.

Policy Statements

In direct response to the actions of some dentists who are circumventing sleep physician examinations and supervision, the AASM has elicited the assistance of the AMA in defining what actions constitute the practice of medicine. AMA resolution H-35.963 states the following:

"It is the policy of our AMA that:

1. Ordering and interpreting objective tests aiming to establish the diagnosis of obstructive sleep apnea (OSA) or primary snoring constitutes the practice of medicine;
2. The need for, and appropriateness of, objective tests for purposes of diagnosing OSA or primary snoring or evaluating treatment efficacy must be based on the patient's medical history and examination by a licensed physician; and
3. Objective tests for diagnosing OSA and primary snoring are medical assessments that must be ordered and interpreted by a licensed physician."

The ADA policy statement specifically states that dentists are to screen all patients for OSA and then refer those patients likely to have an airway issue to a physician for evaluation and diagnosis. The patient is then expected to have a face-to-face examination where the sleep physician determines the medical necessity for a sleep test. If this protocol is ignored, the ADA policy statement could be introduced in a court of law or state board hearing as your standard of care (SOC).

WARNING: If you are screening your patients and ordering HSAT to diagnose whether your patient has an SRBD, you are at risk of being charged with practicing outside your scope of practice and practicing medicine without a license.

Can a dentist use HSAT or pulse oximetry to titrate mandibular advancement devices (MADs)? This question is easier to answer. Both the ADA and AADSM policy statements specifically authorize the use of Type 3 and Type 4 testing for MAD titration purposes. According to section 7 of the ADA policy statement, "Dentists who provide OAT to patients should monitor and adjust the oral appliance (OA) for treatment efficacy as needed, or at least annually. As titration of OAs has been shown to affect the final treatment outcome and overall success, the use of unattended cardiorespiratory (Type 3) or (Type 4) portable monitors may be used by the dentist to help define the optimal target position of the mandible. A dentist trained in the use of these portable monitoring devices may assess the objective interim results for the purposes of

OA titration." Recently, the AADSM published the "DSM Standards for Screening, Treating, and Managing Adults with Sleep-Related Breathing Disorders,"[1] which, for the first time, endorses the use of HSAT for the titration of MADs: "The use of objective data by the qualified dentist to verify the therapeutic position of the OA may be appropriate and used within the scope of practice as defined by the dentist's state dental practice act."

Unfortunately, the ADA and AADSM policy statements appear to be in direct conflict with the AMA and AASM statements. Obviously, restricting the ability of dentists to use testing (oximetry) to titrate appliances greatly limits the success of MAD therapy. Fortunately, the ADA has recognized the need to effectively titrate MADs. The authors proactively discuss HSAT/pulse oximetry use and titration with their referring sleep physicians. Universally, they have all agreed that they want us to effectively titrate our patients and use oximetry when we feel it is necessary. However, you should be aware of this controversy and have a discussion with your referring physicians to determine the protocol they wish you to follow.

Face-to-Face Physician Examination

Patients must have a face-to-face evaluation with a physician prior to undergoing any sleep study, and a physician must write an order for the oral appliance. This regulation is problematic if a dentist is ordering HSAT and a remote sleep physician is diagnosing the patient. Every protocol mandates that a physician must order sleep tests. In the Medicare local coverage determination (LCD), included in the coverage criteria, it is stated: "The beneficiary has a face-to-face clinical evaluation by the treating physician prior to the sleep test to assess the beneficiary for obstructive sleep apnea testing." Additionally, durable medical equipment (DME) suppliers (treating dentists) are responsible for collecting documentation of this evaluation. The LCD further states that "upon request by a contractor, all DMEPOS suppliers must provide documentation of the face-to-face examination." Fortunately, the physician who performed the evaluation prior to the sleep test does not necessarily have to be the same physician who writes the order (or prescription) for the MAD. The LCD states that "the device is ordered by the treating physician following a review of the report of the sleep test. (The physician who provides the order for the oral appliance could be different from the one who performed the clinical evaluation in criterion A.)"

Some dentists fulfill the face-to-face requirements by providing telemedicine examinations. In this situation, a sleep physician sees your patient on a video screen and performs a limited examination to order the HSAT. One silver lining from the pandemic is the relaxation of telemedicine restrictions. With increases in patient convenience, reduction in barriers to care, and parity of payment with in-office encounters, this modality is viable for every dentist.

Can a Dentist Use HSAT or Pulse Oximetry to Screen Dental Patients for SRBDs?

This is a much harder question to answer. This issue has not been adjudicated. Some states have placed dentists on notice that this act may exceed the scope of practice for a dentist in those states. The AMA position paper states that this act involves the practice of medicine. Both the AASM and AADSM policy statements direct a dentist to refer screened patients to a sleep physician.

In response to the position of the AASM, screening products have been developed, such as high-resolution pulse oximetry (HRPO), that are specifically designed to use bruxism and the patient's oxygen desaturation index to screen patients for SRBDs. Here, the argument is that oximetry is not diagnostic of OSA, and therefore these screening tests do not rise to the level of a "sleep test" for the purpose of diagnosing OSA. The legality of these screening devices has NOT been tested in a court of law. Check your state board rulings before using HRPO, HSAT, or similar devices for screening patients for SRBDs or MAD titration. The AADSM website attempts to keep current information posted on individual state's rules on this matter.

In my practice, I have found HRPO to be a very valuable screening and titration tool. This is particularly true for patients with temporomandibular disorders (TMDs) who present with TMD-related discomfort and whom I want to screen for any sleep component. However, make sure your sleep physicians are on board with this protocol.

Must All Dentists Screen for SRBDs?

The ADA policy statement on SRBDs includes the following: "Section 1: Dentists are encouraged to screen patients for SRBD as part of a comprehensive medical and dental history to recognize symptoms such as sleepiness, choking, snoring, or witnessed apneas as an evaluation for risk factors such as obesity, retrognathia, or hypertension. These patients should be referred as needed to the appropriate physicians for proper diagnosis." This policy statement says that all dentists are "encouraged" to screen for SRBDs. Although "encouraged" is not the same thing as "must," a jury could determine that a reasonable and prudent practitioner would screen for SRBDs. Therefore, all risk-averse practitioners should incorporate SRBD screening into their practice. It is not necessary that they treat airway disorders, but it is prudent to screen patients and provide appropriate referrals to a sleep physician.

Informed Consent

To legally provide any service or medical procedure for a patient, the patient must give permission for the treatment. The permission is valid only if it is given with full knowledge of the possible risks and benefits of the treatment. Therefore, appropriate informed consent is mandatory for OAT. Although significant complications are rare, tooth and jaw movement secondary to MAD use is a common long-term result. To minimize risks, patients must be adequately informed before treatment is initiated.

Elements of informed consent

Appropriate informed consent is composed of three elements:

1. Disclosure of information: The patient must be presented with adequate information to decide whether to accept or decline treatment. The information must be presented in a way that the patient can understand, ideally in the native language of the patient.
2. Capacity to consent: The patient must have the mental capacity and be of legal age to consent. Mental capacity is a real concern for DSM practitioners because OSA is closely linked to dementia. Frequently, patients present with obvious neurologic deficits. It is certainly advisable to have a family member present during the consent process. Having the family member cosign the consent document minimizes the risk associated with providing treatment to a patient who presents with obvious neurocognitive deficits.
3. Voluntary consent: The patient must be free to consent voluntarily. This may not seem to be a problem, but male patients are frequently under pressure from their wives or domestic partners to receive treatment for snoring. If in doubt, ask the wife or domestic partner to leave the room and have a frank conversation with the patient in private.

Each of these elements must be satisfied to achieve adequate permission to perform any medical procedure. Generally, if practitioners have a verbal PARQ (procedure, alternatives, risks, and questions) discussion with OAT patients and have each patient sign a well-drafted informed consent document, nothing more is required.

P (PROCEDURE)

The clinician must provide a reasonable description of the procedure that will be performed and how the treatment works (eg, "MAD therapy advances the lower jaw and moves the tongue off the back of the throat to open the airway"). Patients should be shown a model of the appliance that you intend to fabricate so they will know the size and type of appliance they will be wearing. The likelihood of treatment success should be discussed, and the patient must understand that no guarantees can be made.

A (ALTERNATIVES)

Patients should be informed of reasonable alternatives to OAT, including CPAP, surgery, weight loss, airway-directed orthodontic treatment, and positional therapy.

R (RISKS)

The common risks and complications associated with OAT should be discussed with the patient. The complications that could occur over a lifetime of MAD wear are numerous. It would be difficult to include a complete list of all possible issues that could arise. However, some of the possible issues include tooth movement, jaw movement, TMD, injury secondary to appliance breakage, dry mouth, excessive saliva, sore teeth, dental decay, periodontal disease, mobile teeth, fractured teeth and dental restorations, popping and noise in the jaw, acrylic or other (material) allergies, posterior open bite, difficulty chewing, residual sleepiness and symptoms after treatment, and an increased Apnea-Hypopnea Index (AHI) or respiratory disturbance index during follow-up sleep studies.

Q (QUESTIONS)

Patients should be given the opportunity to ask questions regarding any of the above discussions. Do not proceed with OAT until all the patient's questions have been answered.

Once the PARQ discussion is complete, the patient should be presented with a written informed consent for signature. The contents should be explained as needed. After the patient has signed the written consent, the staff member assisting the patient should sign the paper as the witness. The document is dated, and the staff member then enters a note into the record that Doctor X performed a PARQ discussion and the patient executed the written informed consent after all questions were answered. The signed paper can then be scanned into the electronic record, and you can give your patient the original. If you are keeping paper charts, give a copy of the informed consent to your patient and retain the original.

Written consent

Most practitioners believe that a written signed consent form is legally required. This is not the case. Getting a written consent form is only for documentation purposes. Oral consent is legally binding, but proving what information was presented to obtain consent is difficult. Typically, it is wise to have a discussion with the patient outlining the common complications inherent in OAT. Included in the discussion is a time for questions to be answered. Once the discussion is completed, the written consent is presented for signature. Remember, a well-written and executed informed consent document is your most valuable defense tool if your records are ever reviewed by a plaintiff's attorney. A well-written, signed informed consent document will prevent most lawsuits from ever happening.

Product liability

Product liability is the area of law in which manufacturers, distributors, suppliers, retailers, and others who make products available to the public are held responsible for the injuries those products cause. Oral appliances can break. Dorsal fin appliances can fracture, potentially resulting in the aspiration of the posterior fin. Therefore, all patients should be closely examined for signs of lateral bruxism. If the patient presents with excessive wear on the canines, an appliance should be selected that will not significantly restrict lateral movement.

The screws that hold Herbst bars in place can loosen with use and unscrew during sleep. One option to resolve this issue is to place Ceka Bond (Preat) on the screw threads. However, if you need to change the Herbst bars at any point, removing the screws becomes significantly more difficult.

Rubber bands can break during the night and be swallowed or aspirated. Non-latex rubber bands are much more prone to breakage than latex bands. Patients should be warned to change rubber bands regularly to prevent breakage during the night.

Oral appliances are fabricated with materials that can result in allergies. Acrylic, latex, and metal allergies are the most common culprits. Patients should be questioned about known allergies, and appropriate appliances should be selected to avoid exposure to these materials.

Product liability law could make the dentist responsible for any injury to the patient that might occur because of appliance design or breakage. The possible liability would be shared with the laboratory that designed or fabricated the MAD. A good consent form will mention the risk of appliance breakage; however, this might not be adequate to prevent litigation if the appliance design is determined to be flawed or unusually dangerous.

Third-party liability

OSA patients can be dangerously sleepy. Sleepy patients can be a danger to themselves and other innocent individuals. The SOC requires that a practitioner warn all patients about drowsy driving. The bigger legal question is whether a practitioner could be held responsible if a sleepy patient injured himself or another because of the negligence of the treating dentist. In other words, if a sleepy patient caused the injury of an innocent motorist, could a dentist be sued by the innocent motorist if the dentist were negligent in treatment? The good news is that this type of lawsuit has never happened. However, with the growing number of accidents that have been attributed to undiagnosed or uncontrolled OSA, it may be just a matter of time.

All patients should be warned against driving while sleepy. At each appointment, patients should complete an Epworth Sleepiness Scale, and if a patient is showing signs of excessive daytime sleepiness (EDS), refer that patient back to his or her sleep physician for an evaluation and treatment of the EDS. These actions should be well documented.

Stark Law and the federal Anti-Kickback Statute

Over the past few years, some dentists and commercial entities have tried to establish certain financial agreements with referring physicians, where the dentist provides employees to the physician to screen patients and administer HSAT for the physician in return for referrals. The physician is paid for the sleep studies and the dentist receives referrals. This type of arrangement is likely a Stark Law violation.

The Stark Law prohibits physician (dentist) self-referral, specifically a referral by a physician of a Medicare or Medicaid patient to an entity providing designated health services (which include DME) if the physician has a financial relationship with that entity. A financial relationship includes ownership, investment interest, and compensation arrangements.

The federal Anti-Kickback Statute is a criminal statute that prohibits the exchange (or offer to exchange) of anything of value to induce (or reward) the referral of federal health care program business. The Anti-Kickback Statute is the criminal statute designed to prohibit paying for referrals. Conviction for a single violation under the Anti-Kickback Statute may result in a fine of up to $25,000 and imprisonment of up to 5 years. When a private individual has knowledge of a violation of the Anti-Kickback Statute, the citizen can sue on behalf of the federal government. The private citizen sues under the False Claims Act and receives a percentage of any recovery for their "whistleblower" efforts.

Given the severity of these statutes, it is fair to say that a dentist should never offer anything of significant material value to a potential referral source. It should be noted that the Stark Law and Anti-Kickback Statute are applicable to federally funded health insurance (Medicare, Medicaid, Tricare, and Affordable Care Act). However, there are state laws that apply to private commercial medical insurance. The potential liability associated with gifts to physicians far outweighs any referrals that may result. Common in dentistry are holiday gifts from specialists to referring sources. A DSM dentist will find that gift baskets sent to sleep physicians only create uncomfortable situations. The best thank-yous a dentist can send are a heartfelt note about the value of collaboration, excellent care of patients in common, and reciprocal referrals of untested patients.

Litigation in DSM

As of this writing, there have been only a handful of lawsuits in DSM. All of these have been based on TMDs and tooth/jaw movement. The TMD cases currently outnumber those based on tooth movement. However, in the author's opinion, TMD malpractice claims should be the easiest to prevent.

From a risk-management perspective, it is mandatory for all new patients to undergo a complete TMD history and examination prior to treatment. It is imperative to document any signs or symptoms of temporomandibular joint (TMJ) dysfunction prior to seating any MAD. The TMD examination should include range-of-motion measurements, masticatory muscle palpation, and joint auscultation and palpation. The TMD history and examination results should be thoroughly documented as evidence that the patient had existing TMJ damage or dysfunction prior to therapy. The patient should then be informed of the risk of wearing a MAD with a history and examination that are positive for TMD. The patient should be informed that the likelihood of having sore joints, muscle pain, and headaches during MAD therapy is increased due to their existing TMD symptoms. After the discussion, it should be noted in the record that the patient was informed and elected to proceed with therapy and assumed the risk of this complication. It is ideal if the patient signs a TMD release of liability form.

Tooth movement is almost inevitable if the patient wears the appliance long enough. Risks can be minimized with a good consent form and by the fabrication of a morning repositioner. The morning repositioner is an exercise device that can be used to assist the patient in recapturing their centric bite each day. While there is no research at this time that proves that the use of a morning repositioner will prevent tooth movement/mandibular repositioning, the fabrication of this second device should show that the treating dentist took reasonable efforts to prevent unwanted changes. The argument can then be made that the patient did not use the repositioner as directed.

Most malpractice actions that have been filed to date did not have a signed informed consent in the patient's record. It is my professional opinion that the risk of any malpractice case being filed is greatly reduced if the patient executes a well-written informed consent document.

Standard of Care in DSM

SOC is the care that a reasonable and prudent practitioner would provide in the same or similar circumstances. Therefore, a breach of the SOC would be when a practitioner fails to provide reasonable care in any situation. With the AADSM publishing a paper entitled "DSM Standards for Screening, Treating, and Managing Adults with SRBD," it could be argued that this document should be viewed as the current SOC. However, breaches of the SOC for any state must be determined by a jury after expert witnesses testify regarding the care that should have been provided. Additionally, the expert witness will testify how the dentist's breach of the SOC directly caused injury to the patient.

Expert witnesses may use different techniques to establish the SOC of the plaintiff's dentist. First, the expert will deliver his or her professional opinion that the actions of the dentist breached the SOC. However, the most effective technique is to use "learned treatises" in the form of textbooks, articles, and protocols. Once a document is introduced into evidence, juries tend to rely heavily on these documents to determine SOC.

Chapter 3 details the AADSM practice parameters and standards for the treatment of OSA and snoring with OAT (see Box 3-1), and these could be considered the SOC for treating SRBDs. Likewise, we now have the AADSM Policy Statement on Standards for the Practice of DSM. These guidelines are expected to have a positive impact on professional behavior and patient outcomes (and possibly on health care costs), so become familiar with their contents and apply the standards to your practice. Ultimately, each state will determine their SOC for DSM. However, as of this writing, no legal precedence or standards have been established. Nonetheless, if DSM practitioners follow the AADSM parameters and standards, they have a good argument that they followed the SOC.

Reference

1. Levine M, Bennett K, Cantwell MK, Postol K, Schwartz DB. Dental sleep medicine standards for screening, treating, and managing adults with sleep-related breathing disorders. J Dent Sleep Med 2018;5:61–68.

A good laugh and a long sleep are the best cures in the doctor's book.

—Irish Proverb

11

Medical Insurance and Medicare

Ken Berley | Patty Berley

The Times Are Changing

In 1964, Bob Dylan released "The Times They Are A-Changin,'" a song with words that may be eternally true:

> Come gather 'round people, wherever you roam
> And admit that the waters around you have grown
> And accept it that soon you'll be drenched to the bone
> If your time to you is worth saving
> Then you better start swimmin' or you'll sink like a stone
> For the times, they are a-changin'

Sadly, this song accurately describes the current state of affairs as it pertains to medical billing. Dental sleep medicine (DSM) practitioners *are* "drenched to the bone," and we seem to be "swimmin'" like crazy to keep from "sinking like a stone."

The times may be changing, but insurance companies have not. Medical insurance companies follow American Academy of Sleep Medicine (AASM) protocols and Medicare LCD (local coverage determination) parameters when reviewing claims and administrating benefits. They consider sleep medicine to be a medical field controlled by sleep physicians, and as discussed in previous chapters, it is unwise for any dentist to file medical insurance or Medicare for sleep testing. Insurance companies don't follow the protocols of the American Dental Association (ADA) or the American Academy of Dental Sleep Medicine (AADSM). Since the introduction of DSM up until the last 2 years, consistent progress was being made in medical billing, and medical billing of oral appliance therapy (OAT) was becoming easier and more accepted by insurance carriers. That is not the case now. With the introduction of the AADSM position paper on dentists ordering HSATs and the ADA issuing CDT (current dental terminology) codes for OAT, the medical insurance landscape has changed. DSM is under medical review, and we have taken two steps back when it comes to medical billing. Let me explain.

Back in the stone ages (15+ years ago) when I (Patty Berley) first started billing medical insurance for my husband's DSM practice, it was virtually impossible to receive timely payment on any claim. The medical insurance companies were very adept at placing hurdles in our path. There were several reasons for that. First and foremost, medical insurance companies were unfamiliar with the practice of DSM and how effective OAT is for most patients. Our office was the first in the state of Arkansas to file medical insurance for OAT, and it took 9 months of dealing with documentation demands and constant communication with Arkansas Blue Cross and Blue Shield to receive a $468.00 check. It took another 18 months of struggle to get the reimbursement up to $880.00. Every claim resulted in repeated requests for documentation: sleep physician exam notes, diagnostic polysomnography (PSG)/home sleep apnea test (HSAT) results, continuous positive airway pressure (CPAP) trial and failure notes, prescription, dental intake exam, proof of delivery, and the appliance invoice. We spent hours fighting with the insurance companies for every payment. But slowly, with great documentation, billing for OAT became routine.

Now the tables have turned once more. The ADA and AADSM have changed the landscape. The ADA has announced that "as of January 1, 2024, there will be CDT codes for sleep apnea procedures such as screening and home sleep apnea tests, as well as fabrication, delivery and titration of oral appliance therapy devices." According to the Chairman of the ADA Code Maintenance Committee, "These new codes will expand upon the current CDT codes for custom sleep apnea appliance delivery, adjustment, and repair procedures." Additionally, the AADSM recently published a protocol stating that a "qualified dentist" can evaluate a patient for sleep-related breathing disorders (SRBDs) and order HSAT testing. These protocols and coding decisions by the ADA and AADSM have been viewed by some as an attack on the field of sleep medicine and sleep physicians. Remember, physicians and medical insurance companies view sleep-disordered breathing (SDB) as a *medical* condition that should be treated and controlled by a physician. The decision by the AADSM and ADA to encourage dentists to test their patients for SDB will adversely affect sleep physicians and sleep labs because they make their money testing for OSA. Because there are less than 5,000 sleep physicians in this country and over 200,000 dentists, some sleep physicians may worry that dentists will take over the treatment of OSA. They are using their influence with medical insurance companies to demand that dentists follow AASM/Medicare protocols to receive insurance benefits.

Dental Insurance Benefits for OAT

Patients accept treatment more frequently when there is a high probability of securing payment from their insurance providers. Although the ADA is adding CDT codes for OAT and sleep tests, this author is currently unaware of any dental carrier that pays a benefit for OAT and HSAT. Unless and until the CDT codes are benefited, they do not provide any expectation of payment. At this point, the CDT codes exist to allow the dentist to accurately document procedures. Because dental insurance companies do not provide benefits for OAT, medical insurance remains the only reasonable source of benefits for patients.

Medical Insurance Review

Most medical insurance companies review every DSM claim to make sure that the office/dentist filing the claim is following AASM/Medicare protocols. The authors have had significant challenges with UnitedHealthcare and Blue Cross Blue Shield. The good news is that if you follow AASM/Medicare protocols and have all the required documentation, eventually a payment should be received. However, at the time of this writing, you should be prepared for a review (audit) of every claim you file. They *will* ask for your documentation. Make sure you have everything on file, and be ready to provide documentation upon request.

To resolve medical insurance billing problems, one of the authors reached out to some insurance companies for an explanation and was informed that claims for E0486 were being reviewed due to the high percentage of inappropriate claims that were being filed by dentists. The medical review status was a direct result of the fact that many new dentists were filing for OAT without proper documentation and sleep physician supervision. According to Blue Cross Blue Shield, many dentists are dispensing HSATs to their patients without any physician involvement. Blue Cross Blue Shield claims that OAT is being billed without a valid detailed written order (DWO) or prescription and without a face-to-face examination by the patient's physician of record. Therefore, all DSM claims are reviewed, which is a major drain on our time and resources.

Preauthorization

Frequently, insurance companies require a preauthorization/predetermination before you can treat any OSA patient. To receive the preauthorization, you must provide the requested documentation and wait on approval to treat the patient. After the sleep appliance is delivered to the patient and the claim is filed, the insurance company may ask for documentation again. This may come as a complete surprise for many practitioners, but even after receiving a preauthorization prior to treatment, you are not guaranteed payment upon completion. This obstructionist approach is new and is creating ongoing problems. It is time-consuming to obtain preauthorization, and then you may still need to provide additional documentation upon completion of the case. Failure to obtain preauthorization before rendering treatment can result in denial of the claim.

In-network issues

Patients are more likely to accept treatment if you are in-network and have negotiated a payment amount with their insurance carriers. As an in-network provider, you agree to accept the negotiated payment and the patient's out-of-pocket payment is reduced. But because most insurance companies restrict access to in-network health care providers and dentists may struggle to achieve in-network status, OAT is made more expensive for patients.

Documentation requests

The documentation most requested by UnitedHealthcare is for the initial visit/face-to-face physician notes. Blue Cross Blue Shield seems to want all the required documentation, which entails sending 50 to 60 pages of documents for each claim. If you want the patient's medical insurance company to provide a benefit for an oral appliance, you must have documentation of the following events:

1. Each patient must have a physician of record who has performed a face-to-face examination and concluded that there is a reasonable probability of the patient having OSA based on the documented symptoms, physiology, and comorbid conditions. As a result of this examination, an overnight sleep test is ordered by the patient's physician. If the face-to-face examination was more than 6 months prior to writing the DWO, some

insurance companies will reject the DWO. The most common sequence of treatment documentation is as follows: *(1)* Face-to-face examination: Order for PSG/HSAT; *(2)* Face-to-face examination: DWO for CPAP; *(3)* Face-to-face examination: CPAP failure documented, DWO for OAT within 6 months.

2. HSAT/PSG is performed as a result of an order from the physician of record. For insurance companies to provide a benefit for OAT, the sleep study is ideally performed within the last year.
3. If the PSG/HSAT is more than 1 year old, some insurance companies and Medicare will state that the study is too old. Medicare also requires that the study be scored using AASM Rule 1B (4%). Some commercial plans also use the 4% rule. You can check when calling for insurance benefits or by reviewing the medical policy criteria.
4. You can argue against the 1-year rule if the sleep physician who signed the DWO did not request a new sleep study and was willing to write a DWO based on a sleep study that was more than 1 year old and the patient has had continuation of care.
5. The patient's overnight HSAT/PSG must have been reviewed by a board-certified sleep medicine specialist who diagnosed the patient with OSA (Apnea-Hypopnea Index [AHI] > 5). If the patient has mild apnea, most insurance companies and Medicare require that the physician of record document one of the OSA-related comorbid diseases. One of the comorbid conditions associated with OSA is excessive daytime sleepiness (EDS). To successfully document EDS, an Epworth Sleepiness Scale (ESS) screening must result in a score of 10 or greater. Check the patient's medical policy for the treatment of OSA for details.
6. After the sleep physician provides a diagnosis of OSA, the treatment options are discussed with the patient. Options could include weight loss, OAT, hypoglossal nerve stimulation, surgery, and CPAP. For most physicians, CPAP is the initial treatment of choice.
7. Many insurance companies require a CPAP trial before an oral appliance can be ordered. This is particularly true if the patient has an AHI > 30. If an oral appliance is fabricated before the CPAP trial has failed, your claim may be denied. The CPAP failure should be documented by the physician of record in the treatment notes. Always check the patient's medical policy for the treatment of OSA with oral appliances for details regarding eligibility for coverage.
8. Many insurance companies require a preauthorization (see previous section) before an oral appliance can be fabricated. If the patient's insurance company requires a preauthorization and you have not received it

before delivering the oral appliance, your claim may be denied. Some insurance companies may still provide coverage benefits but reduce the coverage amount because a preauthorization was not obtained before treatment. Again, check the patient's medical policy for the treatment of OSA for details.

9. OAT has been categorized as DME (durable medical equipment), so you must have a qualified DWO, a prescription from the patient's physician of record for a mandibular advancement device (MAD; E0486), and a signed LOMN (letter of medical necessity). The DWO should be documented in the notes of the patient's physician of record.
10. Before filing a claim with a medical insurance company, you must be credentialed with that insurance carrier. This is a process where you send the insurance company a W9 and any other identification/tax information necessary for the insurance company to know who you are. The credentialing process does not mean that you are now in-network with that insurance company. In-network status is a contractual agreement between the provider and the insurance company on behalf of the insured and involves a separate negotiation. The American Dental Association participates in a program called CAQH, which is free to all dentists. By entering your information there, any insurance company can access your name, address, school, license, etc, so you don't have to repeatedly fill out credential forms.
11. Do not file medical insurance for E0486 (custom fabricated oral appliance for the treatment of OSA) until the appliance is delivered to the patient. Once the appliance is delivered and the patient is satisfied, you must have the patient sign a proof of delivery (POD). Recently, UnitedHealthcare has started asking for the signed POD, and they are comparing the date on the POD and the filing date on the claim for the sleep appliance (E0486). If the filing date is prior to the POD date, your claim may be denied.

If you have documentation that the preceding prerequisites were satisfied, payment of the claim is more probable. Should a denial occur, check your claim, billing protocols, and documentation for errors. If none are found, you should start the appeals process. Continued refusal to pay is a reason to contact your state insurance commissioner. Once the medical insurance companies realize that you are playing by the rules, any medical review should be lifted.

Remember, filing medical insurance is *not* hard; it is just different. Most dentists who practice DSM come from a restorative dental practice where there are hundreds of procedure codes to wade through to find the one that best describes the dental procedure that was performed for the patient. In DSM, we have one diagnosis code (G47.33, OSA) and only a handful of procedure codes. The most important of these codes is E0486 (custom fabricated MAD for the treatment of OSA). As you approach the information contained in this chapter, do not get discouraged and do not give up. Once you become familiar with the medical insurance form (CMS 1500; see Fig 11-1) and how to fill it out, you will see that it is not hard but does require attention to detail and making sure the documentation is on hand before filing the claim.

Do We Have to File Medical Insurance?

All dentists practicing DSM should strive for a referral-based practice. When physicians consistently refer patients for OAT, dentists can maintain a long-term practice with little or no external marketing. It is the authors' opinion that the only way to achieve a significant referral practice is to file medical insurance and Medicare claims for your patients. We believe that this is one of the pillars of a successful DSM practice and is not optional.

Billing Services

Why not use a billing service? This is certainly an option. There are many medical insurance billing companies who will bill private medical insurance and Medicare for your office. You should be aware that having a billing service does not relieve the obligation of securing information from your patient and tracking down the documentation necessary for filing medical insurance. Billing services will complete the CMS 1500 form and will get preauthorization when required, but you still do the legwork.

Using a billing service can be helpful for the first few months after starting a DSM practice. However, it is imperative that you find at least two employees to undertake the role of insurance coordinator. These individuals will need to be knowledgeable about the documentation required and make sure that it is on file. Educating them will take time and effort but will provide a valuable in-office service. Find a good mentor or coach who can assist with billing during the learning curve. This will make the transition much easier.

If you choose to use a billing company, be careful if they insist on determining the amount that you bill for each procedure. If the billing practices endorsed by your billing company result in an audit, you are responsible for the actions of your biller, and there will be a legal presumption that the claims filed by your billing agency were filed with your full knowledge. Additionally, in the event of a poor outcome, you may not be able to recover from your billing company without legal action.

Types of Insurance

Commercial insurance companies

The most common type of health insurance is commercial insurance, which is any type of insurance policy that is not offered or funded by the federal government. Commercial insurance companies are for-profit, publicly traded corporations, and their goal is to make money for their investors. Generally, commercial insurance companies offer both group and individual policies, and patients enroll through an employer who may pay a portion of the costs. Practitioners are routinely recruited to be in-network with commercial insurance companies. When you become an in-network provider, you agree to a negotiated, often reduced compensation schedule in hopes of treating a larger number of patients.

Affordable Care Act policies

Policies issued under the Affordable Care Act (ACA) constitute a hybrid plan that may be issued by a private insurer under one of the state exchanges or it may be a Medicaid policy. The difference is that these commercial policies are frequently supplemented by the federal government. Therefore, the federal Anti-Kickback Statute and Stark Law likely apply (see chapter 10), as well as federal mail and wire fraud statutes.

Medicare

Medicare is the federal health insurance program for patients who are 65 years old or older, although some younger patients can also have Medicare if they have certain physical or mental disabilities. Medicare typically covers 80% of allowable fees. The patient is expected to pay their yearly deductible and the 20% that is not covered by Medicare.

MEDICARE SUPPLEMENT INSURANCE

Medicare does not cover all medical expenses, so Medicare supplement policies are designed to cover out-of-pocket expenses such as deductibles and copayments. When a patient has Medicare and a supplement policy, you file Medicare first, and if the supplement insurance information is on the claim, then Medicare will file the supplement policy to pay the deductible and the 20% out-of-pocket that is not covered by Medicare.

MEDICARE REPLACEMENT POLICIES

A Medicare replacement policy is another name for Medicare Part C, or a Medicare Advantage Plan. It replaces Medicare Part A and Part B and provides some additional benefits and features. These vary from plan to plan; however, Advantage Plans typically have fewer physicians who participate and frequently require preauthorization for OAT. Some of the plans do not have out-of-network coverage. You can think of these like you do a commercial insurance policy. Call to check benefits and any coverage limitations, out-of-network coverage, preauthorizations, etc.

Medicaid

Medicaid is a government insurance program for persons of all ages whose income and resources are insufficient to pay for health care. Medicaid is jointly funded by the state and federal governments and managed by the states. While it is possible that Medicaid might have coverage for examinations and radiographs, Medicaid does not typically have coverage for sleep appliances in most states. However, if you submit a claim to Medicaid, they may enroll the provider's office as a provider of services that are covered. It is best to check with your state to determine if Medicaid covers the treatment you are providing and if you want to participate with that program.

National Provider Identifier

For your office to file medical insurance, you must have a national provider identifier (NPI) number. This is the number that insurance companies use to identify your practice. It is likely that you already have an NPI, but to apply, go to https://nppes.cms.hhs.gov, and follow the instructions.

The Centers for Medicare & Medicaid Services

The Centers for Medicare & Medicaid Services (CMS) is a branch of the US Department of Health and Human Services and is responsible for creating the form that we must use to file all medical insurance claims and Medicare (CMS 1500 Claim Form; see Fig 11-1). This form is available at most office supply stores or can be found online by searching for "CMS 1500 form." It is the only form that will be accepted when filing medical insurance or Medicare. It is important to note that the ink used on these forms is unique because it allows Medicare to scan the form and upload the information.

Software for Filing Medical Insurance

The more capable dental management software, such as Eaglesoft (Patterson) and Dentrix (Henry Schein), can print your medical insurance claims on the CMS 1500 forms. When printing claim information onto the CMS form, remember that all your information must be correct and inside the appropriate boxes or the claim will be rejected. Dental software programs will not proof your claims for accuracy, but this is the cheapest way to file medical claims. You should be aware that offices that file paper claims frequently suffer delays in receiving payment. In today's digital age, medical insurance companies consistently process electronic claims faster than paper claims.

As your DSM practice grows, you should consider purchasing billing software. Fortunately, there are some medical billing software programs that are free or relatively inexpensive. Speedy Claims (SpeedySoft USA), for example, is relatively inexpensive and can handle all your claim-filing requirements. When filing your claims electronically, you can contract with a claims clearinghouse to proof your claims for accuracy before they are sent for processing. This process results in fewer rejections.

The biggest problem with most medical billing software is that it is not designed to house your chart notes and handle communication letters. Fortunately, there are some DSM practice-management software options that will file your insurance and facilitate your DSM notes and communications. DS3 (Dental Sleep Solutions) and DentalWriter (Nierman Practice Management) are the most common practice-management softwares used in DSM as of this writing, but others may be developed for this growing market. You will have to weigh the costs and benefits of a software investment, especially if you are only doing a few appliances per month.

It is unlikely that most dentists starting a DSM practice can justify purchasing software until the OSA patient flow is established. Most practices just starting out get help filing insurance, either from a coach or billing company, and they maintain separate charts for their patient notes, sleep studies, correspondence, and prescriptions. Correspondence with your referring physicians can always be printed and faxed or emailed, if their security system allows email. (There are secure, HIPAA-compliant email systems, but they must be used by both sender and receiver.) Remember, communication with referring physicians is mandatory. If your office cannot manually keep up with the necessary communications, it is time to invest in specialized software.

In-Network or Out-Of-Network?

When you begin your DSM practice, you will likely be out-of-network with medical insurance companies. Whether you decide to become an in-network provider can depend on many things. It is not always a good thing to be in-network, as some insurance companies have very low benefits for OAT. However, in most cases, being in-network gives you a significant advantage over dentists who are out-of-network. Many insurance companies penalize patients for going out-of-network by increasing deductibles and reducing coverage benefits. Some policies have no out-of-network benefits. Additionally, if you are not in-network, when you call a patient's insurance company to determine benefits, the insurance company may refuse to give you benefit details. This can make it very difficult to estimate your patient's out-of-pocket expenses, and some patients will refuse treatment if you are unable to determine their insurance benefits. The biggest negative of being in-network is that the amount you can charge is a set allowable amount or a negotiated fee that may be close to the amount allowed by Medicare.

If you are out-of-network, it is possible to be granted a gap exception in some areas of the country and be treated as an in-network provider. A gap exception may be possible in areas where there is not a local in-network provider for OAT. Therefore, there is a gap in coverage available to patients in network. Once a gap exception is approved, you are treated as an in-network provider for that one patient and only for the treatment requested. Several factors play into the decision of whether you want to request a gap exception. The first issue is proving that there are no in-network dentists who provide E0486 devices. Frequently, insurance companies will inform you that they have a dentist in-network who treats OSA. In that case you should always ask who the in-network provider is and contact that office to determine if they provide E0486 devices. You will generally find that the in-network provider is an oral surgeon who does not provide these appliances. Documenting this fact opens the door for a gap exception.

Diagnosis and Procedure Codes

ICD-10

The International Classification of Diseases, 10th version (ICD-10) is a list compiled and maintained by the World Health Organization that contains specific codes for diseases, signs and symptoms, abnormal findings, complaints, social circumstances, and external causes of injury or diseases (see Box 11-2). These

TABLE 11-1 Common CPT codes

Procedure	CPT code
Initial examination	99202 or 99203
Recall examination	99211 or 99212
Panoramic radiograph	70355
Tomogram (unilateral)	76100
Tomogram (bilateral)	76102
Cephalometric radiograph	70350
CT scan	70490
MAD (custom)	E0486
MAD (temporary)	E0485
HSAT	95806
Pulse oximetry	94762

are your diagnosis codes. An ICD-10 diagnosis code must be present on each medical claim to alert the insurance company to the disease or condition being treated. The ICD-10 diagnosis code for OSA is G47.33.

CPT codes

The American Medical Association (AMA) maintains the CPT (current procedural terminology) codes, which describe medical, surgical, and diagnostic services and are designed to communicate uniform information about medical services and procedures among physicians, coders, patients, accreditation organizations, and payers for administrative, financial, and analytical purposes. These codes are used to describe a diagnostic procedure, an examination, or radiographic or management services performed by a health care practitioner (Table 11-1). Stay informed of any changes to CPT codes, as they will affect the claim being processed correctly. CPT coding is like ICD-10 coding, except that it identifies the services rendered rather than the diagnosis on a medical claim.

HCPCS codes

HCPCS (Healthcare Common Procedural Coding System) codes are procedure codes that are used for DME. MADs have been classified as DME and are therefore sold as equipment. When filing medical insurance for the appliance, you will need to use the appropriate HCPCS code. E0486 is the HCPCS code for MADs that is recognized by Medicare and commercial insurance companies. However, the Medicare definition for E0486 is specifically defined as an appliance that has a fixed hinge at the sides, front, or palate and that protrudes the mandible and is adjustable by the patient in increments of 1 millimeter or less and maintains that adjustment during sleep and when removed from the mouth. If the appliance being used does not fit the Medicare description, then HCPCS code K1027 is the most accurate code when filing a claim. Examples of a non-hinged appliance that would fit this description would be the SomnoDent MAS (SomnoMed), ProSomnus EVO Sleep and Snore Device (ProSomnus Sleep Technologies), and the Slow Wave DS8 (Slow Wave). Prior to the development of K1027, when filing Medicare claims, HCPCS code A9270 was routinely used. However, A9270 and K1027 are currently not payable codes under Medicare and some commercial insurance companies.

When treating OSA, there is only one diagnosis code (G47.33), and it is used on every claim that we file. After we inform the insurance company that the diagnosis is G47.33 (OSA), then a HCPCS code is used to let them know the procedure that was performed to treat the patient's OSA. The items that we frequently list on our insurance claims are CPT codes for examinations, radiographs, etc, and the HCPCS code for a MAD (E0486). Any time you try to file for anything other than the items listed here, the chance of an audit increases. While many dentists routinely file for HSAT, pulse oximetry, CBCT scans, pharyngometry, rhinometry, and surgical guides, in Ken Berley's legal opinion, filing medical insurance or Medicare for these items places you at a significant risk for an audit.

Dental codes

The ADA has released CDT codes for OAT, including the following:

- D0396: 3D printing of a 3D dental surface scan to obtain a physical model
- D5999: Unspecified maxillofacial prosthesis, by report
- D9947: Custom sleep apnea appliance fabrication and placement
- D9948: Adjustment of custom sleep apnea appliance
- D9953: Reline of custom sleep apnea appliance (indirect)
- D9954: Fabrication and delivery of OAT morning repositioning device
- D9955: OAT titration visit
- D9956: Administration of HSAT
- D9957: Screening for SRBDs

The detailed descriptors provide information of what is included in some codes:

- D5999: This is the CDT code the ADA recommends using when billing a snoring appliance.
- D9953: Resurface dentition side of appliance with new soft or hard base material as required to restore original form and function.
- D9954: Device for use immediately after removing a MAD to aid in relieving muscle/jaw pain and occlusal changes.
- D9955: Postdelivery visit for titration of a MAD and to subsequently evaluate the patient's response to treatment, integrity of the device, and management of side effects.
- D9956: Sleep apnea test, for patients who are at risk for SRBDs and appropriate candidates, as allowed by applicable laws. Also, to help the dentist in defining the optimal position of the mandible.
- D9957: Screening activities performed alone or in conjunction with another evaluation, to identify signs and symptoms of SRBDs.

We are unaware of any dental plan that provides a benefit for OAT at this time. Although these codes have thus far only complicated matters, we are hopeful that this will not always be the case. Dental benefits for OAT would greatly improve therapy acceptance. Well-trained dentists can then make great strides in improving the lives of many patients. However, it would be ideal if any benefit would be in addition to current yearly dental maximums. As we are all painfully aware, most dental plans have a defined annual benefit of $1,000.00 to $2,500.00. Therefore, if OAT were reimbursed under the current yearly dental maximums, most benefits would be used up when OAT is filed. This would make it difficult for some patients if unexpected dental treatment were needed and may induce some to even put off preventive care.

Medical examination and management codes (E/M codes)

The CPT codes that describe the physician/dentist patient encounter are referred to as evaluation and management (E/M) codes. These codes vary depending on whether the examination is an initial examination on a new patient or an established patient visit. In 2021, significant changes were adopted for outpatient evaluation and management coding, making it possible to use either medical decision making or doctor time to determine the appropriate code for the patient's visit. The revision of the coding rules has simplified billing requirements by allowing offices to bill based on the amount of "doctor time" required for each patient visit. Within each type of visit, there are different levels of care and reimbursement. The fifth digit of the CPT code indicates the level

BOX 11-1 Coding based on doctor time

New patient time thresholds	Established patient time thresholds
99202: 15 Minutes	99212: 10 Minutes
99203: 30 Minutes	99213: 20 Minutes
99204: 45 Minutes	99214: 30 Minutes
99205: 60 Minutes	99215: 40 Minutes

of the visit based on time and/or medical complexity. E/M codes end in a number 2 through 5. The number 2 designates the lowest level of care and/or the shortest appointment. The number 5 represents the highest level of care and/or the longest appointment. For example, a new patient's first office visit necessitating a "level 2" examination has an E/M CPT code of 99202. An established patient with a similar level 2 examination would be coded 99212. In 2024, the timing labels were simplified to reflect a threshold time spent (Box 11-1). In other words, when the visit crosses one time amount, it qualifies for that code until the next amount of time is spent.

While the new coding standards indicate that a practitioner can justify various coding levels based on documented time, the patient's records should reflect in detail how that time was spent. Any time you file an E/M code or a CPT code, the insurance company can ask for your documentation to justify billing that code. All time spent on the day of the patient's appointment, including before the patient arrives, during the appointment, and after the patient leaves the office, can be credited to the appropriate level of billing. The record should reflect all reviews conducted and services performed by the doctor. Services and activities that can be included in the total time computation include the following:

- Preparing to see the patient (eg, review of tests)
- Obtaining and/or reviewing separately obtained history
- Performing a medically appropriate examination and/or evaluation
- Counseling and educating the patient, family, or caregiver
- Ordering medications, tests, or procedures
- Referring and communicating with other health care professionals (when not separately reported)
- Documenting clinical information in the electronic or other health record
- Independently interpreting results (not separately reported) and communicating results to the patient, family, or caregiver
- Care coordination (not separately reported)

You cannot include the staff time in this computation. This is doctor time only. When time is used to justify the E/M code, the total time spent for each appointment must be documented in the patient's record for that visit. Failure to document time spent implies that you are using medical decision-making to justify the E/M code used. In this case, your documentation must reflect the appropriate complexity of the medical decision made. An important note is that the time requirement is stated as the "day of the appointment." Preparing for the patient the previous day or completing notes a day later do not count. Be sure to include the timing of your review and write-up in your encounter notes.

CODE 99211 (BILLING FOR STAFF TIME)

CPT code 99211 is used to bill for an office or other outpatient visit for the evaluation and management of an established patient that may not require the presence of a physician/dentist or other qualified health care professional. This code can be extremely valuable for DSM practitioners, particularly when a patient is unable to adjust their appliance. Here the patient can be seen by a staff member, as long as the "presenting problem(s) are minimal." Physicians and dentists can report code 99211, but the code is intended to report services rendered by ancillary members of the medical team, including registered PSG technologists (RPSGTs) and DSM assistants. Code 99212 is the lowest level code that can be used by a physician or dentist.

E/M code 99211 is not billed based on time alone and does not have key component requirements. Documentation should include sufficient information to support the reason for the encounter and any relevant history, physical assessment, and plan of care. Additionally, the service must be incident-to or the completion of OAT. Therefore, the documentation for 99211services must meet the following three incident-to requirements for benefits to be paid:

- The services are rendered under the direct supervision of the physician (dentist).
- The services are furnished as an integral, although incidental, part of the physician's (dentist's) professional services in the course or diagnosis or treatment of an injury or illness.
- When billing incident to the physician (dentist), the physician must initiate treatment and see the patient at a frequency that reflects their active involvement in the patient's case. This includes both new patients and established patients being seen for new problems. The claims are then billed under the physician's (dentist's) NPI.

The documentation associated with a patient visit reported under 99211 should include the patient's vitals, the procedure performed, and any discussion with the patient or with the treating dentist regarding the patient visit. If a new problem is brought up by the patient, such as joint or tooth soreness, this is no longer a 99211 appointment, and the supervising dentist should address those issues.

Filing Medical Insurance

Once a patient is diagnosed with OSA, medical insurance is your best option for receiving benefits. If you have received a referral from a physician, you still may not receive the documentation necessary to file medical insurance. Documents needed include the following:

- DWO/prescription
- LOMN
- Medical records, physician's face-to-face examination notes from when the sleep study was ordered
- PSG/HSAT sleep study
- Sleep physician's diagnosis or interpretation of the sleep study
- Medical records indicating CPAP trial and failure (if applicable)
- Medical records indicating CPAP intolerance (if applicable)
- Medical records indicating any OSA/SDB-related comorbid conditions:
  - Hypertension (high blood pressure)
  - Ischemic heart disease
  - History of stroke
  - EDS (ESS of 10 or greater)
  - Insomnia
  - Impaired cognition
  - Mood disorder

Once all documentation is obtained, perform the following steps:

1. Secure the patient's insurance information.
2. Make a copy of the front and back of the patient's medical insurance card(s).
3. Review the patient's medical insurance policy online for OAT.
4. Call the patient's insurance company to obtain the following information:
   - Verify that the patient has medical benefits for E0486.
   - Ask if a preauthorization is required for E0486.
   - Check if the insurance company follows Medicare guidelines for OAT.

BOX 11-2 Codes for filing medical insurance

Diagnosis Codes
- G47.33 Obstructive sleep apnea (adult, pediatric)
- R06.83 Snoring (no benefit for snoring)

Evaluation and Management Codes
- 99202 Expanded problem-focused evaluation, new patient (15–29 minute appointment)
- 99203 Detailed evaluation, new patient (30–44 minute appointment)
- 99212 Expanded problem-focused evaluation, established patient (10–19 minute appointment)
- 99213 Detailed evaluation, new patient (20–29 minute appointment)

Imaging Codes
- 70259 Radiologic examination, skull, less than four views
- 70320 Radiologic examination, teeth, complete, full mouth
- 70330 Radiologic examination, temporomandibular joint, open and closed mouth
- 70355 Panoramic radiograph

Oral Appliance Codes (includes adjustment appointments for 90 days)
- E0485 oral device or appliance to reduce upper airway collapsibility, adjustable or nonadjustable, prefabricated, includes fitting and adjustment (temporary appliance code) **Note** If this code is used for a temporary appliance, it could nullify any benefits for the permanent appliance (E0486).
- E0486 oral device or appliance to reduce upper airway collapsibility, adjustable or nonadjustable, custom fabricated, includes fitting and adjustment

Modifiers
- NU new equipment, unused
- KX requirements specified in the applicable Medicare LCD have been met

Follow-up Care
- 99212 expanded problem-focused evaluation, established patient

- Ask if a PDAC (Pricing, Data, Analysis, and Coding)–approved appliance is required (https://www.dmepdac.com). Some insurance companies require a Medicare PDAC-approved appliance.
- Verify that the patient has out-of-network benefits for E0486.
- Check the patient's deductible for DME.
- Ask how much of the deductible the patient has met.
- Ask if a network gap exception is available, and if so, how the gap exception is obtained.

Figure 11-1 is an example of a CMS 1500 form completed with the appropriate information for a medical insurance or Medicare claim. Box 11-2 shows the relevant codes for filing. The CMS 1500 form uses a unique red ink that allows the form to be scanned and read by the insurance company. The claim will not be accepted if the claim form does not have the correct ink. The form is separated into information fields that must be completed correctly.

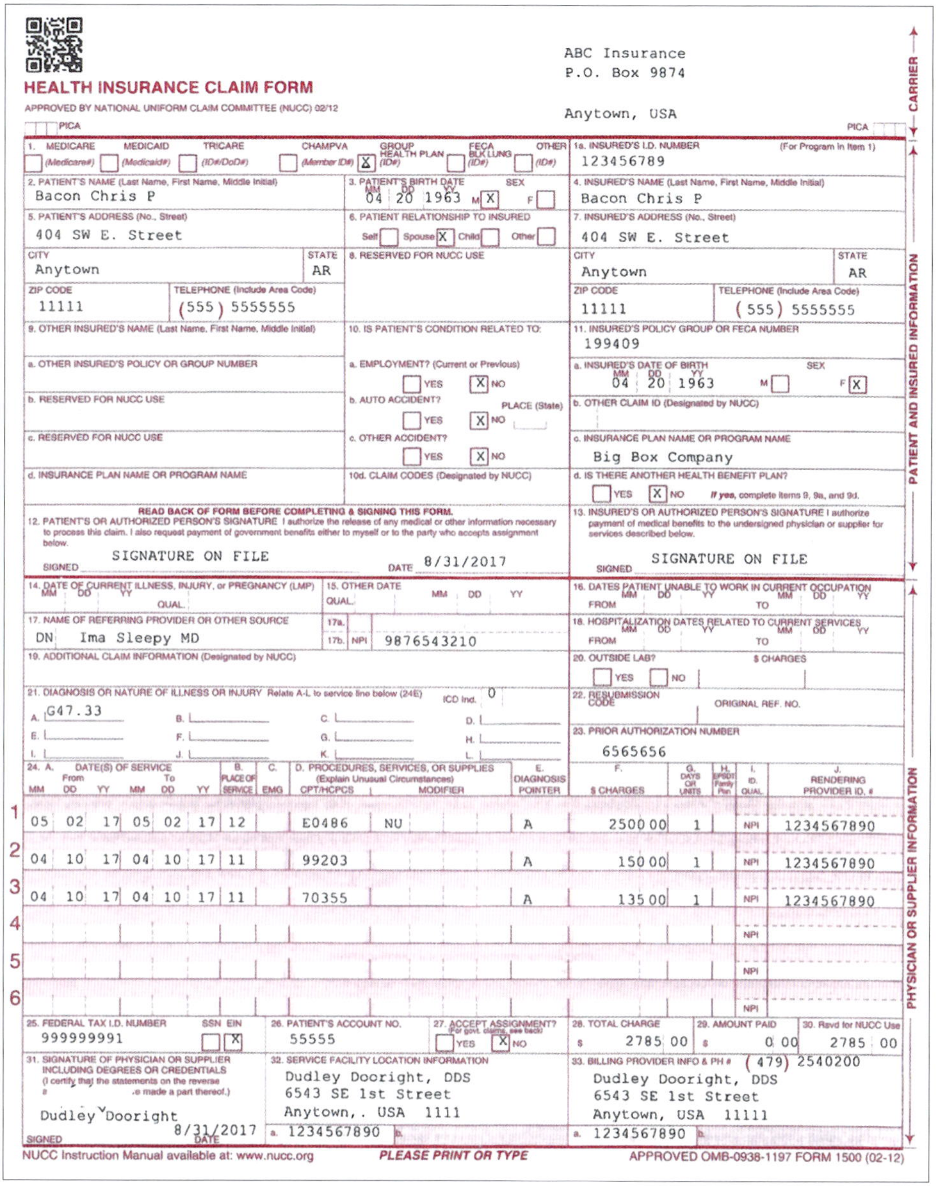
HEALTH INSURANCE CLAIM FORM
APPROVED BY NATIONAL UNIFORM CLAIM COMMITTEE (NUCC) 02/12

ABC Insurance
P.O. Box 9874
Anytown, USA

1. MEDICARE / MEDICAID / TRICARE / CHAMPVA / GROUP HEALTH PLAN [X] / FECA BLK LUNG / OTHER
1a. INSURED'S I.D. NUMBER: 123456789
2. PATIENT'S NAME: Bacon Chris P
3. PATIENT'S BIRTH DATE: 04 20 1963 SEX: M [X]
4. INSURED'S NAME: Bacon Chris P
5. PATIENT'S ADDRESS: 404 SW E. Street
6. PATIENT RELATIONSHIP TO INSURED: Spouse [X]
7. INSURED'S ADDRESS: 404 SW E. Street
CITY: Anytown STATE: AR
ZIP CODE: 11111 TELEPHONE: (555) 5555555
CITY: Anytown STATE: AR
ZIP CODE: 11111 TELEPHONE: (555) 5555555
11. INSURED'S POLICY GROUP OR FECA NUMBER: 199409
10a. EMPLOYMENT? NO [X]
11a. INSURED'S DATE OF BIRTH: 04 20 1963 SEX: F [X]
10b. AUTO ACCIDENT? NO [X]
10c. OTHER ACCIDENT? NO [X]
11c. INSURANCE PLAN NAME OR PROGRAM NAME: Big Box Company
11d. IS THERE ANOTHER HEALTH BENEFIT PLAN? NO [X]
12. PATIENT'S OR AUTHORIZED PERSON'S SIGNATURE: SIGNATURE ON FILE DATE 8/31/2017
13. INSURED'S OR AUTHORIZED PERSON'S SIGNATURE: SIGNATURE ON FILE
17. NAME OF REFERRING PROVIDER OR OTHER SOURCE: DN Ima Sleepy MD 17b. NPI 9876543210
21. DIAGNOSIS OR NATURE OF ILLNESS OR INJURY: ICD Ind. 0 A. G47.33
23. PRIOR AUTHORIZATION NUMBER: 6565656

	From	To	Place of Service	CPT/HCPCS	Modifier	Diagnosis Pointer	$ Charges	Units	NPI
1	05 02 17	05 02 17	12	E0486	NU	A	2500 00	1	1234567890
2	04 10 17	04 10 17	11	99203		A	150 00	1	1234567890
3	04 10 17	04 10 17	11	70355		A	135 00	1	1234567890

25. FEDERAL TAX I.D. NUMBER: 999999991 EIN [X]
26. PATIENT'S ACCOUNT NO.: 55555
27. ACCEPT ASSIGNMENT? NO [X]
28. TOTAL CHARGE: $ 2785 00 29. AMOUNT PAID: $ 0 00 30. Rsvd for NUCC Use: 2785 00
31. SIGNATURE OF PHYSICIAN OR SUPPLIER: Dudley Doorioght 8/31/2017
32. SERVICE FACILITY LOCATION INFORMATION: Dudley Doorioght, DDS, 6543 SE 1st Street, Anytown,. USA 1111 a. 1234567890
33. BILLING PROVIDER INFO & PH #: (479) 2540200 Dudley Doorioght, DDS, 6543 SE 1st Street, Anytown, USA 11111 a. 1234567890
NUCC Instruction Manual available at: www.nucc.org PLEASE PRINT OR TYPE APPROVED OMB-0938-1197 FORM 1500 (02-12)

Fig 11-1 CMS 1500 form.

A common reason for rejection of a claim is when the needed information is not completely contained inside the correct field. For example, if you put an X in a box on the CMS 1500 form, the X must be completely inside the box provided. Table 11-2 describes the information that must be entered into each field on the CMS 1500 form for the typical DSM claim.

TABLE 11-2 Fields on the CMS 1500 form

Field no.	Instructions and comments
1	Select the type of claim you are filing (eg, Medicare, group health, etc).
1a	Enter the patient's ID number assigned by the insurance company.
2–11	Enter the patient information.
12	Patient signature or "signature on file" for release of information to process the claim.
13	If the patient is authorizing payment to the office, then the patient's signature or "signature on file" will go here. If payment is going to the patient, leave blank.
14–16	Not applicable for DSM.
17	This is for the referring or ordering physician's information. For the first box, use "DN" for the referring physician if the claim is a commercial insurance claim. If the claim is a Medicare claim, use "DK" for the ordering physician. The second box is for the physician's name.
17a	Not applicable for DSM.
17b	NPI number of the ordering or referring physician.
18	Not applicable for DSM.
19	Rarely used but is helpful when a corrected claim needs to be submitted. Otherwise nothing goes here.
20	Leave blank. Do not put laboratory fees for the MAD in this box. Insurance companies have been known to pay ONLY the fee placed here instead of the fees on the claim. This is used for lab fees associated with biopsies, etc.
21	Diagnosis code G47.33 (OSA) goes on line A. No other codes are needed for the treatment of OSA. To the far upper right is a box labeled "ICD Ind." A zero (0) is placed here, indicating the diagnosis code is from ICD-10.
22	Not applicable for DSM.
23	If the insurance company requires preauthorization before treatment, then the "preauth" number is placed here.
24A	Date of service will go here. "From" and "To" will usually be the same. When filing radiographs and examinations, use the date the patient had the service done. The date of delivery to the patient is the date for E0486 (MAD).
24B	Where was the treatment done? Code 11 indicates services that are performed in the office (ie, 70355, 99202, etc). Code 12 indicates that the service is for use at home (ie, E0486). MAD appliances are used at home, so 12 is used.
24C	Not applicable for DSM

TABLE 11-2 (cont) Fields on the CMS 1500 form

Field no.	Instructions and comments
24D	Procedure (CPT/HCPCS) codes are used in the first part of the box (ie, 70355, E0486, etc). The next section is for modifiers. Modifiers are used to further describe the treatment. NU modifier is used after E0486 to signify that you are supplying new DME, a new (not reused) appliance. The NU is used on all medical claims for E0486. KX modifier is used in addition to the NU modifier for E0486 on Medicare claims to indicate that you have followed all of Medicare's guidelines AND that you have all the appropriate documentation required by Medicare, including but not limited to the prescription/written order, LOMN, and proof of delivery.
24E	Diagnosis pointer cross references the date and service code on the claim form to diagnosis code in box 21A.
24F	Charges for the services provided on the line of the claim form.
24G	For the E0486, a one (1) would be placed for one unit delivered. For most of the other services, a one (1) will be used also.
24H	Not applicable for DSM.
24I	Nothing is needed here. This space already has "NPI" listed, indicating that the number following it in 24J is the NPI number of the rendering provider of the service.
24J	Identification number of the dentist providing the services. Usually the NPI number.
25	Federal tax ID number for the dentist providing the service(s).
26	Patient's account number used in the provider's office.
27	A selection must be made. If "YES" is selected on a Medicare claim, then Medicare will send the check to the provider, and the provider is agreeing to accept what the Medicare allowable is for that service. If "NO" is selected, then the check will be sent to the patient, and you will need to collect from the patient. If you are a nonparticipating Medicare provider, you can choose on a case-by-case basis if you want to accept the Medicare payment for the claim. If you are a participating DME provider, then select "YES."
28	Total charges for the claim.
29	Leave blank.
30	Leave blank.
31–33	Signature of provider, facility information, and billing provider information.

MEDICARE

History of Medicare DME for OAT

DSM took a giant leap forward in 2011, when CMS opened the door for dentists to participate in Medicare by offering OAT for the treatment of OSA. At the urging of the AASM, OAT was classified as DME, which is a subcategory of Medicare Part B. As a result, when dentists provide OAT for Medicare patients, they are functioning as a medical equipment supplier. We do not issue canes or wheelchairs, but dentists providing OAT are not viewed by Medicare as health care providers. The decision to place OAT within DME ensured that sleep physicians would maintain oversight of OAT and remain in control of patient care. This is because all DME requires a physician's prescription before the equipment can be dispensed. Therefore, no dentist can legally fabricate an oral appliance for the treatment of OSA without a prescription from a supervising prescribing physician. However, Medicare did include language that limited the fabrication of an oral appliance to a licensed dentist. Therefore, any physicians that are fabricating oral appliances for Medicare patients are in direct violation of the current CMS regulations.

For a beneficiary (patient) to qualify for OAT benefits, a sleep physician must diagnose the patient's OSA, and the supervising physician must write a prescription for OAT, which must then be filled (provided) by a licensed dentist. The diagnosing sleep physician's notes must reflect the OSA diagnosis. Dentists get their authority to treat OSA patients from the diagnosing and prescribing physicians and must rely on the notes of these practitioners to document the appropriateness and medical necessity of OAT for reimbursement.

Medicare Regulations

The local coverage determination (LCD) L33611 and related policy article A52512 outlines what is necessary for OAT to be a covered service under Medicare. Some of the more commonly misunderstood criteria are the following:

- The beneficiary must have a face-to-face examination with a physician prior to the diagnostic PSG/HSAT. A copy of this summary should be readily available should Medicare request the diagnosing physician's notes. Therefore, it is a good idea to obtain copies of these notes prior to providing MAD therapy.
- The DWO must be issued (signed and dated) by the prescribing physician within a 6-month period from the date of the required face-to-face examination visit. This will be before the sleep study was ordered.

- The diagnosis of any SRBD must be made by a sleep physician, and any diagnostic testing for SRBDs must be ordered by a physician. The LCD specifies that a dentist may not order the diagnostic test; it is the responsibility of the supervising physician to determine the appropriate treatment based on the severity of the beneficiary's SRBD.
- It is acceptable if the physician that ordered the diagnostic test is not the physician that signs the DWO for OAT. An example would be a beneficiary who sees a primary care physician (PCP) and discusses sleep-related issues, and then the PCP orders a PSG/HSAT that is then interpreted by a board-certified sleep physician. The beneficiary may see the PCP or another physician qualified to treat SRBDs after an OSA diagnosis, who then determines the appropriate therapy for the treatment of the patient's OSA. It should be noted that a postdiagnosis appointment with a physician is not mandatory under the LCD.

The oral appliance must be issued (provided) by a licensed dentist as a medical supplier; this makes it possible for dental offices to enroll as DME suppliers (physicians cannot legally provide OAT and bill Medicare). OAT is a covered Medicare benefit if appropriate for the patient and medically necessary. Once an OSA diagnosis is made by a physician, the treating dentist is provided a signed DWO (prescription) for OAT. Custom-fabricated oral appliances for OSA will be eligible for Medicare reimbursement by the DME Medicare Administrative Contractor (MAC) only if the devices have been listed or reverified by PDAC according to the revised guidelines. To see complete Medicare policy details gathered in one place, visit: https://www.cgsmedicare.com/jb/mr/oralappliances.html.

Readers should refer to LCD L33611 and the related oral appliance policy articles (A52512 and A55426) for documentation requirements for OAT for the treatment of OSA. A thorough understanding of the LCD and related articles is mandatory for any dentist filing Medicare. Therefore, keep these articles available as a reference.

Discussing Medicare can easily start a heated argument. There is significant disagreement within DSM on how Medicare should be approached. What is universally agreed upon is that when dentists provide OAT for patients with Medicare, we are DME providers. To become a DME provider, a dentist must complete a CMS-855S form and apply as a Medicare durable medical equipment, prosthetics, orthotics, and supplies (DMEPOS) provider to the DME MAC administrator for their jurisdiction. As stated previously, DME is medical equipment (think wheelchair). Additionally, Medicare requires that DMEPOS providers secure a $50,000.00 bond for each practice location as security against Medicare billing fraud. Dentists can ask their insurance brokers for a surety bond policy, which is not expensive. This $50,000.00 bond is available to auditors in the event of an adverse ruling or overpayment demand.

As a medical equipment provider, we dispense the equipment, and there is NO provision for examinations, adjustment, radiographs, or recall appointments—Medicare pays a single bundled fee for OAT. Medicare pays the "universal" fee that is meant to include all fitting and adjustments for a period of 90 days. The medical directors at Medicare have consistently stated that radiologic services, examinations, and adjustments should not be billed separately to Medicare Part B. After 90 days, the MAD is supposed to be effective, with no further appointments required. When you file HCPCS code E0486, the payment provided for the MAD will include any and all required adjustments but no examinations, radiographs, or subsequent recalls.

Some practitioners opine that when treating a Medicare patient, dentists are both a health care provider (Medicare Part B provider) AND a Medicare DME supplier. To become a Medicare Part B provider, you must complete a CMS-855I form and send this document to the Medicare Part B administrator for your state. Once approved as a Part B provider, a dentist may be able to bill for evaluation and management procedures, office visits, and testing procedures such as pharyngometry, rhinometry, and radiography. The argument used to justify filing Part B for the initial examination and radiographs is that these processes are performed before the decision is made to fabricate the MAD and are necessary to determine if the patient is dentally healthy enough for OAT. Therefore, if the examination and radiographs are performed prior to determining if the patient is a candidate for OAT, then the examination and radiographs are not part of the MAD therapy and can be billed separately. The AADSM has recently issued a statement that dentists should not be filing Medicare Part B for E/M examinations, recall visits, or radiography.

The question that haunts this author (Ken Berley) regarding Part B practitioners is that Medicare specifically prohibits a Part B practitioner from recommending DME equipment when the practitioner has a financial interest in the recommendation. If you are a Part B practitioner, you cannot recommend that the patient's MAD needs to be replaced because you will make money from that recommendation. This would likely be a Stark Law violation, although to date this has not been tested in court.

Medicare Participating or Nonparticipating Provider

When you complete an application to become a Medicare provider (Part B or DME), you must decide if you want to be a participating Medicare provider or nonparticipating provider. If you wish to be a participating Medicare provider, you will need to complete a CMS-460 form and submit this form with your application. As a participating provider, you are committed to accept what Medicare allows for OAT. If you wish to be a nonparticipating provider, you do not have to submit any additional documentation, and Medicare will register you as a nonparticipating provider by default. As a nonparticipating provider, you can balance bill the Medicare patient for your usual fee that exceeds the Medicare allowable. However, you are always free to accept assignment of benefits when you deem that to be appropriate, essentially acting, for that individual patient, as if you are a participating provider. This allows the dentist to be flexible for some Medicare recipients while preserving the ability to bill the full fee when that is more appropriate.

Reasonable Useful Lifetime for DME

Under federal regulation 42 CFR 414.210(f), the Reasonable Useful Lifetime (RUL) of any piece of DME is to be not less than 5 years. Under the RUL, Medicare will not benefit multiple pieces of DME that are used to treat the same condition. For example, Medicare would likely refuse benefits for a motorized battery-powered wheelchair and a standard wheelchair. The "same or similar" provision is an attempt to prevent the payment of duplicate therapy (you only get one wheelchair). Therefore, if Medicare has paid for a piece of DME for the treatment of OSA, any new claim that you submit within 5 years for the treatment of OSA will be denied. A beneficiary cannot have two pieces of DME that have been determined to be the "same or similar" to treat OSA. Unfortunately, CMS has determined that CPAP and OAT are "similar" pieces of DME used to treat OSA.

Medicare will pay for the replacement of a piece of DME during the first 5 years of use if the item is lost (due to extenuating circumstances such as flood, hurricane, or other natural disaster) or irreparably damaged or if the beneficiary's medical condition changes such that the current equipment no longer meets the beneficiary's needs. Replacement due to irreparable wear during the period of RUL is not covered. Additionally, replacement due to extensive dental work is not covered. Therefore, we need to perform a detailed dental examination with radiographs prior to OAT to determine the health of the dentition and the potential need for significant restorations soon. Any pressing dental problems should be addressed prior to fabricating an oral appliance.

Because CPAP and OAT have been classified by CMS as same or similar devices, under the RUL guidelines, Medicare will pay for only one of these therapies every 5 years for the treatment of OSA. If a new sleep appliance is needed, then a new DWO/prescription and LOMN will need to be obtained from a physician.

"Same or Similar" Denials

Until March 2018, dentists could file Medicare claims for OAT without any significant problems. However, in March 2018, CMS updated their system in response to the increased payments for OAT resulting from some patients using both CPAP and OAT, which violates CMS regulations. Medicare's system is now fully updated and programmed to automatically deny any claim for OAT if Medicare has paid for CPAP within the last 5 years, linking the OAT code with the CPAP code as similar devices for the treatment of OSA. The enforcement of the CMS "Same or Similar"/RUL policy has significantly affected many DSM practices. Now if a Medicare beneficiary has had CPAP therapy for more than 90 days within the last 5 years, any claim submitted for OAT will be denied.

Why is 90 days the magic number? During the initial 90 days of PAP rental, the treating physician is expected to evaluate whether CPAP is the best therapy to treat the beneficiary's OSA. Once satisfied with the patient's compliance and the efficacy of CPAP therapy, the treating physician signs a Medicare CPAP certification. Certification is appropriate whenever the beneficiary used CPAP for 4 hours or more per night for a minimum of 21 days out of any 30-day period within the first 90 days of CPAP usage. If a Medicare patient has had a CPAP for more than 90 days, you can be sure that Medicare has funded the PAP therapy. Once the certification is signed and Medicare pays for the PAP therapy, any oral appliance claim submitted for Medicare reimbursement will be denied due to the RUL policy.

The good news is that repeated letters to the medical directors at CMS have finally resulted in some concessions. It is now the position of the CMS that if a dental practitioner can provide documentation showing that CPAP usage has been discontinued by the treating physician, all Medicare regulations were followed to the letter, and all payments for PAP therapy have ceased, then, and only then, will Medicare cover OAT.

What if the patient fails PAP after 91 days of use?

If the beneficiary "fails" PAP therapy after day 91, the probability of overturning a denial significantly decreases. The claim will be denied due to the RUL regulation. The treatment timeline must be well documented, and the ordering physician must enter an order to "discontinue PAP therapy" and order OAT. If the ordering physician's notes do not show that CPAP was discontinued, Medicare will not benefit OAT. As a side note, these requirements are problematic from a legal standpoint, as no reasonable sleep physician should discontinue any therapy without an alternative therapy in place. In other words, if PAP has been prescribed by a physician, it might be a breach of the standard of care to discontinue this therapy before a MAD has been delivered. Additionally, the beneficiary's DME PAP supplier must discontinue billing Medicare for PAP expenses, and the supplier's notes must reflect that PAP was discontinued. The PAP supplier's notes should be included in any denial reconsideration and show that all PAP expenses have ceased. The ordering physician's treatment notes must document why the Medicare beneficiary failed PAP and show that a valid attempt was made to comply with therapy. The treating dentist cannot provide this documentation; it MUST come from the ordering physician.

What if the patient fails CPAP before certification?

If the ordering sleep physician determines that the beneficiary has not met the requirements for PAP certification, it is extremely important that the sleep physician's notes document that the PAP was discontinued and why it was ineffective. A MAD fabricated and delivered prior to the certification of PAP will be paid with no denial. Therefore, it is ideal if the diagnosing physician can determine the most appropriate treatment for the beneficiary's SRBD as soon as possible to give DSM practitioners adequate time to deliver a MAD within the first 90 days of treatment. Unfortunately, DSM providers will likely have a difficult time delivering a MAD within the first 90 days of OSA therapy if PAP is dispensed initially due to scheduling and fabrication time. Therefore, most Medicare beneficiaries who are referred for OAT will likely have a claims history that will include a payment for PAP within the last 5 years, and OAT denial is likely.

You received your first denial: Appeal

The first level of the appeals process requires that you submit a "redetermination." The Medicare redetermination request form is available at https://www.cms.gov/ or on your DME jurisdiction's website. When filing a redetermination, include as much documentation as you have to support overturning the denial of your claim, such as the physician's DWO (which must be dated within 6 months of the original face-to-face office visit before diagnosis), the diagnosing physician's office notes for the face-to-face examination, a copy of the sleep test (PSG or HSAT), the PAP prescription, the physician's office notes regarding PAP failure, the PAP discontinuance order, the treating dentist's clinical intake examination and delivery appointment notes, and a copy of the denial. The redetermination must include all supporting documentation necessary to prove medical necessity for OAT after discontinuation of PAP therapy. Include the PAP supplier notes, if available, to show that PAP expenses are no longer being billed to Medicare. This will show that the beneficiary is not using combination therapy, which would be a violation of Medicare regulations. Include the physician's notes to explain any lapse in the continuation of care (eg, PAP machine returned 12 months ago and there has been a lapse in treatment). Your dental intake examination and the ordering sleep physician's notes should document how the beneficiary's symptoms have worsened, making OAT "medically necessary."

The more medical justification you provide, the better the chance of overturning the denial. The more time that the rental of the PAP machine is past day 91, the less chance you have of a successful outcome.

WHAT IF THE REDETERMINATION IS DENIED?

A level 2 appeal is your next course of action, which is known as a "reconsideration" of the claim. Again, the appeal must be requested in writing, and the necessary form can be obtained at https://www.cms.gov/. It is essential to include all supporting documents that you have available. Explain why the denial of your redetermination was inappropriate. The reconsideration request will be reviewed by the qualified independent contractor for your jurisdiction. This is the last level of the appeals process that allows you to submit supporting documentation; therefore, it is imperative to include all the information you have that can support overturning the case.

Advanced Beneficiary Notice

Given the system update and restrictions associated with the "same or similar" policy, it is vitally important to determine whether this restriction will apply for any Medicare beneficiary. If you determine that a patient's Medicare claim for OAT will be denied under RUL, it may be advisable to execute an Advanced Beneficiary Notice (ABN) to inform the patient that the Medicare claim will likely be denied. The ABN places the beneficiary on notice that if the Medicare claim is denied, the beneficiary is personally responsible for the charges for OAT. If you fail to obtain a signed ABN from the patient prior to rendering the service, your practice will not be able to collect any amount due from the patient when Medicare denies the claim. Therefore, a signed ABN may be useful when an RUL denial is expected. Participating and nonparticipating Medicare suppliers should execute an ABN prior to impressions/scans when a Medicare denial is anticipated. When presented with the probability of a denied Medicare claim, the beneficiary can make an informed decision.

Unfortunately, if an ABN is signed, the appropriate modifier must be used when filing to inform Medicare that an ABN has been executed. This act ensures that your Medicare claim will be denied and makes a reversal of this denial more difficult. When submitted with the appropriate ABN modifier, Medicare is placed on notice that "the supplier feels the item will not be a covered service, and the beneficiary has been informed of this fact and understands why the item will not be covered by Medicare." Refer to the LCD for more information regarding correct coding for oral appliances that do not meet Medicare guidelines.

If an ABN is on file and the office is instructed to submit to Medicare, when the claim is submitted correctly, the resulting denial will indicate that the beneficiary is responsible for the charges. Providers should be aware that they are then required to collect the fee that was submitted (eg, if you file for $6,500.00, you are required to collect that amount).

If the beneficiary is willing to forego filing the claim to Medicare, a cash discount may be possible. The patient becomes a cash patient when an ABN is executed, and option B is selected on the ABN document. If option B is selected, the patient must understand why no Medicare coverage is expected and that you will not file a claim with Medicare for the OAT.

Extra tip: Most offices are unaware that some medical insurance companies may refuse to allow you to collect from a patient on denied claims if you are in-network. Therefore, prudent practitioners may want to start using an advanced patient notice for services that a private payer might not cover. Some payers will accept the Medicare ABN, but some have their own form. If you are in-network with one or more medical insurance companies, you should check with those payers and see if they have an ABN-type notice for your use.

What if a physician orders OAT as the first line of treatment and it is not effective?

If OAT is the first line of treatment, the ordering physician is responsible for evaluating and documenting the effectiveness of the therapy. Once the sleep physician determines that OAT is inadequate, PAP may be ordered if the beneficiary qualifies under LCD L33718. Again, a claim for PAP will automatically be denied as not reasonable and necessary when submitted. The PAP will be classified as "same or similar treatment within the 5-year RUL." Timing is of the essence; if PAP is initiated immediately after failing OAT, the denial would have the possibility of being overturned at first-level appeal. PAP will always receive preferential treatment.

It is possible that DSM may have received an unexpected benefit because of a Medicare update that may make it easier to document that OAT is ineffective than it is to document the ineffectiveness of PAP. If your referring sleep physicians are willing to prescribe OAT as the first line of treatment, it should be easier to get Medicare to agree to a CPAP in case of OAT failure. Only time will tell, however; under RUL, OAT may be the best choice as first-line therapy for mild to moderate cases. A discussion with your referring physicians could prove beneficial to your DSM practice. Readers should be aware that this is a fluid situation. Therefore, it is vital that practitioners stay abreast of current Medicare notifications.

*Many things we need can wait.
The child cannot. Now is the
time his bones are formed, his
mind developed. To him we cannot
say tomorrow; his name is today.*

—*Gabriela Mistral*

12

Pediatric Airway Problems

Who wouldn't be disturbed by watching a child struggle to breathe? Health care providers, therapists, school professionals, and parents all want to see children grow to maximum health and potential, yet there are uncountable numbers of children who are falling short simply because a compromised airway prevents them from getting a great night's sleep.

Pediatric airway disorder warrants an entire text of its own, and indeed, many are available for comprehensive consideration. This chapter gives readers enough information to orient themselves in the field and the skills to identify children at risk in their practice, community, and family. One fact we must establish immediately is this: There is no consensus about how to treat children with an airway disorder. What is known about pediatric airway disorder is rapidly expanding.

Two critical points need to be made upfront: *(1)* The disorder is not a sleep problem; rather, it is an airway problem with several consequences, including disrupted and unrefreshing sleep. *(2)* Nearly everything we are comfortable with in the discipline of adult dental sleep medicine must be modified when considering children's health issues. It is often said that "children are not just little adults," and the authors cannot imagine an area of health care where this statement is more accurate. Readers are cautioned to avoid applying the same thinking that is used to treat adult sleep-related breathing disorders (SRBDs) to children's airway problems.

Growth and development of the craniofacial respiratory complex is over 90% complete by the time a child reaches 10 years of age in the absence of a genetic anomaly that affects the area, such as Down or Williams syndrome.[1]

This chapter addresses the care of non-syndromic, typically developing (TD) children between 4 and 13 years old. The airway is critical at every age, of course, but discussion of neonates to age 4 is for another text, and the airways of children over 13 years old are more like adult airways than those of growing children.

Evidence-Based Treatment

Most clinicians make treatment decisions based on the best clinical evidence available as applied to the individual patient, which allows for use of clinical wisdom. Standards for this evidence include randomized controlled trials, meta-analyses, and carefully managed cohorts. Creating such trials in children, who are growing over any study time frame, is challenging. Similarly, no one would expect an industrial review board to approve of any study that withholds treatment from a diagnosed, growing child, considering the grave lifetime consequences of such a choice. There is considerable evidence available that supports early intervention, with the continuous addition of new data. This field is far from unsupported in decision-making, as even a cursory search through PubMed will show. The conscientious provider is a constant learner who will wield new understanding with wisdom and solid clinical judgment.

Today, it is unacceptable for a child to achieve permanent dentition with a mouth full of cavities; soon, it will be just as unacceptable for that child to finish growth with an underdeveloped airway.

A recent systematic review of risk factors related to obstructive sleep apnea (OSA) that looked for publications focused on prevention of the disease found only four papers, compared to the nearly 24,000 articles related to treatment.[2]

Pediatric Airway Insufficiency

Why do children experience nocturnal airway issues? Several theories have been proposed to explain this phenomenon. The most accepted theories hypothesize that the craniofacial respiratory complex in many children is underdeveloped due to the Western culture of soft diets (baby food), bottle feeding (as opposed to breastfeeding), and pacifiers and sippy cups (which result in nonproductive sucking). These actions collectively result in the lack of lateral and anterior development of the maxillary and mandibular bones. When skeletal supports fail to develop, the tongue is displaced posteriorly, resulting in nocturnal airway insufficiency. Complicating matters is the fact that children seem to be more susceptible to airway compromise than adults. Pediatric airway insufficiency starts with poor daytime breathing habits, continues with nocturnal flow limitations, and ends with full obstructive sleep apnea on the other end of the spectrum. Children seem to be extremely sensitive to even small reductions in oxygenation during sleep and can display various airway-related symptoms with very small changes in airflow. Once a child starts snoring, the airway is already compromised.

Problems Related to Airway Underdevelopment

The human body at birth is dependent, with many immature physiologic systems that gradually develop into a functioning, efficient, complexly interactive organism capable of being self-sustaining for decades. From infancy to adolescence to adulthood, the body depends on the growth and development of every cell type and organ system to achieve maturity. In turn, cells require proper nutrition, a daily period of sleep, and unrestricted respiration to maximize their genetic potential. Even fully supported systems are influenced by environmental conditions. Adulthood, the end of growth, is the sum of all controlling factors.

Disruption of any of the fundamental needs during times of rapid growth logically leads to a different endpoint of growth than would be achieved without disruption. The earlier parents and medical professionals recognize off-track growth in a child, the sooner the developmental curve can be redirected. There is never a time that poor breathing produces a better outcome than fully capable respiration.

How a restricted airway affects the individual will vary according to when in life the disruption began. For example, normal tongue function is necessary for maxillary arch development. Some children are born with an inability to nurse due to a severely restricted tongue or lip frenum. Correction immediately after birth can allow for normal breastfeeding, sucking, and swallowing behavior to proceed. Surgical release of the frenum will allow the tongue to rest within the palatal vault, which helps develop the nasal airway. Without treatment, children as young as 2 years old are more likely to show signs of an SRBD and, by age 11 years, are more likely to show abnormal facial structure growth patterns.[3] As outlined in the American Dental Association's Policy Statement on the Role of Dentistry in the Treatment of Sleep Related Breathing Disorders: "In children, undiagnosed and/or untreated OSA can be associated with cardiovascular problems, impaired growth, as well as learning and behavioral problems."

It is imperative that children with a compromised airway are identified as soon as possible. Medical providers have a responsibility to assess airway competency in children. Dentists are likely to see kids more frequently, and with more of a preventive emphasis, than pediatricians or primary care providers. Dental and dental hygiene training programs focus on the growth and development of the craniofacial respiratory complex in greater detail than any part of medical training. Otolaryngologists have a deeper understanding of the area but tend to be interested in surgery, not how the tissues achieve their full-grown shape.

How does the dentist identify a child at risk for a compromised airway? The most validated screening tool is the Pediatric Sleep Questionnaire (PSQ).[4] Using this or another tool, such as BEARS (**B**edtime problems, **E**xcessive daytime sleepiness, **A**wakenings during the night, **R**egularity and duration of sleep, and **S**noring),[5] in a dental office, administered and discussed by trained auxiliary staff, is a straightforward way to guide families into discovering the connection between airway problems and observed behavior. The most reliable source of information for whether a child is thriving or at risk is the parent, usually the mother. There are several resources that can be used by guardians to learn what to "look for." Some of those resources are included in the reference list at the end of this chapter.

Dentists are the only medical professionals specifically trained to assess growth and development of the maxilla and mandible. Often in dental school and even orthodontic graduate programs, training is focused on achieving a straight-tooth smile with an occlusion in harmony with temporomandibular joint function and muscle comfort. While these are laudable goals, dentists must expand their scope of awareness to the airway that lies immediately adjacent to, and is heavily influenced by, the orofacial structures. The term *craniofacial respiratory complex*, coined by pediatric dentist Dr Kevin Boyd, is gaining popularity. Considering all the anatomy that is implied in such a title, it becomes apparent that airway-aware dentists must maintain familiarity with the developing anatomy of the airway while observing arch shape, palate depth, anteroposterior alignment of the jaws, and orientation to the common planes of reference. As is true with all types of learning, once a problem or pattern becomes recognizable, it becomes widely noticed.

Once the trained dentist notices signs of an underdeveloped craniofacial respiratory complex, many children will be screened. Those identified to have a compromised airway can be guided into several treatment pathways. Children may have tethered oral tissues, meaning the lingual, labial, or buccal frenula do not allow proper movement of the tissues. These tissue ties are bits of fascia that did not undergo full apoptosis before birth, leaving residual restrictions. Children with tethered oral tissues should be evaluated by a speech and language pathologist or a dental hygienist who has become certified in myofunctional therapy (see chapter 13). These professionals are trained not only in assessment but also in the critical movements that are required following any surgical correction. No matter who in the community performs the release surgery—be it you, an oral surgeon, periodontist, otolaryngologist, or another kind of surgeon—the clinical outcome will not be optimal without proper postsurgical movements. These can be challenging for the patient and the family, so connection with a dedicated provider is a key to success. Go to www.Myofunctional-Therapist.com to find a trained provider in your area.

There is always a question about whether the child needs to have an adenotonsillectomy and/or maxillary expansion to address an airway problem. There are too many variables to be able to display a decision tree, and the research is ongoing. Papers have been written that show value for both expansion and surgery. Recent research has shown a reduction in the volume of lymphoid tissue following expansion alone.[6] There is no consensus on which should come first or which has the greater influence to achieve optimum airflow. Clinicians can assess each child as an individual and create a treatment plan involving the family, available providers, and insurance coverage details with the confidence that any step forward to achieve an open airway during sleep will help that child. No single treatment is likely to be completely curative, so proper medical oversight must be emphasized as the child continues to grow.

One aspect of early airway therapy that can be addressed by any provider and must be emphasized at home is mouth breathing. There are two pathways to fill the lungs, but only nasal breathing delivers properly cleaned, warmed, and humidified air to the respiratory system. Nitric oxide, a powerful antibacterial and anti-inflammatory gas, is produced by the nasal mucosa and has important functions in a wide range of physiologic and pathophysiologic processes.[7] Children with nasal breathing habits have smaller and narrower maxillae, vaulted palates, malocclusion, gingivitis, and other ills; dental professionals are perfectly poised to encourage healthier breathing habits (see chapter 14).[8] Dentists committed to airway health can seek information and training in these areas according to their interest, commitment, and willingness to incorporate significant behavior-based interventions into their service mix. A leading thinker in this area, Dr Barry Raphael, points out that the shape and position of the skeletal structures are highly influenced by soft tissue function. Any variance from optimal skeletal structures has its origin in soft tissue dysfunction—think of mouth breathing versus nasal breathing. Dr Raphael says, "First, make it easy for them to breathe, then teach them to breathe easily."

Expansion of the maxilla and guidance of the growth of the mandible are beyond the scope of this text. Strategies include exercises, fixed and removable custom expansion devices, and prefabricated growth guidance systems that combine coaching, exercises, and mouthpieces for day and night use. Recent meta-analysis reports have verified positive effects on commonly measured breathing parameters, as well as patient and family quality of life, using functional appliances to correct growth patterns and poor habits.[9]

Every dental professional is required to be able to recognize children at risk for SRBDs and guide them and their families to the appropriate providers. It is up to dentists to lead the way in changing the medical culture until no child reaches adulthood with a crowded, insufficient airway.

References

1. Villa MP, Malagola C, Pagani J, et al. Rapid maxillary expansion in children with obstructive sleep apnea syndrome: 12-month follow-up. Sleep Med 2007;8:128–134.
2. Correa E, Conti DM, Gozal D, O'Connor-Reina C. Preventive medicine in OSA—A systematic review and a call to action [epub ahead of print 23 July 2024]. Sleep doi: 10.1093/sleep/zsae164.
3. Huang Y, Quo S, Berkowski JA, Guilleminault C. Short lingual frenulum and obstructive sleep apnea in children. Int J Pediatr Res 2015;1:1–4.
4. Chervin RD, Hedger K, Dillon JE, Pituch KJ. Pediatric sleep questionnaire (PSQ): Validity and reliability of scales for sleep-disordered breathing, snoring, sleepiness, and behavioral problems. Sleep Med 2000;1:21–32.
5. Owens JA, Dalzell V. Use of the 'BEARS' sleep screening tool in a pediatric residents' continuity clinic: A pilot study. Sleep Med 2005;6:63–69.
6. Yoon A, Abdelwahab M, Bockow R, et al. Impact of rapid palatal expansion on the size of adenoids and tonsils in children. Sleep Med 2022;92:96–102.
7. Maniscalco M, Bianco A, Mazzarella G, Motta A. Recent advances on nitric oxide in the upper airways. Curr Med Chem 2016;23:2736–2745.
8. Lee SY, Guilleminault C, Chiu HY, Sullivan SS. Mouth breathing, "nasal disuse," and pediatric sleep-disordered breathing. Sleep Breath 2015;19:1257–1264.
9. Bernardes R, Ferreira LMDB, Machado AJ Jr, Jones MH. Effectiveness of functional orthopedic appliances as an alternative treatment among children and adolescents with obstructive sleep apnea: Systematic review and meta-analysis. Sleep Med 2023;105:88–102.

Make sure I'm chewing, swallowing, and breathing. My whole body is working together. I can just find a rhythm and keep going and going and going.

—Joey Chestnut

13

Myofunctional Therapy

Samantha Weaver | Joy L. Moeller

When I was a young girl, my father and stepmom set out to build their dream house on Telegraph Hill in San Francisco. I remember the months of planning, the visits from the architect to firm up the design, and finally, the big day when ground was broken and construction began. It felt like a long time until the building was finally complete. The day we passed inspections, we had a celebration and started moving our things inside as the fog rolled in and the city lights glinted off the bay. We were eager to settle into our new home and live in the space that had been a construction site for so long.

But it didn't take long before problems began to arise. Within a few months, cracks appeared in the walls. Several leaks emerged with the autumn rains. Further inspection revealed that the footings were pulling away from the structure itself. To everyone's dismay, we had to vacate the property immediately because the foundations proved to be unstable.

Building a house is complex to say the least, and within that complexity lies a metaphor for how imperative strong foundations are for any structure. In the field of myofunctional therapy and sciences, we consider strong oral foundations to be the key to long-term dental stability. Simply put, how you breathe, chew, and swallow will make or break even the best treatment planning and execution. This chapter focuses on the practice of myofunctional therapy and how it can support optimal outcomes in dental and overall health.

What is Myofunctional Therapy?

Myofunctional therapy is a method for optimizing the oral physiology of the stomatognathic system and the interaction between the teeth, jaws, and associated tissues. Also known as *neuromuscular re-education of the oral facial muscles*, myofunctional therapy promotes the stability of the stomatognathic system by training the muscles of the orofacial and pharyngeal complex. A primary function of the tongue is to protect the airway, but improper oral resting posture of the tongue during growth years will have a negative influence on the development of the oral cavity.[1] When the tongue is resting against the hard palate (thus maintaining the proper oral volume), it enhances and/or creates stability for the temporomandibular joints (TMJs). If the tongue is habitually resting down and forward in the mandible (as may happen with a lack of airway patency and/or the excessive use of bottles,[2] pacifiers, and digit sucking, or a restricted frenum[3]), normal form and function may be disrupted.[4] A smaller oral volume may not provide proper support for the upper airways, the stability of the TMJs, or the development of optimal dental arches.[5,6] Added to that problem is the modern diet of processed foods; soft foods may lead to low muscle tone by diminishing the frequency and intensity of mastication.

Myofunctional therapy targets the muscles of the orofacial and pharyngeal complex through a series of techniques to optimize the muscles in terms of strength, range of motion, accuracy of motion, rest position, and coordination. Unlike skeletal muscles, most orofacial muscles perform multiple functions. This means that targeting a single muscle is nearly impossible because these muscles work in concert with each other to perform specific actions.[7] For example, if one were to focus on "strengthening the lips" due to lip incompetence (open mouth posture) with the muscles recruited in a technique such as the "button pull" (in which resistance is exerted against an opposing force that engages the orbicularis oris muscles), one would find that not only are the orbicularis oris muscles engaged but also the lower lip by way of interdigitation.[8]

Whereas the term *myofunctional* refers to the function of muscles alone, it is important to understand the interdependence these muscles have with other structures, including bones, teeth, and soft tissues such as the salivary glands and frenula. All these structures interplay as early as gestation and interact with the environment through epigenetic factors. These factors may be internal, such as breathing and nutrition, or external, such as traumas or orthodontic appliance therapy.

Cascading Effects

Understanding how muscles and hard structures interact explains how a condition such as deficient nasal breathing or a restricted lingual frenulum may create a cascading effect on the body, which eventually influences breathing during sleep. When a child mouth breathes, ingested pathogens may trigger sensitivities or allergies that cause the nasopharyngeal lymphoid tissues to enlarge, leading to other dysfunctions. Regular mouth breathing, even if part time, can influence facial growth patterns and have skeletal postural implications beyond the craniofacial respiratory complex. Poor head posture creates compensatory responses throughout the musculoskeletal system of the entire body.

Hypertrophic lymphoid tissues, such as palatine tonsils, prevent nasal breathing during the daytime and nighttime. This causes an immediate and usually chronic compensatory position of the jaw, in which the tongue is lowered and sitting within the mandible as opposed to against the hard palate. This in turn allows the natural tension of the cheeks to push medially with a force that lacks any counterbalance by the tongue against the palate. The result is a narrow, ogival (pointed, or gothic) palate with reduced transverse maxillary dimension.[9] Because the growth of the maxilla guides the growth and development of the mandible, when this dynamic is suboptimal, both dental arches will be vulnerable to malocclusion.[10] Hypertrophic tonsils also reduce the space for the posterior portion of the tongue and restrict the airway. The tongue, in turn, pushes forward (tongue thrusting) to accommodate breathing.

A collapsed maxilla also impacts the tongue. As mentioned previously, a tongue with reduced space can't rest comfortably in the palate. This may contribute to a low tongue resting posture and vertical growth of the mandible. Chewing, speaking, and swallowing could even be affected as the tongue adapts to this reduction of the retrolingual space.

Ankyloglossia

Tight lingual frenula have a critical impact on the normal function and development of the orofacial complex. Restricted frenula not only affect the oral resting posture of the tongue but also disrupt the intrinsic and extrinsic tongue muscles. If the frenum is restricted, the genioglossus muscle cannot function normally. As the tongue adapts to this restriction, it may impact airway patency and contribute to sleep-disordered breathing (SDB).[11] Furthermore, the attachment of the tongue to the mandible may restrict forward growth and development.

In cases of ankyloglossia, a lingual frenectomy is essential to allow full-range mobility. Even more essential is preoperative and follow-up myofunctional therapy.[12] A myofunctional therapist will work with the patient to repattern the muscles, ensure full range of motion of the tongue, and make sure the tissues do not reattach after surgery. It is ideal to release the restricted frenum as early as possible (ie, at birth) because the tongue will achieve optimal function through the activity of breastfeeding.[13] Breastfeeding promotes tongue-palate contact and requires the back of the tongue to activate by making a suction seal. These actions promote the optimal muscle function of the entire orofacial complex.

Orofacial Myofunctional Disorders

A myofunctional evaluation is required to determine which (if any) orofacial myofunctional disorders (OMDs) are present. OMDs are related to the disruption of functions inside the stomatognathic system, mostly related to mouth breathing, tongue resting posture, atypical swallowing, and chewing dysfunction. Like any good clinician, the trained myofunctional therapist carefully identifies the disorder before choosing therapy. A complete list of the 32 clinical markers, or phenotypes, of OMDs describes these disorders at length.[14] Here, a partial list is provided:

- Mouth breathing
- Open mouth posture
- Anterior or bilateral tongue thrust
- Tongue tie (ankyloglossia)
- Lip tie
- Atypical swallowing
- Disruptive oral habits
- Chewing disorders
- Hypotonic masseters
- Speech misarticulations
- Hypertrophic tonsils/adenoids
- Sleep disorders
- Snoring
- Bruxism/clenching
- Cavities and/or gum disease
- Restricted maxilla/high arched palate
- Malocclusion
- Changes in saliva

- Venous pooling
- Craniofacial dysfunction
- Macroglossia
- History of infant feeding challenges
- Tinnitus
- Esthetic changes
- Abnormal breathing
- Forward head posture
- Eustachian tube dysfunction
- Tongue scalloping
- Craniofacial dysfunction

Screening for OMDs includes checking for mouth breathing; mentalis strain when swallowing; tonsil hypertrophy; tongue, lip, or cheek restrictions; and indications of clenching or grinding. Open-ended questions can be used to probe into functions from birth to present day to discover early feeding practices and daily nutritional patterns, with attention paid to the substance of the food regularly eaten. A skilled therapist will form a therapeutic alliance with the patient that allows for information to be openly exchanged between the two to gain a detailed relevant medical and dental history and use validated protocols to assess the behaviors, structures, and oral motor functions related to the stomatognathic system.

With clinical markers identified, a myofunctional therapist then triages them by severity and priority for treatment. Some phenotypes (such as tongue thrust) are directly treated, whereas others (Eustachian tube dysfunction) are treated indirectly. Improving the functions around chewing, swallowing, and jaw and tongue posture can have an indirect influence on how the Eustachian tube clears. Similarly, forward head posture would be influenced by optimizing breathing and tongue posture.[15] In all cases where OMDs are active, working collaboratively with allied health providers has an enormous influence on how efficiently a person might change an existing function and habituate new functional patterns.

Treatment

Myofunctional therapy involves a combination of behavioral guidance on habits, sleep hygiene, eating, and exercises that optimize tongue posture, nasal breathing, balanced chewing, and optimal swallowing. Some techniques are active, and others are passive in nature. Passive techniques promote integration on a subcortical level as the brain repatterns to support function without active participation by the patient. A combination of active and passive treatment can have a beneficial influence on neurologic integration. Typically, both approaches are used, depending on the needs of the patient.[16]

While there is no hard rule for the length of time required for neurologic integration, it is important to consider the principles of neuroplasticity, which drives automaticity. The principles of neuroplasticity describe the ways in which the brain learns and automates functional patterns.[17] These principles include the following:

- "Use it or lose it." Movement patterns that are practiced will persist.
- Plasticity is experience specific, so practicing the right skills is important.
- Repetition matters because frequent and consistent practice improves performance.
- The intensity of practice matters. Push for better performance.
- Time matters. Not all skills are learned at the same rate.
- Salience matters. The goal someone is shooting for must be meaningful to them.
- Age matters, as younger brains learn more easily.
- Transference applies because learning one skill can improve others.
- Interference from stress loads influences learning. In other words, every part of our lives matters and has the potential to affect therapy.

These principles are why therapeutic techniques are employed, often several times a day. Repetition is at the heart of learned behaviors. These principles also explain why it is so important for the therapist to get a full picture of a patient's lifestyle. The stress levels people live with can limit a patient's capacity to learn new patterns. Interference by stress hormones can have a direct impact on neuroplasticity.[18]

It is also important to generalize the patient's ability to perform functions in a multitude of environments, not just in the treatment room. Furthermore, the age of the patient will drive how long treatment times may take. Generally, younger cases move faster because habits and patterns are not as engrained; however, the awareness that comes with an adult's behavior could also promote more self-correction. Interference can play a huge role in the duration of treatment too, not just school and vacation schedules but, as mentioned above, the stress loads on family systems. A family that is doing too much will need to prioritize therapy to ensure the focus, commitment, and the neurologic ability to learn new patterns. This could not be more critical for success.

The Future of Myofunctional Therapy

Myofunctional therapy first appeared in the dental literature in the early 1900s, when it was connected mainly to orthodontics. In fact, the term was first coined by orthodontic pioneer Alfred Paul Rogers, DDS, who emphasized the critical nature of the position of the tongue at rest and in movement on craniofacial morphology and subsequent orthodontic and occlusal stability.[4] Even though myofunctional therapy has been around for over a hundred years, it is only now becoming a vital part of comprehensive care. Don't disparage clinicians who operated with their best knowledge at the time, but vow to bring your practice as far to the front of what we know today as possible, and keep moving forward as we all learn more.

Since 2009, research on the benefits of myofunctional therapy and SDB has increased.[19] A meta-analysis by Camacho et al[20] reported that myofunctional therapy lowered the Apnea-Hypopnea Index (AHI) by 62% in children and 50% in adults. Other meta-analyses have shown that myofunctional therapy "improved the AHI, minimum oxygen saturation, ESS, and snoring intensity in patients with mild and moderate OSA."[21] Early myofunctional intervention has been found to be an adjunctive treatment for the prevention and treatment of malocclusion,[22,23] obstructive sleep apnea,[24] orofacial pain,[25] and developmental disorders.

Conclusion

Excellent health of the craniofacial respiratory complex depends on properly functional breathing, chewing, swallowing, habit awareness, and mouth clearing (elimination). By revising restricted oral tissues and retraining poor habits, optimal function is possible. Myofunctional therapy improves the probability of long-term occlusal stability. Proper growth guidance induces the best skeletal support of the airway. Nasal breathing aids in periodontal health and healthy sleep patterns. And proper chewing and swallowing support normal digestion and the development of muscle patterns that reduce the risk of orofacial pain and enhance esthetics. Myofunctional therapy is a powerful treatment that can provide the foundations for oral health for years to come. Screening for OMDs should be part of every comprehensive evaluation, with therapy included in any treatment plan if OMDs are present.

Oral foundations are much like those in our homes. When the foundations are substandard, the walls crack. When the foundations for oral health are substandard, therapeutic success is not sustainable—we call that relapse.

Good foundations are critical for long-term peace of mind and health. When you find a therapist in your area (or online) who will partner with you, your patients' outcomes will improve.

Patient testimonial

"If my tongue would have been left untreated, the quality of my life would have been forever compromised. My travails began in the early 1970s, when a respected orthodontist overlooked a profound deviant swallowing pattern and numerous lingual restrictions that caused malocclusion, misaligned teeth, and a narrow airway. Instead of correcting the root cause of my orofacial posture, the doctor exacerbated the clinical picture by pulling four healthy teeth, shrinking my dental arches, and constricting my airway, crowding an already compromised tongue space. It took decades of physical pain, sleep disturbance, and improper breathing before finding clinicians to correct the swallow; reshape my face, jaw, and teeth; and improve my sleep patterns. Myofunctional therapy is a small miracle that can restore good health. Thank you, Joy, for giving me back my life and restoring my faith in the healing arts." —Philip D. 5-31-23

References

1. Yoon A, Gozal D, Kushida C, et al. A roadmap of craniofacial growth modification for children with sleep-disordered breathing: A multidisciplinary proposal. Sleep 2023;14:46.
2. Romero CC, Scavone H Jr, Garib DG, Cotrim-Ferreira FA, Ferreira RI. Breastfeeding and non-nutritive sucking patterns related to the prevalence of anterior open bite in primary dentition. J Appl Oral Sci 2011;19:2:161–168.
3. Northcutt M. The lingual frenum. J Clin Orthod 2009;43:557–565.
4. Rogers AP. Exercises for the development of muscles of the face with a view to increasing their functional activity. Dental Cosmos LX 1918;59:857–876.
5. Lieberman DE, Krovitz GE, Yates FW, Devlin M, St Claire M. Effects of food processing on masticatory strain and craniofacial growth in a retrognathic face. J Hum Evol 2004;46:655–677.
6. Rapley G, Musket T. Baby-Led Weaning. Vermilion, 2008.
7. Ito J, Moriyama H, Shimada K. Morphological evaluation of the human facial muscles. Okajimas Folia Anat Jpn 2006;83:7–14.
8. Blair C, Smith A. EMG recording in human lip muscles: Can single muscles be isolated? J Speech Hear Res 1986;29:256-266.
9. Kim JH, Guilleminault C. The nasomaxillary complex, the mandible, and sleep-disordered breathing. Sleep Breath 2011;15:185–193.
10. Camacho M, Li D, Kawai M, et al. Tonsillectomy for adult obstructive sleep apnea: A systematic review and meta-analysis. Laryngoscope 2016;126:2176–2186.
11. Mathur R, Mortimore IL, Jan MA, Douglas NJ. Effect of breathing, pressure and posture on palatoglossaland genioglossal tone. Clin Sci (Lond) 1995;89:441–445.
12. Ghaheri BA, Cole M, Fausel SC, Chuop M, Mace JC. Breastfeeding improvement following tongue-tie and lip-tie release: A prospective cohort study. Laryngoscope 2017;127:1217–1223.

13. Zaghi S, Valcu-Pinkerton S, Jabara M, et al. Lingual frenuloplasty with myofunctional therapy: Exploring safety and efficacy in 348 cases. Laryngoscope Investig Otolaryngol 2019;4:489–496.
14. OMD Matrix: 32 Clinical Markers of an Orofacial Myofunctional Disorder. Academy of Orofacial Myofunctional Therapy, 2016.
15. Okuro RT, Morcillo AM, Ribeiro MAGO, Sakano E, Conti PBM, Ribeiro JD. Mouth breathing and forward head postural effects on respiratory biomechanics and exercise capacity in children. J Bras Pneumol 2011;37:471–479.
16. Chuang LC, Lian YC, Hervy-Auboiron M, Guilleminault C, Huang YS. Passive myofunctional therapy applied on children with obstructive sleep apnea: A 6-month follow-up. J Formos Med Assoc 2017;116:536–541.
17. Robbins J, Butler SG, Daniels SK, et al. Swallowing and dysphagia rehabilitation: Translating principles of neural plasticity into clinically oriented evidence. J Speech Lang Hearing Res 2008;51(suppl):S276–S300.
18. Pittenger C, Duman RS. Stress, depression, and neuroplasticity: A convergence of mechanisms. Neuropsychopharmacology 2008;33:88–109.
19. Guimarães KC, Drager LF, Genta PR, Marcondes BF, Lorenzi-Filho G. Effects of oropharyngeal exercises on patients with moderate obstructive sleep apnea syndrome. Am J Respir Crit Care Med 2009;179:962–966.
20. Camacho M, Certal V, Abdullatif J, et al. Myofunctional therapy to treat obstructive sleep apnea: A systematic review and meta-analysis. Sleep 2015;38:669–675.
21. Zhang F, Tian Z, Shu Y, et al. Efficiency of oro-facial myofunctional therapy in treating obstructive sleep apnoea: A meta-analysis of observational studies. J Oral Rehabil 2022;49:734–745.
22. Van Dyck C, Dekeyser A, Vantricht E, et al. The effect of orofacial myofunctional treatment in children with anterior open bite and tongue dysfunction: A pilot study. Eur J Orthod 2016;38:227–234.
23. Smithpeter J, Covell D Jr. Relapse of anterior open bites treated with orthodontic appliances with and without orofacial myofunctional therapy. Am J Orthod Dentofacial Orthop 2010;137:605–614.
24. Amat P, Tran Lu Y É. The contribution of orofacial myofunctional reeducation to the treatment of obstructive sleep apnoea syndrome (OSA): A systematic review of the literature [in French]. Orthod Fr 2019;90:343–370.
25. Melis M, Di Giosia M, Zawawi KH. Oral myofunctional therapy for the treatment of temporomandibular disorders: A systematic review. Cranio 2022;40:41–47.

The missing pillar in health is breath. It all starts there.

—*James Nestor*

14

A Multidimensional Approach to Addressing Breathing and Sleep Disorders

Patrick McKeown

Conflict of interest: Patrick McKeown is a Buteyko Breathing Educator, the founder of MyoTape, and the owner of MyoTape.com and The Oxygen Advantage.

The way you breathe affects every system, organ, and cell in your body. It can boost your immunity, support the movement of your joints right from your core, and impact cognition, mood, cardiovascular health, athletic performance, craniofacial development, and sleep. Quite simply, breathing optimally can enrich quality of life in every domain. Unfortunately, many people develop daily and nightly breathing patterns that are less than ideal, meaning they miss out on the myriad benefits of breathing functionally. Dysfunctional breathing may manifest as over-breathing, mouth breathing, noisy breathing, yawning or sighing regularly, or breathing primarily into the upper chest. It is estimated that between 6% and 10% of the general population have symptoms of dysfunctional breathing.[1,2] The figure is higher for those with asthma (29%–36%)[3,4] and higher still for those with anxiety disorders (up to 75%).[5]

Dental practitioners are uniquely positioned to raise awareness of the importance of functional breathing. Adopting healthy breathing practices and eliminating dysfunctional breathing habits has enormous potential to benefit the health and well-being of you and your patients. In this chapter, I draw on my 20-plus years of experience researching breathing to outline the

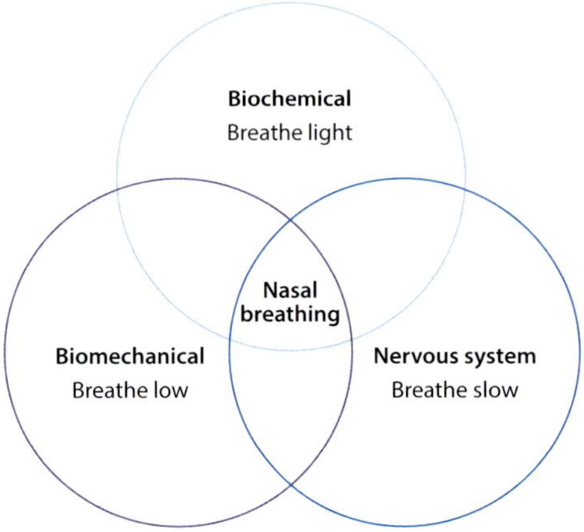

Fig 14-1 Dimensions of functional breathing: Breathe light, breathe low, and breathe slow.

three dimensions of functional breathing, stressing the importance of nasal breathing throughout. I also describe ways to assess dysfunctional breathing in your clinical practice (in both adults and children) and provide simple exercises that can be employed to address it.

THE FOUNDATION: BREATHE LIGHT, LOW, AND SLOW

Functional breathing is underpinned by biochemical, biomechanical, and psychophysiologic dimensions (Fig 14-1). Understanding the multidimensional nature of breathing and the impact of each dimension on mind and body is key. The *biochemical dimension* refers to the balance of carbon dioxide (CO_2) in the blood, which can become too low during chronic hyperventilation. When CO_2 is depleted, cells and organs struggle to get enough oxygen and can become hypoxic. The *biomechanical dimension* refers to the proper functioning of the breathing muscles, especially, though not exclusively, the diaphragm. The *psychophysiologic dimension* refers to the two-way connection between breathing and the nervous system. For example, anxiety causes breathing to become fast and shallow. In turn, fast and shallow breathing perpetuates anxiety. The foundation of healthy breathing patterns is breathing in and out through the nose in a light, slow, and regular breathing pattern, driven by the diaphragm.

Breathe Light: Functional Breathing from a Biochemical Perspective

Many people habitually and unconsciously over-breathe, either via an increased respiratory rate or increased respiratory volume. This impacts the body's biochemistry. To breathe optimally, the body requires the correct homeostatic balance of oxygen (O_2) and CO_2. From a biochemical perspective, breathing too quickly or too deeply—essentially hyperventilating—results in too much CO_2 being expelled. As the partial pressure of CO_2 in the blood decreases, the alkalinity of the blood increases and respiratory alkalosis ensues. In 1904, the physiologist Dr Christian Bohr discovered that if blood CO_2 levels are below the usual range, it makes it more difficult for red blood cells to release O_2 to where it is needed throughout the body, resulting in hypoxia.[6,7]

Because CO_2 is the primary driver to breathe, low levels both cause and perpetuate over-breathing. A person who over-breathes may experience a variety of symptoms, including shortness of breath, cold hands and feet, and feeling panicked or anxious, and they likely have disrupted sleep.[8,9] The tendency to over-breathe can become chronic. It is exacerbated by stress, hormonal changes, overeating, alcohol, and the mistaken belief that prevails in the Western world of the importance of taking a deep breath. Long-term, chronic hyperventilation can have serious consequences; it can contribute to heart disease, high blood pressure, sleep-disordered breathing (SDB), and even early death.[9] You can see why the instruction "take a deep breath," which is pervasive throughout sports, yoga, media, and even medicine, may be detrimental. The respiratory physician Dr Claude Lum, known for his research in hyperventilation, called hyperventilation syndrome the "fat folder" syndrome in reference to the fact that patients are often passed from one specialist to another without getting a clear diagnosis.[10]

Breathing exercises that target the biochemistry of breathing involve manipulating the body's levels of CO_2 to achieve and maintain optimal levels. The Breathe Light exercise (described later in this chapter) involves reducing the volume of air breathed in with light nasal breathing by softening and slowing the breath and by holding the breath to create slight air hunger. Regularly practicing reduced volume breathing reduces the body's sensitivity to CO_2 accumulation. With improved tolerance to CO_2 in the body, the correct balance of O_2 and CO_2 is restored. The respiratory rate slows down, breathing becomes lighter, and circulation and O_2 delivery improves to tissues and organs throughout the body, including the heart and brain.

Practicing the Breathe Light exercise is what got me hooked on breathing techniques. Within a couple of minutes of performing the exercise, I could intrinsically feel the difference it was making in my body. I could feel the temperature increase in my hands, a sign that my circulation had improved. I could also feel increased saliva in my mouth, a sign that my body had shifted into a parasympathetic "rest and digest" state. The effects on my cardiovascular and nervous systems were apparent and immediate. Breathe Light has been a staple of my daily practice ever since.

Breathe Low: Functional Breathing from a Biomechanical Perspective

The biomechanical dimension of optimal breathing encompasses the functioning of the breathing muscles. Lungs are like sponges; they cannot get bigger on their own. Muscles in the chest and abdomen contract to create intra-abdominal pressure, the diaphragm moves downward, and there is lateral expansion of the lower two ribs, causing air to flow in. Upon exhalation, the muscles relax, and the lungs deflate on their own, much like a balloon. Breathing muscles include the diaphragm, the intercostal muscles, and the abdominal muscles. The muscles of the face, mouth, and pharynx also play a role; these control the lips, tongue, soft palate, and other structures to help with breathing.[11] Problems with any of these muscles can narrow the airway, make it more difficult to breathe, and contribute to sleep apnea.

Poor breathing from a biomechanical dimension manifests as upper chest breathing instead of breathing low and engaging the diaphragm. Spending long hours working at a computer, leaning over the dentist's chair, or staring at a smartphone can cause the body to slump forward, compromising the amount of space available and restricting diaphragmatic movement. Upper chest breathing requires effort from smaller breathing muscles. These accessory muscles are useful for lifting the ribs up and out but are not designed to be active all the time. Just as muscular imbalance in the joints can lead to repetitive strain injury, this overuse contributes to the development of trigger points and back and neck pain and strain.

Functional breathing patterns also play an important role in the mechanical stability and mobility of the spine and trunk. When you breathe from your diaphragm, the resulting intra-abdominal pressure supports your spine and pelvis, and this is integral to core strength. Breathing low uses the diaphragm and enhances breathing efficiency, improving arterial oxygenation as more air gets to the alveoli in the lungs, enhancing O_2 and CO_2 exchange with the blood, and bringing benefits throughout the body.

Breathing exercises to help improve the biomechanics of breathing involve light and low nasal breathing with lateral expansion and contraction of the lower ribs. Optimizing the biomechanics of breathing may be achieved by

Fig 14-2 The cycle of stress and dysfunctional breathing.

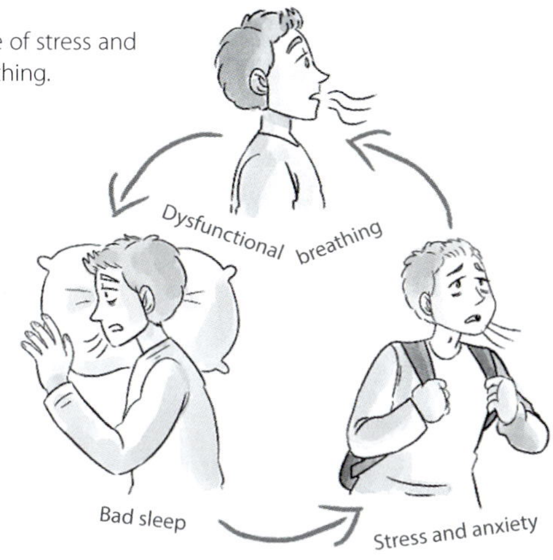

wearing a Buteyko Belt or simply by practicing breathing exercises while lying down and placing a sandbag or book on the diaphragm to bring awareness to the area. These exercises result in greater diaphragmatic recruitment and efficient functioning of the breathing muscles. Benefits include improved stabilization of the spine, breathing efficiency, a calmer mind, shifting the body into "rest and digest" mode, and better sleep quality.

Breathe Slow: Functional Breathing from a Psychophysiologic Perspective

Breathing slowly can have considerable physiologic effects on the mind and body, impacting mood, heart rate, respiratory rate, blood pressure, digestion, concentration, energy levels, and sleep. There is a bidirectional relationship between breathing and emotions. When we feel stressed or anxious, breathing becomes faster, harder, irregular, and predominantly limited to the upper chest. When breathing is dysfunctional, you're more likely to experience anxiety, chronic stress, and negative, repetitive thoughts. There is also a bidirectional relationship between breathing and sleep. When breathing is faster, harder, into the upper chest, or through an open mouth, sleep quality and quantity will suffer; a bad night's sleep will subsequently leave you anxious, stressed, and dehydrated[12]— all states that perpetuate dysfunctional breathing (Fig 14-2).

Slow breathing can be employed to modulate the stress response and switch states as required. The sympathetic branch of the autonomic nervous system is responsible for the "fight-or-flight" stress response, such as an increase in heart rate and pupil dilation. This system functions as a short-term stress response, but daily stressors such as financial pressures, a busy work schedule, and family commitments can cause the fight-or-flight reaction to stay turned on, with the body remaining in a constant state of physiologic arousal. Long-term activation of the stress response system results in overexposure to cortisol and other stress hormones, affecting virtually every system in the body, either directly or indirectly. When stressed, we may find it difficult to concentrate and think clearly. We likely also feel anxious and irritable, find it hard to relax, and can experience headaches or other body pains, changes in appetite, upset stomach, or trouble sleeping.[13] When symptoms of stress become persistent and affect daily functioning, they can have a detrimental impact on health and well-being. Chronic stress can worsen preexisting health problems, such as heart disease, hypertension, diabetes mellitus, and irritable bowel syndrome,[14] and has also been shown to induce inflammation in the body, both peripherally and centrally.[15]

Breathing provides a powerful and direct gateway to the autonomic nervous system, allowing you to modulate internal states by maintaining parasympathetic-sympathetic balance.[16] Slow, diaphragmatic breathing stimulates the vagus nerve, the main nerve of the parasympathetic nervous system. The vagus nerve controls organ functions including digestion, heart rate, respiratory rate, perspiration, and muscle sensations. On exhalation, the vagus nerve secretes the neurotransmitter acetylcholine, which causes blood vessels to dilate and slows heart rate. Studies have shown that slow breathing can result in increased comfort, relaxation, a feeling of pleasantness, vigor and alertness, and reduced symptoms of arousal, anxiety, depression, and anger.[17]

Ideally, the nervous system is resilient and adaptive, upregulating into sympathetic mode only when a period of focused, alert attention is required or to cope with an unexpected stressor and then swiftly downregulating into parasympathetic mode and returning to a calm or relaxed state. To optimize breathing from a psychophysiologic perspective, simply breathe more slowly, reducing the respiratory rate to between 4.5 and 6.5 breaths per minute. This slower breath balances the autonomic nervous system, dampening the stress response activated by chronic hyperventilation and activating the parasympathetic relaxation response, thereby calming body and mind—and improving sleep quality.

The Importance of Nasal Breathing

Breathing through the nose is fundamental to functional breathing. As far back as 1954, ENT (ear, nose, and throat) specialist Dr Maurice Cottle, who founded the American Rhinologic Society, wrote that the human nose has 30 functions. I was unable to locate Dr Cottle's list, so more recently, I embarked on compiling a list myself (found at the end of this chapter). No doubt, the functions I list are different than Dr Cottle's, as the science has developed. That withstanding, the numerous functions of the nose are a testament to how important this organ is for health and well-being.

The nose is designed to help you breathe most efficiently. It filters, warms, and humidifies the air we breathe. We can extract about 10% to 20% more oxygen breathing through the nose than we can with equivalent breaths through the mouth.[18,19] Nasal breathing is slower and draws the air into the lower parts of the lungs. As a result, air stays in the lungs longer, and the body has more time to extract O_2 from that air. Breathing nasally can also help to maintain the strength and function of the breathing muscles and reduce breathlessness.

Nasal breathing protects against airborne viruses, bacteria, allergens, and other pathogens, and it opens the blood vessels in the lungs, allowing better O_2 diffusion. During nasal breathing, nitric oxide (NO) is produced in the nasal cavity and carried into the lungs. This provides many important functions. NO has antiviral and antibacterial qualities, so it protects against infections. The high concentration of NO in the sinuses is instrumental in keeping the nose, throat, and lungs free of disease and inflammation. NO also helps to widen blood vessels, so it can lower blood pressure and significantly increase the oxygen-absorbing capacity of the lungs. It can also widen the airways and relax the muscles in the lungs, making breathing easier and minimizing symptoms for those with asthma and rhinitis. When nasal breathing is combined with slow breathing, this allows an even greater concentration of NO to be carried into the lungs, yielding greater benefits.

Adult breathing patterns may be assessed using a measurement tool called the Control Pause (described later in this chapter). As the Control Pause score increases, breathing becomes slower, and it is likely that a higher Control Pause score leads to improved uptake and use of NO. Regardless of your current Control Pause score, you should breathe only through your nose during rest, physical exercise, and sleep.

Unfortunately, many people breathe habitually through an open mouth during wakefulness and/or sleep, which can have many negative consequences, including poor craniofacial development, crooked teeth, and dental caries.[20] Studies estimate the incidence of mouth breathing in children to be between 25% and 50%.[21–23] In the adult population, a 17% incidence of mouth breathing is reported.[24,25] Mouth breathing promotes over-breathing and upper chest breathing. As already discussed, dysfunctional breathing impacts the body's physiology; blood circulation and O_2 delivery are reduced throughout the body, and the body's stress response is activated.

Despite the knowledge of nasal functions dating back 70 years and the many benefits of nasal breathing, there is still a lack of general awareness of the importance of breathing in and out through the nose in dentistry, medicine, and healthcare. This is partly due to the difficulty in diagnosing mouth breathing. Another obstacle is that health care professionals are so often stretched with busy workloads that they simply do not have time to educate and train patients in respiratory rehabilitation.

Sleep-Disordered Breathing

Sleep disorders affect the quality, timing, and amount of sleep on a regular basis. There are different types of sleep disorders, including insomnia, obstructive sleep apnea (OSA), and narcolepsy. Every year, problems with falling asleep or daytime sleepiness affect approximately 35% to 40% of the US adult population.[26] Sleep disorders often co-occur with other medical and/or mental health conditions and have a deleterious effect on energy, mood, concentration, memory, and overall health. Disrupted sleep has serious adverse short- and long-term health consequences because sleep plays such a vital role in brain function and many body systems.

Sleep (like ideal breathing) has a powerfully positive, restorative effect on the brain. Just like our body has a lymphatic system that helps remove waste products from our tissues, our brain has a similar system called the *glymphatic system*. The glymphatic system works by using a network of specialized cells called *astrocytes* that surround the blood vessels in the brain, forming a network of tunnels that allows cerebrospinal fluid to flow freely around the brain tissue. This cerebrospinal fluid flushes out the waste and toxins that have accumulated during the day.

A 2015 study found that when participants slept well throughout the night, the cellular waste by-products that accumulated in and around the brain cells during the day were thoroughly removed. The researchers concluded that one of the primary purposes of sleep is as a sort of "garbage disposal for the brain." When sleep is denied, the active process of the glymphatic system does not have time to remove waste products, so potentially neurotoxic waste products, such as amyloid beta (which is known to accumulate in conditions like Alzheimer disease), can build up. Short-term, these effects are apparent in poor cognitive abilities, behavior, and judgment. Long-term, it has been suggested that sleep deprivation could have more serious negative consequences on brain health.[27]

Many sleep disorders are characterized by abnormal breathing patterns, particularly mouth breathing. Mouth breathing makes sleep lighter, and the risk of sleep apnea is higher. In a study of 95 persons with established sleep apnea, only 37% breathed solely through the nose. The remaining 63% either breathed solely through the mouth or switched between nose and mouth breathing during sleep.[28] The study found that mouth breathing was significantly associated with worse oxygen desaturation and an increased degree of upper airway collapse. Breathing through an open mouth activates the stress response, and it leaves the airways more vulnerable to collapse, which can trigger snoring and even cause breathing to periodically stop altogether.

Breathing exercises can help significantly reduce symptoms of snoring, insomnia, and sleep apnea. Integrating light, low, and slow nasal breathing into everyday habits can help you to achieve a restful night's sleep and awaken feeling refreshed and energized. Above all, it is vital to restore nasal breathing during sleep. The following sections describe how to assess and address dysfunctional breathing in adults, children, and teens. The chapter closes with a list of the functions of the nose, illustrating just how fundamental nasal breathing is.

ASSESSING AND ADDRESSING DYSFUNCTIONAL BREATHING IN ADULTS

So, how might you tell if a patient or client has dysfunctional breathing patterns? Chronic hyperventilation can present in a far less dramatic way than acute hyperventilation, thereby evading detection. Dysfunctional breathing patterns can manifest in a variety of ways. You may notice that your patient is breathing through an open mouth, or they may be breathing a little fast and hard, or into their upper chest. They may report having fast, audible breath during rest or gentle movement, along with yawning regularly and feeling tired during the day.

Assessing Breathing Using the Control Pause

The Control Pause is a simple measurement tool to assess adult breathing patterns. You may use it to assess your own breathing and that of your patients. The Control Pause measures the number of seconds a person can comfortably hold their breath after exhalation. It will increase as breathing improves and can be used to track progress. When measuring the Control Pause, it is important not to push beyond the first distinct urge to breathe. This isn't a competitive challenge, nor is it a measure of willpower.

How to measure the Control Pause

Although the Control Pause may be measured at any time of the day, to get the most accurate measurement, the Control Pause should be performed in the morning, before the day begins. A timer or stopwatch that counts seconds will be needed. The steps are as follows:

1. Sit upright in a straight-backed chair or on a mat.
2. Allow your breathing to settle.
3. When you feel your breathing is quiet and steady, take a normal silent breath in and out through your nose.
4. After the exhalation, pinch your nose to hold your breath.
5. Time in seconds until you feel the first reaction by the body to resume breathing.
6. When you feel that first definite desire to breathe, let go of your nose and breathe in through it.

After the breath-hold, breathing should immediately be calm and quiet. The first definite desire to breathe may be a contraction in the diaphragm or throat or just a psychologic need for air. This is not a perfect measure of breathing, and it is not a "test" to be done competitively. It simply indicates how functional your breathing is today. If you find yourself (or your patients) getting obsessed with the Control Pause score, forget about it for a few weeks.

The Control Pause score gives feedback about breathlessness and sensitivity to CO_2. A Control Pause score ≥ 25 seconds equates to ease of breathing. A Control Pause score < 25 seconds, especially between 10 or 15 seconds, indicates breathing that is fast, hard, and into the upper chest. The breathing exercises that follow work by increasing tolerance to changes in CO_2 in the blood. This makes breathing slower, easier, and steadier.

Exercises for Dysfunctional Breathing Patterns

Because breathing is regulated by the autonomic nervous system, it is largely an automatic and involuntary action; however, it can also be subject to voluntary control. The first step is identifying and bringing awareness to the habits or breathing practices that may have crept in that are less than ideal. Once dysfunctional habits are identified, it is possible to retrain dysfunctional breathing patterns by consistently practicing a handful of simple breathing exercises. The instructions for breathing exercises found in the rest of this chapter can be shared with patients who are interested in correcting compromised breathing patterns.

Nose Unblocking exercise

If the nose is congested, you are likely to revert to mouth breathing, and this will inhibit a restful night's sleep. To decongest the nose, practice the following exercise. Take care, as this exercise involves holding the breath until a strong air hunger is experienced. This exercise is not suitable for people with high or low blood pressure, anxiety, panic disorder, or cardiovascular issues, or during pregnancy. If you do have any of these conditions, hold your breath for a maximum of only 15 seconds.

1. Take a normal breath in and out through your nose.
2. Pinch your nose with your fingers to hold your breath.
3. As you hold your breath, move your body, or gently nod your head up and down.
4. Hold your breath for as long as you can, until you feel moderate to strong air hunger.
5. Let go of your nose, and breathe through it as calmly as possible.
6. Repeat six times, resting for 30 to 60 seconds between each repetition.

Practice the Nose Unblocking exercise as often as necessary, and try wearing a nasal dilator during rest, exercise, and sleep to alleviate the feeling of air hunger. In time, with sustained practice of the breathing exercises and an improved Control Pause score, the feeling of nasal congestion will dramatically reduce. Until that happens, you can use this exercise whenever you need to, even when you have a stuffy nose because of a bad cold!

Breathe Light exercise

The goal of this exercise is to gently soften your breathing rate and volume to generate a feeling of air hunger that makes you feel like taking in a slightly bigger breath. After a short while practicing this exercise, CO_2 will accumulate in your blood, creating the feeling that you would like to take in more air. This is valuable feedback that you are performing the exercise correctly and reducing your breathing volume toward normal.

The air hunger you feel during this exercise should be tolerable. If you notice that your breathing rhythm is becoming fast or chaotic, or if the need for air is too much, stop the exercise and breathe normally for half a minute, then resume gentle, light breathing to create a tolerable need for air once more. As you practice the exercise, pay attention to whether you feel drowsy, have warmer hands, or have increased watery saliva in the mouth. These signs indicate that you have activated the rest (feeling drowsy) and digest (increased watery saliva) response.

Breathe Light is the most important exercise to help improve breathing patterns during wakefulness and sleep. Using it will help with insomnia, snoring, and sleep apnea.

1. Place one hand on your chest and one hand on your abdomen.
2. Gently soften and slow down your breathing to create a slight hunger for air.
3. Slow down the speed of air as it enters your nostrils.
4. Allow the breath out to be slow and relaxed.
5. The goal is to breathe softly so that about 30% less air enters your lungs.
6. You are performing the exercise correctly when you feel a tolerable air hunger.
7. If the air hunger is too much, rest for 15 seconds and start again.
8. Practice this exercise for 5 minutes, four times daily.

Breathe Slow exercise

Insomnia and obstructive sleep apnea exert stress on the body and mind. Slowing down breathing helps to bring balance to the automatic functioning of the body. Research over the past 30 years reports that slowing the breathing rate to between 4.5 and 6.5 breaths per minute helps to bring the body and mind into balance.

1. Breathe in silently through your nose for a count of 5 seconds.
2. Breathe out silently through your nose for a count of five seconds. This Breathe Slow practice amounts to a respiratory rate of six breaths per minute.
3. Practice this exercise for 10 minutes daily.

Nose, Slow, and Low exercise

To improve breathing patterns, practice this exercise for 5 minutes, one to two times daily. An ideal time to practice is when you first go to bed.

1. Lie on your back with knees bent (this helps to engage the diaphragm).
2. Place your hands on the sides of your lower ribs.
3. As you breathe in through your nose, feel your lower ribs moving out.
4. As you breathe out through your nose, feel your lower ribs gently moving in.

The goal is for about 20% of the movement to be driven by the diaphragm and 80% from the upper chest. Ideally, breathing is nasal, light, slow, and deep. Breathe deeply and lightly at the same time. Note that there is no need to fill your lungs with air. The key to good breathing is breathing softly, silently, and through the nose into the lower regions of the lungs.

Breathing exercises for insomnia

A racing mind and breathing irregularities both contribute to insomnia. When you find yourself lying awake in the middle of the night, this can be partly due to dysfunctional breathing during sleep. However, the hyperarousal caused by overstimulation of the mind is also to blame. To tackle insomnia, it is necessary to activate the body's relaxation response. It is also essential to improve breathing patterns during sleep so that the airway can function without causing the breath to stop or adding resistance to breathing.

DIFFICULTY FALLING ASLEEP

- Make sure you breathe only through your nose during rest, physical exercise, and sleep.
- Practice the Breathe Light exercise for 15 minutes before sleep.

FREQUENTLY WAKING UP AFTER 4 OR 5 HOURS OF SLEEP

Waking up after a few hours of sleep is challenging. You're not quite fully alert to get up and start the day, but you're not tired enough to fall back asleep easily. Disturbances to breathing during sleep, including partial or total collapse of the throat, can cause awakening. If you experience this, practice the steps below.

- Bring your attention to your breathing to help calm racing thoughts.
- Practice the Breathe Light exercise to activate your body's relaxation response.
- Improve your Control Pause by continuing with daily practice. Once your Control Pause score is greater than 20 seconds, air turbulence in your nose and throat will reduce. You will sleep more deeply and be less likely to wake during the night.
- Listen to the 20-minute guided breathing and relaxation for insomnia, spoken by Patrick and available on YouTube and Spotify. Google "Patrick McKeown guided insomnia." It works, and you are likely to be asleep by the end of the track.

Breathing exercises for snoring

Mouth snoring is the result of a large volume of air passing through a collapsible airway, causing the soft palate to vibrate. It stops when the mouth is closed during sleep. Nose snoring is caused by turbulent airflow in the nasal airway, where the nose meets the throat (the nasopharynx). Obstruction of the nose caused by nasal stuffiness, a deviated septum, or an anatomically smaller nose can increase resistance to breathing. However, hard and fast breathing also contributes to nasal snoring.

To illustrate the impact of faster and harder breathing during nasal snoring, I often ask my students to make the sound of a snore through the nose. To do this, it is normal to tighten the throat at the back of the nose and speed up breathing. Now, begin to slow down the speed of your breathing, in and out through the nose. Slow down your breathing until it is almost imperceptible. Breathe hardly any air in and out of the nose. Now, try to snore when your breathing is light and slow. You will find it more difficult. Snoring is not solely due to a compromised nasal airway. Breathing patterns can also play a role. Having a low Control Pause score with a faster respiratory rate and increased volume of air per minute contributes to turbulence in the upper airway. While most interventions target the airway, the missing piece of the puzzle is flow. Any engineer investigating resistance to flow in a pipe will consider not only the diameter of the pipe but also the speed and volume of the flow.

It's important to get snoring under control, not only for the sake of a better night's sleep (and the sake of your sleeping partner) but also because if left untreated, it can become more severe and progress to OSA.

To stop mouth snoring:

- Use MyoTape (or similar medical-grade tape for the skin) to keep the mouth closed during sleep. You simply cannot snore through the mouth when breathing is through the nose.

To significantly reduce nasal snoring:

- Decongest your nose using the Nose Unblocking exercise.
- Practice nasal breathing during wakefulness and sleep.
- Reduce the flow of breathing by practicing Breathe Light for 10 minutes, four times a day.
- Increase your Control Pause score to above 20 seconds.

For many people, nasal snoring can be eliminated altogether. For others, particularly those with a narrow airway, nasal snoring will continue but at a lower intensity, meaning it won't be so loud and problematic.

Breathing exercises for OSA

People with OSA tend to snore very loudly, and they experience frequent episodes of shallow breathing (hypopnea) and pauses in breathing (apnea) lasting 10 seconds or more. The first step in treating OSA is to make the switch to nasal breathing during sleep. This is important even for those who use a continuous positive airway pressure (CPAP) machine or mandibular advancement device (MAD) to treat sleep apnea. Mouth breathing is a common factor for CPAP noncompliance because air that is meant to keep the airway open leaks out through your open mouth instead. A more recent study of 21 persons with sleep apnea (Apnea-Hypopnea Index [AHI] between 10 and 50 events per hour) that investigated the application of mouth tape with a MAD found that this combination is more effective than the MAD alone.[29]

Mouth taping by itself, however, is not sufficient to address sleep apnea. People with a low Control Pause breathe more into the upper chest with a harder and faster breathing pattern. Exhalations are not slow and prolonged, due to the faster breathing rate. Enforced nasal breathing could add additional resistance to breathing on the exhalation simply because there is not enough time for the exhalation to take place. Hence, the exhalation may take place through the mouth in a mouth-puffing phenomenon, a characteristic more common in mouth breathers during sleep. Persons with severe sleep apnea are more likely to experience intermittent mouth puffing in comparison to those with mild or moderate sleep apnea.[30] In this vein, it is important for people with sleep apnea to improve their functional breathing patterns during wakefulness.

To help reduce the severity of OSA, there are two considerations:

1. You need to open your airway so that it is less likely to collapse during sleep.

- Breathe through your nose during wakefulness and sleep, with the tongue resting on the roof of your mouth.
- Breathe low, with optimal recruitment of the diaphragm.
- Lose some weight (if appropriate), as this helps to reduce fat deposits in the throat, allowing for a wider airway.

2. You need to normalize your breathing volume.

- Improve your everyday breathing as reflected by a higher Control Pause. Every 5-second improvement to your Control Pause indicates that your breathing volume is normalizing.
- With improved breathing patterns, breathing becomes lighter, slower, and deeper through the nose. Also, with a higher breath hold time, breathing is more stable during sleep.
- Breathing lightly and slowly during sleep reduces negative pressure in the airway, thereby reducing the risk of collapse.

Breathing Through the Nose During Sleep

We've already described why it is vital to breathe through your nose during sleep, but how can you make sure it happens? When you wake up in the morning, your mouth should be naturally moist. If you have been breathing through your mouth at night, you will wake up with a dry mouth. You may also find that you have smelly breath. Mouth breathers have a higher incidence of gum disease, halitosis, and tooth decay than nasal breathers.

If you tend to mouth breathe during the night, you can try mouth taping, following these guidelines. Taping the mouth at night may seem like a scary prospect at first. However, the method has been used with great success by Oxygen Advantage trained instructors and in Buteyko Breathing Clinics around the world. It may be reassuring to know that it does not take long to get used to. I have no doubt that the single best thing I ever did to improve my sleep was to tape my mouth at night. For persons with OSA, it is important that the tape does not cover the mouth, as this prevents mouth puffing and may worsen the severity of OSA. Ideally, the tape is placed surrounding the mouth, bringing the lips together to help ensure nasal breathing while at the same time allowing mouth puffing if necessary. There are different tape options available, including MyoTape, which allows mouth puffing and is available from MyoTape.com.

To overcome any initial anxiety about having your mouth taped, try wearing the tape for 20 minutes before you go to bed. Also, be aware that if you are accustomed to breathing through your mouth, the tape is likely to fall off during the first couple of nights. This will resolve fairly quickly. Within a few days, your body will relearn its natural nasal breathing pattern, and the tape will remain in place. You may then begin to experience the best sleep you have ever had.

If your nose is partially blocked before going to bed, use the Nose Unblocking exercise to clear it before taping your mouth. Rest assured, however, that if you are wearing the lip tape at night, your nose will never become completely blocked. This is because nasal breathing helps to dilate the nasal passages. If you breathe heavily during the night while wearing the tape, your nose may partially block. If this is the case, you may also find it helpful to wear a nasal dilator, which can be purchased online. This small plastic dilator is placed inside the nose to open the nasal passages and alleviate snoring. In time, if you follow the breathing exercises and techniques in this book and as your nasal congestion improves, you will be less likely to require a nasal dilator.

If, during the night, you find it difficult to breathe while using the tape, gently reduce your breathing until you feel comfortable. Try to acclimatize to the tape rather than removing it. Without it, you are likely to revert to mouth breathing during sleep, and this will only make your symptoms worse. For a more detailed explanation of the link between everyday breathing and OSA, read McKeown et al.[31]

Do NOT use MyoTape or any other lip tape at night if you are feeling nauseated or have been drinking alcohol. If your child has an upset stomach or is likely to vomit, do NOT tape his or her mouth during sleep.

Daily Practice Instructions for Adults

- Breathe only through your nose during rest, physical exercise, and sleep.
- Adopt the correct tongue resting posture. Three-quarters of your tongue should rest on the roof of your mouth, with the tip of your tongue placed behind, but not touching, your top front teeth.
- Achieve a minimum Control Pause score of 20+ seconds.
- Practice Breathe Light for 5 minutes, four to six times daily. Schedule the 5-minute intervals throughout the day, and schedule a full 10 minutes of this practice before sleep.
- Walking or any physical exercise with the mouth closed is a tremendous practice for improving sleep quality. Walk for 30 minutes to 1 hour daily at an intensity where you feel comfortably breathless. If you need to breathe through an open mouth, slow the pace of your walk.
- To ensure you're breathing through your nose, tape your mouth closed while sleeping. A dry mouth signifies open-mouth breathing during sleep, so if your mouth is naturally moist in the morning, there is no need for the tape.

The Oxygen Advantage app is available for healthcare professionals and patients free of charge and includes all breathing exercises and a daily plan.

Assessing and Addressing Dysfunctional Breathing in Children and Teens

To help children and teens change their breathing habits, they need to understand the importance of breathing through the nose. When I work with young people, I ask them which reasons they consider to be the most important when it comes to breathing nasally. The most popular replies tend to focus on athletic performance and the development of a good-looking face. I find it best not to highlight the negative features of mouth breathing when talking to children. Instead, I find they respond well to hearing about the many benefits of nasal breathing. The following ideas may be helpful.

- **Nasal breathing makes you more intelligent:** Explain that intelligent people breathe in and out through their noses. Nasal breathing improves cognition, concentration, alertness, and energy levels because it promotes better sleep and delivers more oxygen to the brain. This helps children to focus better in class, so learning will be easier and more enjoyable.
- **Nasal breathing improves sports performance:** When children habitually mouth breathe, they tend to become breathless quickly during sports or physical exercise. This might make them reluctant to take part in healthy activities they would otherwise enjoy. Professional athletes, Olympians, Special Forces, and military personnel all use breathing techniques to improve their performance during training.
- **Mouth breathing causes crooked teeth and bad breath:** No teenager wants to have bad breath. Nasal breathing helps to maintain a healthy mouth and prevent smelly breath.[32] It can also avert problems in the development of the face, such as narrow jaws; crooked, overcrowded teeth; and small upper airways.
- **Breathing through the nose helps you sleep better and gives you more energy:** Mouth breathing interferes with a good night's sleep, and you will have less energy to enjoy life.
- **Mouth breathing is bad for posture:** Persistent mouth breathing during early childhood can lead to changes in posture as the head is thrust forward to optimize the oral airway.[33] This, along with a tendency to breathe into the upper chest, will have a detrimental effect on the stability of the spine. These things may not be particularly motivating for children, but parents will understand their importance.
- **Nasal breathing leads to good table manners:** If the child has a blocked nose, he or she may have difficulty eating. Nasal congestion makes it tricky to coordinate breathing and swallowing, so the child may need to stop chewing or chew faster to breathe through the mouth. This breathlessness may look like bad table manners as the child sniffs and gulps his way through each meal.

In all cases, the best place to start is by encouraging nasal breathing both day and night. Children under 5 years of age may find it difficult to practice breathing exercises, so parents of young children must take preventative action to avoid the factors that contribute to over-breathing. Children tend to mirror their parents, even in their breathing habits. If mom or dad tends to walk around the house with their mouth open, puffing and panting and not paying attention to their breathing, children will do the same. Likewise, a child will struggle to learn if everybody else in the house continues with their own bad habits. I often see the behavior of parents interfering with the progress of their children in this way. Parents need to lead by example. Only then can you ensure success with breathing reeducation. Luckily, this is a win-win situation because everybody involved will enjoy the benefits.

Help the child to understand what "breathing too much" means and that over-breathing is what causes tiredness, wheezing, coughing, and a stuffy nose. The best way to do this is by giving a physical demonstration. Ask the child to hold out a finger and blow a large puff of air onto their finger. Let them feel the strength and quantity of air on their finger. Explain that this is "big breathing." Then, ask the child to blow a tiny amount of air onto their finger. This should be so light they can hardly feel it at all. Explain that this is correct breathing. You can also ask the child to explain the ideas behind good breathing to other people in the household. This will allow the child time to reflect on his or her breathing. By listening to the storytelling and description the child gives, you will be able to tell how well the theory has been understood.

Assessing Children's Breathing Using the Steps Exercise

The Steps exercise is both a main exercise and a measurement of progress for children. The exercise is simple and safe for the vast majority of children. A child's Steps score, though not a perfect measurement, provides some feedback about breathing patterns. It may be useful to place tape across the child's lips during the Steps exercise (a suitable tape is 1-inch Micropore tape from 3M or similar). This will help to ensure the child maintains nasal breathing during the exercise. It is also useful to ascertain how comfortable nasal breathing is for the child after doing the exercise. Holding the breath to achieve a moderate to strong air hunger has no reported risks for healthy children, and as I discovered during my teaching time, taping to bring the lips together is an invaluable tool in breathing reeducation.

Warning: If a child, teen, or adult has pulmonary hypertension, epilepsy, or any serious medical condition, they must NOT practice the Steps exercise.

If the child has diabetes mellitus, be aware that breath-holding exercises can lower blood sugar levels. Give the child a snack before practicing the exercise and monitor blood sugar levels frequently during the Steps exercise. If the child is wheezy or coughing, limit the Steps exercise to between 10 and 20 paces. The Steps exercise will help improve asthma and reduce the child's symptoms, but it is important that breathing at the end of the exercise remains controlled. Heavy breathing after a breath hold can exacerbate symptoms.

The following Steps exercise is practiced by children to help open their airways and improve breathing patterns:

1. Exhale through the nose.
2. Pinch the nose with fingers to hold the breath.
3. Walk or run while holding the breath.
4. When the air hunger is relatively strong, let go of the nose and breathe in.
5. Walk a few paces to recover breathing.
6. Try to get breathing under control within a few breaths.
7. Rest for about 1 minute, and whenever you feel comfortable, repeat.

It is best to avoid practicing this exercise right after meals. The Steps exercise should be performed six times per set, with about 30 to 60 seconds of rest between each repetition. Sets of Steps are to be practiced two times per day. Count the Steps out loud, and record the child's score so that progress can be monitored from week to week. Compare each week's Steps with the previous scores to evaluate improvement and encourage the child to increase the number of steps they take. Some children can be motivated with star charts and rewards. The Steps exercise can also be incorporated into other activities, such as skipping or running.

Breath hold exercises such as the Steps exercise can be very effective for decongesting the nose. However, if the child repeatedly removes the tape due to a feeling of air hunger despite having practiced six repetitions of the Steps exercise, there may be an obstruction at the back of the nose due to enlarged adenoids. If the adenoids and tonsils are enlarged, seek advice from a doctor or health care professional. It may be beneficial to explore maxillary expansion, myofunctional therapy, and the other exercises contained in this chapter to help develop the airway and restore nasal breathing patterns.

Young children have a relatively strong response to the build-up of CO_2 in the blood, although this will lessen as they get older. With this in mind, the Steps exercise should be adapted according to the child's age. Children between 5 and 7 years should aim to achieve 50 to 60 paces during Steps. For children between 8 and 9 years, the goal is to reach 60 to 70 paces. And for children 10 years and over, 80 paces is optimal.

Physical Exercise with the Mouth Closed

The following exercise conveys the importance of breathing through the nose during physical activity. It is also a good exercise to improve respiratory muscle strength, as an extra load is added to the diaphragm. Nasal breathing imposes a resistance to breathing during wakefulness that is two to three times that of the mouth. This helps maintain diaphragm function and strength.

1. Have the child or teenager walk for 1 minute with lips together (preferably with tape) and the tongue in the roof of the mouth.
2. After 1 minute of continuous walking, have the child jog lightly for 1 minute, followed by walking with lips together for 1 minute. Continue to alternate, first jogging and then walking to recover.

SDB in Children and Teens

A restful night's sleep is key to the overall health and emotional well-being of children. Unfortunately, studies estimate that between 4% and 11% of children experience SDB.[34,35] Daytime symptoms of SDB include inattentiveness, difficulty focusing, behavioral and mood problems, morning headaches, fatigue, excessive daytime sleepiness (EDS), and in severe cases, failure to thrive.[36] For parents or caregivers, it can be heartbreaking to see children struggle with this problem, knowing that it's affecting their ability to learn and develop. It can also be frustrating to try to manage a child's behavior when they are tired and irritable.

Children with SDB experience recurrent awakenings throughout the night, resulting in non-restorative sleep. With lighter and poorer quality sleep, slow wave sleep (the most restorative form of sleep) is interrupted. This can have considerable negative consequences, impacting mood, attention, cognition, and behavior.[36,37] Multiple studies report an association between SDB and impulsivity, hyperactivity, aggressive behavior, and decreased attention.[35,38–41] In a study involving over 11,000 British children between the ages of 6 and 57 months, it was reported that children with SDB, if untreated by 5 years of age, had a 40% increased risk of having special educational needs by age 8.[42]

The gold standard of treatment for sleep disorders in children is removal of the adenoids and tonsils. Although practiced since the 1970s, the effectiveness of this procedure was not systematically studied until 2010.[43] Data from 578 children was reviewed, and results showed a significant decrease in sleep apnea severity following removal of the adenoids and tonsils. Disappointingly, only 27% of children had their sleep apnea cured. The remaining 73% continued to have sleep apnea, despite removal of the adenoids and tonsils.

Until 2017, little was known about the long-term health consequences of tonsillectomy and adenoidectomy. These tiny organs in the body, often thought of as just small lumps of flesh in the back of the throat and nose, play a crucial role in a child's immune system, and there can be long-lasting effects if they are removed. A large-scale study was conducted in Denmark with over 1 million people who had undergone either adenoidectomy, tonsillectomy, or adenotonsillectomy.[44] The research subjects had undergone this surgery during the first 9 years of their lives, and the study focused on the health risks they faced 30 years later, specifically those related to the 28 diseases to which this surgery could have exposed them. To effectively weigh the cost-benefit ratio of these surgeries, the study also contrasted the relative risks for these 28 diseases with the absolute risks for the conditions these surgeries were supposed to treat. The findings were quite eye-opening.

First, the study reported that these surgeries significantly impacted people's breathing and overall respiratory health:

> "Tonsillectomy nearly triples the risk of diseases of the upper respiratory tract and adenoidectomy doubles the risk of chronic obstructive pulmonary disorder (COPD) and diseases of the upper respiratory tract and nearly doubles the risk of conjunctivitis."[44]

Overall, when all 28 disease groups were considered, there were significant and consistent, though small, increases in relative risks for at least 78% of them. This suggests that the tonsils are extremely important in normal development. When surgeons remove them, they interfere with many processes necessary for the child's future health.

The study concluded the following:

> "The short-term health benefits of these surgeries for some conditions may not continue up to age 30 years. Indeed, apart from the consistently reduced risk for tonsillitis (after any surgeries) and sleep disorders (after adenoidectomy), longer-term risks for abnormal breathing, sinusitis, chronic sinusitis, and otitis media were either significantly higher after surgery or not significantly different."[44]

Notably, for abnormal breathing, there was no significant change in relative risk up to 30 years of age after any surgery, and only adenoidectomy was beneficial in reducing sleep disorders. This means that whatever short-term benefits the surgery provided, it didn't have a lasting effect on most of these conditions.

Though this study reflects findings in only one country, the conclusions were novel in the health discipline and have certainly challenged the orthodoxy of early removal of the tonsils and adenoids in children. The study also suggests that these tissues, far from being accessories, are essential biologic components of the body that significantly contribute to a child's optimal development. The study also indicated that mild disturbances to children's bodies could have severe and long-term consequences. As the body of research in this field grows, the conversation will become more interesting.

A pertinent question regarding the described study is whether the individuals continued breathing through their mouth after surgery. Mouth breathing, irrespective of tonsillectomy and adenoidectomy, would increase the risk of upper and lower airway disease. Unfortunately, the researchers didn't seem to consider whether the children were breathing through their mouth or nose. In another paper,[45] tonsillectomy and adenoidectomy were found to offer only short-term improvements, unless nasal breathing was restored. Continued breathing through the mouth will affect airway growth, predisposing the patient to airway collapse or sleep apnea later in adulthood. The researchers wrote that the "elimination of oral breathing, ie, restoration of nasal breathing during wake and sleep, may be the only valid 'finish line' in pediatric sleep disordered breathing."[45]

Based on this discussion, SDB in children is both complex and multifactorial. There is no easy solution, and it is imperative for healthcare providers to offer a multidisciplinary approach. Dentists are in an opportune position both to recognize the risk factors for sleep disorders and to provide a long-term solution. Combining maxillary expansion to develop width and forward growth of the face, myofunctional therapy, and functional breathing practices is a safe and noninvasive way to intervene. However, even when the nose is treated and the nasal airway is expanded, it does not always guarantee nasal breathing, which highlights the necessity of functional breathing training. Conversely, dysfunction of the nasal muscle and throat, along with poor posture and faulty breathing patterns, contribute to mouth breathing, highlighting the need for myofunctional therapy.[46]

To gain an understanding of how everyday breathing influences SDB, it is worth taking a look at the association between asthma and sleep apnea in children.[47] Asthma involves narrowing of the lower airway due to chronic inflammation and mucus production. It is one of the most common childhood conditions, affecting 7 million children (8%) in the US.[48] It is a fallacy to differentiate the upper airway from the lower airway; both are linked, and whatever takes place in the lower airway travels to the upper airway and vice versa.[49] Children with asthma often experience a stuffy nose and are tired much of the time. It is common to observe children, especially those with poorly controlled asthma, breathing through an open mouth in a faster and harder, upper chest breathing pattern. This same breathing pattern reduces upper airway space, which increases resistance to breathing during sleep. In addition, habitual open mouth posture during formative years contributes to craniofacial alterations, increasing the risk of OSA. Traits of asthma that promote OSA include nasal obstruction, a narrow upper airway, and an increase in upper airway collapsibility.[50] Not all children with sleep apnea have asthma, but it is important to understand the link between the lower and upper airways and how poor breathing patterns can impact breathing during sleep. More importantly, breathing exercises are an effective tool for improving overall respiratory function.

Using Mouth Tape in Children

During my work with children and parents, I occasionally encountered a child who persistently breathed through an open mouth, no matter how many times we emphasized the importance of nasal breathing. In most cases, these children were able to unblock their noses by practicing the Steps exercise, so it became apparent that their habit of mouth breathing was not due to a nasal obstruction. The parents felt as if they were constantly nagging to no avail, and the child would become frustrated and upset by the constant pressure to breathe through the nose, and I couldn't figure out why this mouth breathing habit continued, despite all our combined efforts. Then I began working much more with lip tape, ensuring that the children wore paper tape across their lips for set periods during the day. This simple but profoundly effective technique was a game changer, resulting in an immediate improvement in nasal breathing habits for those children.

An easy way to ensure consistent and ongoing nasal breathing is to ask children to wear medical-grade paper tape or MyoTape around their lips for at least half an hour each day. It is helpful to combine this with an activity that distracts the child, such as reading, watching TV, or playing on a tablet or phone. If parents have reservations about using tape, you can suggest they try it and see for themselves how taping works and that it will still allow the child to speak. Simply search for my free children's breathing program on YouTube, where you will find my daughter, Lauren, modeling the lip tape.

The best approach when helping children to improve their breathing habits is to be consistent and patient. The idea that it takes 21 days to form or change a habit is unrealistic and outdated. Scientists have found that, on average, a new habit takes 66 days to build, and it can even take as long as 254 days.[51] This time is necessary for new neural connections to become established and for breathing behavior to change. If you are trying to change your own breathing habits, you will need to be equally patient.

- Ask the child to wear MyoTape across the lips for at least half an hour each day. It is best to do this when the child is distracted.
- Use games to introduce the techniques to small children. Be as creative as you like!
- Perform nose clearing/unblocking as needed (using the Steps exercise).
- Practice the Steps exercise while walking, jogging, or running. Do this for six repetitions, two to three times a day. Record the number of steps reached in a diary (or use ButeykoClinic or Oxygen Advantage apps).
- Breathe through the nose at all times!

It is important for parents to be mindful of their child's breathing throughout the day. If at any time they can hear their child breathing or see them breathing with their mouth open, parents should remind the child to breathe gently through the nose with their tongue on the roof of the mouth. Ensure that your child does not let any air sneak in through the mouth. This too can be made into a game, reinforcing the importance of keeping the mouth closed by telling off the "sneaky" air for trying to get in. Children have short attention spans, so games can really help. If a child becomes bored with practicing the exercises, you can replace the Steps exercise with breath holding while playing, jogging, running, hopscotch, performing jumping jacks, or jumping on a trampoline.

To conclude, children can benefit enormously from breathing exercises that promote nasal breathing and help prevent SDB. I believe passionately that this is absolutely vital for each child to reach their full potential. All of my children's breathing programs will always be free of charge. You can find a wealth of tutorial videos on YouTube by searching for "Patrick McKeown children." Exercises for both adults and children are available on the ButeykoClinic and Oxygen Advantage apps. For further information, please visit https://buteykoclinic.com or https://oxygenadvantage.com.

FUNCTIONS OF THE NOSE

As long ago as 1954, ENT specialist Dr Maurice Cottle wrote that the human nose has 30 functions. Over the years, I compiled a list myself. So far, I have also found 30 functions—highlighting just how important nasal breathing is for health and well-being.

Everyday Performance

1. Helps to induce relaxation

Nasal breathing introduces resistance that slows the breathing rate. The nasal passages are smaller than the mouth, which means that air has to pass through them more slowly. This natural resistance helps regulate breathing and promotes relaxation.[52]

2. Improves cognitive function

People with normal nose function also have improved cognitive function and energy levels compared to those with chronic nasal issues. In a study of 100 persons (50 with chronic rhinosinusitis) to investigate cognitive function, participants with nasal congestion were found to have significantly more cognitive dysfunction and fatigue on validated instruments and had worse reaction times on computerized testing.[53]

3. Influences partner choice

The sense of smell is important when choosing a mate.[54] Scientists have discovered that certain signals are picked up via olfaction. Two people with very similar genetic makeup could be related, and inbreeding increases the risk of unfavorable genes being passed down from one generation to another. The influence of body odor in mate selection was confirmed in experiments by Wedekind in 1975, and findings show that women prefer the odor of men who are dissimilar to themselves.

4. Increases visuospatial awareness

In 2019, researchers at the Weizmann Institute in Israel suggested that nasal inhalation could be linked to cognition as part of an evolutionary survival mechanism.[55] A sense of smell is, after all, equated with sniffing out danger. For our distant ancestors, this meant accurately assessing their surroundings to make life-or-death decisions. The Weizmann team theorized that this ancient sensory system might benefit from nasal inhalation and that, in modern life and competitive sports, nasal inhalation might automatically trigger conditions in the brain that optimize visuospatial focus. They demonstrated that nasal breathing synchronized electrical activity in the brain on a wavelength that helped to maximize visuospatial awareness.

5. Mediates olfactory-induced behavioral responses

The sense of smell, a primary function of the nose, plays a significant role in aiding behavioral responses by activating the amygdala and the hippocampus. The amygdala is responsible for the emotional processing of odorant molecules, with odors being able to serve as rewards or punishments in the associative learning process. This means that odors associated with positive states reinforce behaviors that lead to more of the positive state, and vice versa for the negative states. Brain imaging studies have found that activation of the amygdala correlates with pleasant and unpleasant odors, reflecting the link between odors and emotions.[56]

The hippocampus, which is also closely linked to the sense of smell, assists with the learning process and is associated with episodic memory. This is why an odor can lead to the retrieval of a memory from a specific time or place, highlighting the complex interplay between the sense of smell, emotion, and our cognitive processes. You might have experienced a time when a particular scent brought you back to some event years ago.

The nose and its functions shape our behavior, memory, and emotional responses.

6. Reduces vocal effort

Professional singers engage in prolonged periods of breathing through the mouth. This increases the minimum pressure required to initiate and sustain vocal fold oscillation. Compared to oral breathing, nasal breathing can naturally humidify and filter incoming air, which can help prevent irritation and inflammation of the vocal cords, leading to improved voice quality and a lower risk of developing voice disorders. Thus, breathing through the nose can help reduce the vocal effort required during speech. It is important for singers to maintain nasal breathing during their everyday life, including during exercise, rest, and sleep. Breathing through the nose helps to prevent dryness of the larynx.[57]

7. Contributes to nasal resonance

The nose plays a crucial role in speech by creating nasal resonance. This occurs when sound waves from the vocal cords resonate in the nasal cavity, lending a unique quality to the voice. Without the nose, the voice would sound monotone and lack depth. Additionally, nasal resonance helps to add emphasis and nuance to our speech, allowing us to communicate effectively with others. Conversely, too much nasal resonance decreases speech intelligibility and impairs social interaction.[58]

Breathing

8. Improves recruitment of the diaphragm

The diaphragm, which separates the chest from the abdomen, is the main breathing muscle. Breathing through the mouth causes reduced movement of the diaphragm. Conversely, breathing through the nose increases recruitment of the diaphragm.[59] For persons with upper chest breathing, switching to habitual nasal breathing is an important part of rehabilitation. This is relevant to all disciplines dealing with the biomechanical dimension of breathing (eg, physiotherapy, physical therapy, yoga, Pilates, etc).

9. Increases oxygen uptake in the blood

Nose breathing is more effective at increasing oxygen uptake than breathing through the mouth. When our nose is blocked, the oxygen uptake in the blood is reduced. In a study of individuals who continuously breathed through their noses, arterial pressure of oxygen increased by nearly 10%.[60]

10. Produces nitric oxide

The nose produces a molecule known as nitric oxide, which plays a role in maintaining healthy lung function and may help to protect against certain respiratory infections.[61]

11. Dilates blood vessels in the lungs

Breathing through the nose helps dilate blood vessels in the lungs and improves arterial oxygenation.[61]

12. Redistributes blood throughout the lungs

Because human beings stand upright, the gas exchange in the lungs could be negatively impacted in the upper regions of the lungs, but by breathing through the nose, nitric oxide redistributes blood throughout the lungs and increases blood flow by as much as 24% in the upper regions. Nitric oxide from the nose not only improves oxygen transfer from the lungs to the blood in bipedal mammals but also protects the body against infection.[62]

13. Defends against inhaled pathogens

Another crucial function of the nose is to act as a line of defense against inhaled pathogens. When we breathe, the air passes through the nasal passages, which are lined with mucus, hairs, and immune cells. These mechanisms trap and remove harmful particles, such as bacteria and viruses, from the air we breathe, preventing them from entering the lungs.[63] The nose also plays a critical role in the chemical inactivation of pathogens. The nasal cavity contains enzymes and other chemical agents that can destroy harmful substances before they enter the respiratory system. For example, lysozyme is an enzyme found in the nasal mucus that can break down the cell walls of bacteria, rendering them harmless. This chemical defense mechanism is essential to our body's immune system, helping protect us from various airborne threats. Breathing through the nose harnesses nitric oxide, which is produced in the paranasal sinuses. Higher levels of nitric oxide are associated with fewer cold symptoms and airway infections following periods of stress in daily life.[63]

14. Helps maintain lung elasticity

Breathing through the nose imposes resistance to both inspiration and expiration, which in turn helps to maintain normal elasticity of the lungs to ensure optimal conditions for gas exchange.[64]

15. Contributes to thermoregulation

The nose plays a vital role in the body's ability to maintain its core temperature within a specific range. The nasal passages are filled with blood vessels that help dissipate heat from the body. As we inhale, the air passing through the nose is warmed by these blood vessels, helping to regulate our body temperature. The nose can also help prevent overheating in hot environments by increasing blood flow to the skin.[65,66]

16. Humidifies incoming air

The major function of the nose is to humidify air before it reaches the lungs for gas exchange. Conditioning inspired air is achieved through the evaporation of water from the internal surface of the nasal airway. Drawing moist and warm air helps to protect the lungs from drying out and becoming inflamed.[67,68]

17. Regulates water balance

The nose helps regulate water balance in the body by conserving water during exhalation. The air we breathe contains moisture from our respiratory tract as we exhale. The nasal mucosa helps to capture and recycle this moisture, reducing water loss from the body.[69]

Sleep Quality

18. Improves oxygenation during sleep

The nose is critical during sleep for breathing well to improve oxygenation levels. Studies have shown that nasal breathing during sleep leads to more oxygen uptake than mouth breathing. This is particularly important for people with sleep apnea. Proper nasal breathing can reduce the severity of sleep apnea symptoms and improve overall sleep quality.[70]

19. Improves deep sleep

Nasal breathing has been shown to contribute to deeper and more restful sleep. This is because breathing through the nose reduces the severity of snoring and OSA. It is important to wake up with a moist mouth in the morning, which is an important indicator of nasal breathing during sleep.[71,72]

Smell and Taste

20. Smell

Humans have approximately 450 types of olfactory receptors. The nose is a complex and multifaceted organ that performs various critical functions. Its most well-known function is olfaction, which involves detecting and processing odorant molecules in the air. This intricate process involves a series of receptors and nerve pathways that allow us to distinguish between countless scents, from pleasant aromas to unpleasant odors.[73]

21. Sense of smell as a test for neurologic injury

The sense of smell is a sensitive test for neurologic injury associated with traumatic brain injury. In one study, impaired ability to smell was the most common neurologic deficit found in 65 veterans.[74]

22. Taste perception

The nose plays a crucial role in accurately tasting things. This is because the nose communicates with the orbitofrontal cortex, which is the part of the brain responsible for taste perception. This brain center receives taste and smell signals and processes them together, coupling smell and taste. Additionally, the orbitofrontal cortex is responsible for odor perception and discrimination and creating a spatial odor map to recognize specific odors.[75]

Asthma and Rhinitis

23. Controls asthma

Asthma is characterized by inflammation and narrowing of the airways, which can lead to breathing difficulties and other symptoms. Studies have shown that nasal breathing can reduce the severity and frequency of asthma symptoms, mainly asthma that is triggered by exercise. Additionally, some asthma medications are delivered through the nose.[76]

24. Controls allergic rhinitis

Allergic rhinitis, commonly known as hay fever, is a condition that affects millions of people worldwide. It is an allergic reaction to environmental triggers, such as pollen, dust, or animal dander. Symptoms of allergic rhinitis include sneezing, a runny nose, itchy eyes, and nasal congestion. The nose plays a vital role in controlling allergic rhinitis, as it acts as a filter, trapping allergens before they can enter the respiratory system. Additionally, the nasal passages produce mucus, which can help remove allergens from the body. Proper management of allergic rhinitis can significantly improve quality of life, and the nose plays a crucial role in achieving this goal.[66]

25. Nasal dilation

The nose can dilate, or open wider, to allow for increased airflow during exercise or stress. This is a natural response to an increased demand for oxygen and helps to ensure that the body receives enough oxygen during periods of exertion. Holding the breath for 30 seconds or longer has been found to open up the nose to make breathing easier in most subjects who have been tested. Furthermore, it was found that physical exercise decreases nasal resistance.[77]

Physical Exercise

26. Decongests the nose during exercise

Nasal resistance decreases linearly as expired CO_2 levels and exercise levels increase.[78] The constant relationship between nasal resistance and minute ventilation during hypercapnia and exercise suggests that nasal resistance is regulated by the respiratory center to match the level of respiratory demand.

27. Prevents exercise-induced bronchoconstriction

Breathing through the nose during physical exercise markedly reduces post-exercise airway narrowing as compared to breathing through the mouth. This is relevant to all people, whether diagnosed with asthma or not.[79]

28. Contributes to better use of oxygen during exercise

Breathing through the nose during physical exercise reduces the pressure of oxygen expired from the body. This indicates that breathing through the nose is more efficient at extracting O_2 from the lungs and blood to be used by the working muscles.[80]

29. Reduces ventilation

At first, when one switches to breathing through the nose during exercise, the sensation of air hunger is stronger. With sustained practice of nasal breathing during exercise, however, the body adapts to a higher tolerance to the accumulation of CO_2. This is in turn leads to a reduction in ventilation, leading to reduced breathlessness and greater economy. In one study, ventilation (volume of breathing) was reduced by 22% with nasal breathing.[81]

Facial Development

30. Development of the Face

In one study, the breathing mode (nose or mouth) in 47 children was assessed, along with measurements of facial development. The researchers attempted to correlate the effects of nasal obstruction on development of the face. In comparison to nose breathing, mouth breathing in children was more likely to be associated with longer facial structure.[82]

References

1. Thomas M, McKinley RK, Freeman E, Foy C, Price D. The prevalence of dysfunctional breathing in adults in the community with and without asthma. Prim Care Respir J 2005;14:78–82.
2. Kiesel K, Rhodes T, Mueller J, Waninger A, Butler R. Development of a screening protocol to identify individuals with dysfunctional breathing. Int J Sports Physical Ther 2017;12:774.
3. Thomas M, McKinley RK, Freeman RK, Foy C. Prevalence of dysfunctional breathing in patients treated for asthma in primary care: Cross sectional survey. BMJ 2001;322:1098–1100.
4. Martínez-Moragón E, Perpiñá M, Belloch A, De Diego A. Prevalence of hyperventilation syndrome in patients treated for asthma in a pulmonology clinic [in Spanish]. Arch Bronconeumol 2005;41:267–271.
5. Courtney R. Multi-dimensional model of dysfunctional breathing and integrative breathing therapy—Commentary on the functions of breathing and its dysfunctions and their relationship to breathing therapy. J Yoga Phys Ther 2016;6:257.
6. Video Translation of Professor Buteyko from ButeykoClinic.com. Buteyko Clinic, Moscow, 2007.
7. Buteyko Clinic International. The Life of Konstantin Pavlovich Buteyko. https://buteykoclinic.com/about-dr-buteyko/. Accessed 1 March 2024.
8. Dysfunctional Breathing—What Is It and How Can I Manage It? https://londonchestspecialist.co.uk/2021/11/03/dysfunctional-breathing-what-is-it-and-how-can-i-manage-it/. Accessed 1 March 2024.
9. McKeown P. The Breathing Cure: Exercises to Develop New Breathing Habits for a Healthier, Happier and Longer Life. OxyAt Books, 2021.

10. Lum LC. Hyperventilation: The tip and the iceberg. J Psychosom Res 1975;19:375–383.
11. National Heart, Lung, and Blood Institute. How Your Body Controls Breathing. https://www.nhlbi.nih.gov/health/lungs/body-controls-breathing. Accessed 1 March 2024.
12. Rosinger AY, Chang AM, Buxton OM, Li J, Wu S, Gao X. Short sleep duration is associated with inadequate hydration: Cross-cultural evidence from US and Chinese adults. Sleep 2019;42(2).
13. World Health Organization. Stress. https://www.who.int/news-room/questions-and-answers/item/stress. Accessed 1 March 2024.
14. Verywell Mind. How Chronic Stress Impacts Health. https://www.verywellmind.com/chronic-stress-3145104. Accessed 1 March 2024.
15. Liu YZ, Wang YX, Jiang CL. Inflammation: The common pathway of stress-related diseases. Front Hum Neurosci 2017;11:316.
16. Russo MA, Santarelli DM, O'Rourke D. The physiological effects of slow breathing in the healthy human. Breathe 2017;13:298–309.
17. Zaccaro A, Piarulli A, Laurino M, et al. How breath-control can change your life: A systematic review on psycho-physiological correlates of slow breathing. Front Hum Neurosci 2018;12:353.
18. Barelli PA, Loch WE, Kern EB, Steiner A. Rhinology: The Collected Writings of Maurice H. Cottle, MD. American Rhinologic Society, 1987.
19. Lee KJ, Park CA, Lee YB, Kim HK, Kang CK. EEG signals during mouth breathing in a working memory task. Int J Neurosci 2020;130:425–434.
20. Lin L, Zhao T, Qin D, Hua F, He H. The impact of mouth breathing on dentofacial development: A concise review. Front Pub Health 2022;10:929165.
21. Felcar JM, Bueno IR, Massan ACS, Torezan RP, Cardoso JR. Prevalence of mouth breathing in children from an elementary school. Cien Saude Colet 2010;15:437–444.
22. Abreu RR, Rocha RL, Lamounier, Guerra AFM. Prevalence of mouth breathing among children. J Pediatr (Rio J) 2008;84:467–470.
23. De Menezes VA, Leal RB, Pessoa RS, Pontes RMES. Prevalence and factors related to mouth breathing in school children at the Santo Amaro project-Recife, 2005. Braz J Otorhinolaryngol 2006;72:394–399.
24. Izuhara Y, Matsumoto H, Nagasaki T, et al. (2016). Mouth breathing, another risk factor for asthma: The Nagahama Study. Allergy 2016;71:1031–1036.
25. Zaghi S, Peterson C, Shamtoob C, et al. Assessment of nasal breathing using lip taping: A simple and effective screening tool. Int J Otorhinolaryngol 2022;6:10–15.
26. Hossain JL, Shapiro CM. The prevalence, cost implications, and management of sleep disorders: An overview. Sleep Breath 2002;6:85–102.
27. Eugene AR, Masiak J. The neuroprotective aspects of sleep. MEDtube Sci 2015;3:35.
28. Cai Y, Goldberg AN, Chang JL. The nose and nasal breathing in sleep apnea. Otolaryngol Clin North Am 2020;53:385–395.
29. Labarca G, Sands SA, Cohn V, et al. Mouth closing to improve the efficacy of mandibular advancement devices in sleep apnea. Ann Am Thorac Soc 2022;19:1185–1192.
30. Jau JY, Kuo TB, Li LP, et al. Mouth puffing phenomena of patients with obstructive sleep apnea when mouth-taped: Device's efficacy confirmed with physical video observation. Sleep Breath 2023;27:153–164.
31. McKeown P, O'Connor-Reina C, Plaza G. Breathing re-education and phenotypes of sleep apnea: A review J Clin Med 2021;10:471.
32. Motta LJ, Bachiega JC, Guedes CC, Laranja LT, Bussadori SK. Association between halitosis and mouth breathing in children. Clinics 2011;66:939–942.
33. Okuro RT, Morcillo AM, Ribeiro MÂ, Sakano E, Conti PB, Ribeiro JD. Mouth breathing and forward head posture: Effects on respiratory biomechanics and exercise capacity in children. J Bras Pneumol 2011;37:471–479.
34. Lumeng JC, Chervin RD. Epidemiology of pediatric obstructive sleep apnoea. Proc Am Thorac Soc 2008;5:242–252.

35. Di Carlo G, Zara F, Rocchetti M, Venturini A, et al. Prevalence of sleep-disordered breathing in children referring for first dental examination. A multicenter cross-sectional study using pediatric sleep questionnaire. Int J Environ Res Public Health 2020;17:8460.
36. Trosman I, Trosman SJ. Cognitive and behavioral consequences of sleep disordered breathing in children. Med Sci (Basel) 2017;5:30.
37. Jung JY, Kang CK. Investigation on the effect of oral breathing on cognitive activity using functional brain imaging. Healthcare (Basel) 2021;9:645.
38. Gozal D. Sleep-disordered breathing and school performance in children. Pediatrics 1998;102:616–620.
39. Ali NJ, Pitson D, Stradling JR. Sleep disordered breathing: Effects of adenotonsillectomy on behaviour and psychological functioning. Eur J Pediatr 1996;155:56–62.
40. Goldstein NA, Fatima M, Campbell TF, Rosenfeld RM. Child behavior and quality of life before and after tonsillectomy and adenoidectomy. Arch Otolaryngol Head Neck Surg 2002;128:770–775.
41. Bourke R, Anderson V, Yang JS, et al. Cognitive and academic functions are impaired in children with all severities of sleep-disordered breathing. Sleep Med 2011;12:489–496.
42. Bonuck K, Rao T, Xu L. Pediatric sleep disorders and special educational need at 8 years: A population-based cohort study. Pediatr 2012;130:634–642.
43. Bhattacharjee R, Kheirandish-Gozal L, Spruyt K, et al. Adenotonsillectomy outcomes in treatment of obstructive sleep apnea in children: A multicenter retrospective study. Am J Respir Crit Care Med 2010;182:676–683.
44. Byars SG, Stearns SC, Boomsma JJ. Association of long-term risk of respiratory, allergic, and infectious diseases with removal of adenoids and tonsils in childhood. JAMA Otolaryngol Head Neck Surg 2018;144:594–603.
45. Guilleminault C, Sullivan S. Towards restoration of continuous nasal breathing as the ultimate treatment. Goal in pediatric obstructive sleep apnoea. Enliven: Pediatr Neonatol Biol 2014;1:1.
46. Levrini L, Lorusso P, Caprioglio A, et al. Model of oronasal rehabilitation in children with obstructive sleep apnea syndrome undergoing rapid maxillary expansion: Research review. Sleep Sci 2014;7:225–233.
47. Min YZ, Subbarao P, Narang I. The bidirectional relationship between asthma and obstructive sleep apnea: Which came first? J Pediatr 2016;176:10–16.
48. Trivedi M, Mallah ME, Bailey E, et al. Pediatric obstructive sleep apnea and asthma: Clinical implications. Pediatr Ann 2017;46:e332–e335.
49. Bartley J, Wong C. Nasal pulmonary interactions. In: Önerci M (ed). Nasal Physiology and Pathophysiology of Nasal Disorders. Springer, 2013:559–566.
50. Alkhalil M, Schulman E, Getsy J. Obstructive sleep apnea syndrome and asthma: What are the links? J Clin Sleep Med 2009;5:71–78.
51. Lally P, Van Jaarsveld CH, Potts HW, Wardle J. How are habits formed: Modelling habit formation in the real world. Eur J Social Psychol 2010;40:998–1009.
52. Russo MA, Santarelli DM, O'Rourke D. The physiological effects of slow breathing in the healthy human. Breathe (Sheff) 2017;13:298–309.
53. Soler ZM, Eckert MA, Storck K, Schlosser RJ. Cognitive function in chronic rhinosinusitis: A controlled clinical study. Int Forum Allergy Rhinol 2015;5:1010–1017.
54. Ihara Y, Aoki K, Tokunaga K, Takahashi K, Juji T. HLA and human mate choice: Tests on Japanese couples. Anthropolog Sci 2000;108:199–214.
55. Bergland C. Breathe in! Nasal inhalations are linked to laser-like focus. Weizmann Institute of Science, 2019.
56. Kadohisa M. Effects of odor on emotion, with implications. Front Syst Neurosci 2013;7:66.
57. Sivasankar M, Fisher KV. Oral breathing increases Pth and vocal effort by superficial drying of vocal fold mucosa. J Voice 2002;16:172–181.
58. Young A, Spinner A. Velopharyngeal insufficiency. In: StatPearls [Internet]. StatPearls Publishing, 2023.

59. Trevisan ME, Boufleur J, Soares JC, Haygert CJ, Ries LG, Corrêa EC. Diaphragmatic amplitude and accessory inspiratory muscle activity in nasal and mouth-breathing adults: A cross-sectional study. J Electromyogr Kinesiol 2015;25:463–468.
60. Swift AC, Campbell IT, McKown TM. Oronasal obstruction, lung volumes, and arterial oxygenation. Lancet 1988;1(8577):73–75.
61. Lundberg JO, Settergren G, Gelinder S, Lundberg JM, Alving K, Weitzberg E. Inhalation of nasally derived nitric oxide modulates pulmonary function in humans. Acta Physiol Scand 1996;158:343–347.
62. Sánchez CA, Hallberg J, Lundberg JO, et al. Nasal nitric oxide and regulation of human pulmonary blood flow in the upright position. J Appl Physiol (1985) 2010;108:181–188.
63. Nonrespiratory functions of the lung. In: Lumb AB (ed). Nunn's Applied Respiratory Physiology, ed 8. Elsevier, 2017.
64. Nasal Breathing. https://www.sciencedirect.com/topics/medicine-and-dentistry/nasal-breathing. Accessed 29 March 2023.
65. Widdicombe J. Microvascular anatomy of the nose. Allergy 1997;52(40 suppl):7–11.
66. Geurkink N. Nasal anatomy, physiology, and function. J Allergy Clin Immunol 1983;72:123–128.
67. Naclerio RM, Pinto J, Assanasen P, Baroody FM. Observations on the ability of the nose to warm and humidify inspired air. Rhinology 2007;45:102–111
68. Rundell KW, Jenkinson DM. Exercise-induced bronchospasm in the elite athlete. Sports Med 2002;32:583–600.
69. Svensson S, Olin AC, Hellgren J. Increased net water loss by oral compared to nasal expiration in healthy subjects. Rhinology 2006;44:74–77.
70. Hsu YB, Lan MY, Huang YC, Kao MC, Lan MC. Association between breathing route, oxygen desaturation, and upper airway morphology. Laryngoscope 2021;131:E659–E664.
71. Olsen KD, Kern EB, Westbrook PR. Sleep and breathing disturbance secondary to nasal obstruction. Otolaryngol Head Neck Surg 1981;89:804–810.
72. Petruson B. Increased nasal breathing decreases snoring and improves oxygen saturation during sleep apnoea. Rhinology 1994;32:87–89.
73. Nagappan PG, Subramaniam S, Wang DY. Olfaction as a soldier—A review of the physiology and its present and future use in the military. Mil Med Res 2017;4:9.
74. Ruff RL, Riechers RG 2nd, Wang XF, Piero T, Ruff SS. A case-control study examining whether neurological deficits and PTSD in combat veterans are related to episodes of mild TBI. BMJ Open 2012;2:e000312.
75. Rolls ET. Taste, olfactory, and food reward value processing in the brain. Prog Neurobiol 2015;127–128:64–90.
76. Peterson B, Theman K. Reduced nocturnal asthma by improved nasal breathing. Acta Otolaryngol 1996;116:490–492.
77. Hasegawa M, Kern EB. The effect of breath holding, hyperventilation, and exercise on nasal resistance. Rhinology 1978;16:243–249.
78. Mertz JS, McCaffrey TV, Kern EB. Role of the nasal airway in regulation of airway resistance during hypercapnia and exercise. Second-Place Resident Award at 1982 Research Forum. Otolaryngol Head Neck Surg 1984;92:302–307.
79. Shturman-Ellstein R, Zeballos RJ, Buckley JM, Souhrada JF. The beneficial effect of nasal breathing on exercise-induced bronchoconstriction. Am Rev Respir Dis 1978;118:65–73.
80. Morton AR, King K, Papalia S, Goodman C, Turley KR, Wilmore JH. Comparison of maximal oxygen consumption with oral and nasal breathing. Aus J Sci Med Sport 1995;27:51–55.
81. Dallam GM, McClaran SR, Cox DG, Foust CP. Effect of nasal versus oral breathing on vo2max and physiological economy in recreational runners following an extended period spent using nasally restricted breathing. Int J Kinesiol Sports Sci 2018;6:22–29.
82. Baumann I, Plinkert PK. Effect of breathing mode and nose ventilation on growth of the facial bones [in German]. HNO 1996;44:229–234.

Take care of your body;
it's the only place you
have to live.

—*Jim Rohn*

15

Physical Therapy

Brad Gilden | Bill Esser

Physical therapists are trained to recognize and treat faulty postural and movement patterns involving the human musculoskeletal and neuromuscular systems. When skeletal alignment or movement efficiency is compromised, compensations occur that affect the health of the entire system. Two of the areas most impacted by these compensatory activities are the stomatognathic and respiratory systems, which extend from the nasopharyngeal region down to the diaphragm. The thoracic diaphragm, the primary driver of inhalation, becomes hypertonic when the rib cage is misaligned over the pelvis, leading to cervical accessory muscle-driven breathing patterns. When the neck becomes excessively involved in breathing, tension develops in the craniofacial, orofacial, craniomandibular, cervical, and thoracic regions, often resulting in upper airway resistance. This increased resistance can manifest as further compensations leading to nasal congestion, mouth breathing, excessive tongue activity, and altered pressure systems, which may contribute to increased demands on the cardiovascular system. Symptoms that arise from these compensations may include headaches, tinnitus, dry mouth and throat, vestibular/balance deficits, scoliosis, temporomandibular joint (TMJ) pain, neck pain, gastroesophageal reflux disorder (GERD), ankyloglossia, and the development of malocclusion.

The role of an airway-centric physical therapist (ACPT) is to correct inefficiencies in postural and movement patterns to prevent or reverse these compensatory tendencies. By restoring efficient posture and body mechanics, ACPTs can reduce or eliminate painful symptoms and support dental work, reducing the risk of relapse.

When a patient presents to a medical professional with suspected nasopharyngeal abnormalities, there are both intrinsic and extrinsic factors contributing to the problem. Intrinsic factors may include anatomical anomalies that increase resistance to airflow, such as a narrow maxilla, swollen tonsils/adenoids, a retruded mandible, malocclusion, and ankyloglossia. Extrinsic factors that can increase airway resistance may include forward head posturing, parafunctional habits (such as nail biting), poor workstation or sleeping positions, an inflammatory diet, or poor stress management skills. A multidisciplinary approach with appropriate referrals to trusted colleagues can be the difference between treatment success and failure. Building a team that includes an ACPT to help identify and treat intrinsic and extrinsic factors is paramount. Interdisciplinary collaboration between dentists and physical therapists is crucial for the holistic management of patients with airway and sleep disorders, such as obstructive sleep apena (OSA) and chronic snoring. Dentists play a pivotal role in the early identification and diagnosis of these disorders through oral examinations and evaluation of dental occlusion. Physical therapists then contribute by addressing musculoskeletal imbalances and postural dysfunctions that exacerbate the condition. Working together, these professionals develop a comprehensive treatment plan to improve airway function and enhance overall patient wellbeing. This collaborative approach ensures that patients receive well-rounded care, addressing both the anatomical and functional aspects of their condition, ultimately leading to better treatment outcomes and improved quality of life.

In this text, an *ACPT* is defined as a physical therapist with specialized postgraduate education focused on the evaluation and treatment of patients with disorders related to the nasal and oral airway, including OSA and other sleep-related breathing disorders. However, you will not find a specific degree associated with this designation. ACPTs use a multidisciplinary approach to provide medical and therapeutic interventions that alleviate airway obstruction and improve patient quality of life. ACPTs work closely with other health care professionals, including dentists, otolaryngologists, myofunctional therapists, and pulmonologists. See the end of this chapter for guidance on locating an ACPT in your area.

Temporomandibular Joint Disorder

Evaluation and treatment of the TMJs occupies something of a "no man's land." In 1934, an article by otolaryngologist J.B. Costen implicated occlusion as the primary cause of temporomandibular disorder (TMD). A second article 10 years later further solidified the framework that malocclusion is the cause of TMDs. This led the medical profession to avoid diagnosing and treating TMDs and instead lean on the physical therapy and dental professions. At best, however, physical therapists receive a few hours of training on the TMJs in their doctorate programs and learn very little regarding the occlusion. Most dentists we've worked with also report learning little about the TMJs, and even less about the cervical spine.

To successfully evaluate and treat patients with TMD, the relationship between the head and trunk must be considered. Research over the past 25 years has shown that most of the associations between occlusion and TMD are incorrect. Night parafunction, facial muscle pain, and even TMJ capsular pain have not shown a direct correlation with TMD. In one systematic review, the authors concluded that "there were very few associations reported between malocclusions, functional occlusion, and TMD ... and even these associations were not uniform between studies."[1] Continuing to practice alteration of the occlusion as a treatment or prevention of current or future TMD issues may risk exacerbating the condition or lead to additional complications. TMD is most likely *not* a result of occlusal discrepancies but is secondary to complex interactions between the individual's biology, psychology, and environment.

Screening for ACPT Referral

The first step to adding physical therapy to your patient's plan of care is to properly identify when a referral is appropriate. Many of your patients may already be working with a rehabilitation professional (physical therapist, chiropractor, occupational therapist, osteopath). It is a good policy to ask if they enjoy working with this professional. This could be an opportunity to add a qualified professional to your team whom your patient already values and trusts. In any case, there are specific parameters to determine the appropriateness of a referral to an ACPT. Box 15-1 includes qualifying questions that may lead you to consider making a referral. The forms provided at the end of this chapter can also be used as customizable templates when performing screening.

Dentists can perform a quick screen to determine whether a patient should be referred to an ACPT. You should expect asymmetric craniofacial patterns in every patient during this screen, but a large clustering of asymmetries combined with subjective complaints of pain or the loss of stomatognathic function should lead to consideration of a referral. First, instruct the patient to stand with their back to a blank wall (a graphing grid on the wall can be very helpful). Ask the patient to relax and look straight ahead. Take pictures with a digital camera to measure facial symmetry and track changes throughout the course of care.

BOX 15-1 Qualifying questions for referral to an ACPT

- Are you experiencing pain or stiffness in any part of your body that is affecting your mobility, posture, or range of motion?
- Have you recently been injured or undergone surgery that has limited your ability to perform daily activities?
- Do you notice any changes in your posture, gait, or balance that may be affecting your overall movement and functionality?
- Do you have increased pain upon waking in the morning?
- Do you snore or gasp for air during sleep?
- Do you breathe through your mouth during either the day or night?
- Do you have fullness or ringing in your ears?
- Do you experience dizziness/lightheadedness when changing position (eg, sit to stand)?
- Do you experience tension headaches and/or migraines?
- Do you experience jaw pain and/or clicking?

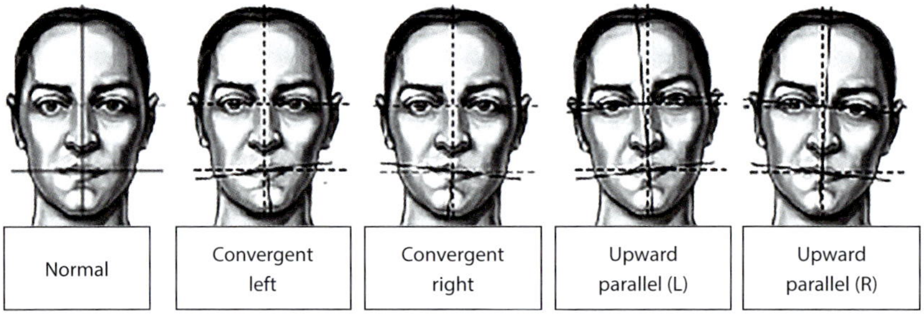

Fig 15-1 Frontal plane assessment.

Static postural assessment

- Determine if convergence and a mandibular shift are present (Fig 15-1). First, draw a line through the pupils and across the lip line. Then, determine if the lines converge to one side. This is a sign of decreased development of the condyle and ramus on that side, which is correlated clinically with injury to the disk/condyle, decreased blood supply, and hampered development of the condyle on that side.
- Determine altered chin position from midline:
  1. Mark a point between the eyes and the middle of the bridge of the nose (nasion).
  2. Mark a point in midline just under the nose (subnasion).
  3. Mark a point in the middle of the chin.
  4. Drop an imaginary vertical line to see if the chin is in line or shifted to one side.

     ❑ Right mandibular shift ❑ Left mandibular shift

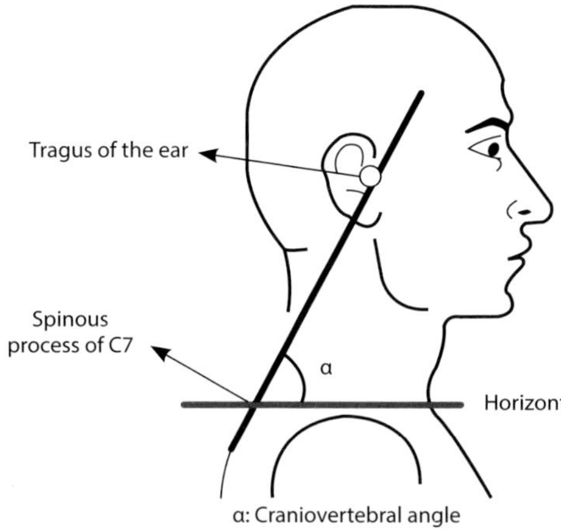

Fig 15-2 Measuring the CVA.

- Correlate chin deviation with the labial frenulum and convergence to that side.
- Evaluate the probability of an atlas or upper cervical dysfunction. Check for parallel lines sloping upward on the same side (this is the probable direction of atlas rotation). The flexion rotation test is used to confirm probable atlas rotation. Parallel lines sloping upward that are high on the left are indicative of a left atlas rotation. In the majority of cases, the flexion rotation test is limited when checking for rotation to the right.
- Make additional observations in the frontal plane:
  Ear Height: ❑ Level ❑ Right higher ❑ Left higher
  Ear show: ❑ Equal ❑ Right higher ❑ Left higher
  Eyebrow height: ❑ Level ❑ Right higher ❑ Left higher
  Lip seal: ❑ Sealed no chin strain ❑ Sealed chin strain ❑ Apart
  Pupil Height: ❑ Level ❑ Right greater ❑ Left greater
  Nasal bone: ❑ Midline ❑ Right deviated ❑ Left deviated
  Chin: ❑ Midline ❑ Right deviated ❑ Left deviated
  Throat: ❑ Midline ❑ Right deviated ❑ Left deviated
  Shoulder Height: ❑ Level ❑ Right higher ❑ Left higher
- Next, have the patient turn to the side for sagittal plane assessment.
- Evaluate the forward head position by determining the craniovertebral angle (CVA)—the acute angle formed from the tragus of the ear to C7, with a horizontal line at C7 (Fig 15-2).
  ❑ > 50 degrees ❑ < 50 degrees (indicates forward head posture)
- Evaluate the position of the mandible by asking the patient to lightly close their lips. Look at the position of the chin in relation to the lower lip.
  ❑ Class I ❑ Class II ❑ Class III

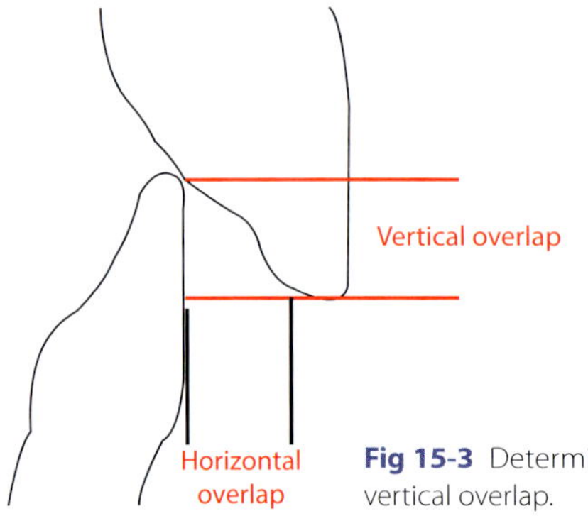

Fig 15-3 Determine whether the patient exhibits horizontal or vertical overlap.

- Evaluate the shoulder position.
  ❑ Level ❑ Right forward ❑ Left forward
- Evaluate the relationship of the sternum to the floor.
  ❑ Perpendicular to floor ❑ Elevated ❑ Depressed

Soft tissue and intraoral inspection

- Take note of any scar(s) on the face/chin. These could be signs of previous macrotrauma to the face. Scars are often opposite the side of disc displacement.
  ❑ Scar on right of chin ❑ Scar on left of chin
- Look for scalloping of the tongue. Scalloping usually indicates a low tongue resting posture, or the patient may be using the tongue to brace against or between the teeth at night. This is an indication of airway compromise.
  ❑ No scalloping ❑ Mild scalloping ❑ Moderate scalloping ❑ Severe scalloping
- Perform a labial/buccal inspection. With the teeth lightly touching, lift the upper and lower lips away from one another and inspect the alignment of the lower frenulum.
  ❑ Lower frenulum in line with upper frenulum
  ❑ Lower frenulum to the right of upper frenulum
  ❑ Lower frenulum to the left of upper frenulum
- Is frenulum/buccal tie limiting lip mobility?
  ❑ No ❑ Yes (upper) ❑ Yes (lower)
  ❑ Yes (upper and lower)
- Evaluate the relationship between the maxillary and mandibular teeth (Fig 15-3).

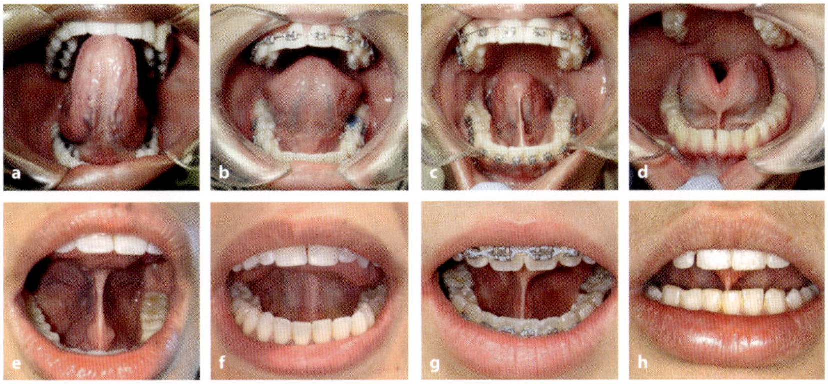

Fig 15-4 Assessment of tongue range of motion. *(a to d)* Determining anterior tongue mobility by measuring the ability to touch the tongue tip to the incisive papilla at total jaw opening. *(e to h)* Determining mid-tongue mobility by measuring the ability to maintain lingual palatal suction while opening the mouth. (Reprinted with permission from Zaghi et al.[2])

a. Vertical overlap (overbite): How far do the maxillary incisors extend over the mandibular incisors in the superior/inferior dimension? (ideal is 2 to 3 mm) ________ mm

b. Horizontal overlap (overjet): How far do the maxillary incisors extend over the mandibular incisors in the anterior/posterior dimension? (ideal is 2 to 3 mm) ________ mm

c. Tori: Assess for extra bone at the center of the hard palate and inside the anterior mandible. Extra bone deposition in the maxilla/mandible may be a sign of excessive clenching activity.
❑ None ❑ Maxillary tori ❑ Mandibular tori

- Check for clench lines (horizontal lines on the insides of the cheeks).
  ❑ Not present ❑ Present
- Note any other findings that may be relevant (eg, tooth wear and gum health).

Tongue position and mobility

- Determine the tongue resting position by asking the patient where the tongue is at rest.
  ❑ Roof of mouth ❑ Bottom jaw ❑ Front of teeth ❑ Not touching anything
- Measure jaw and tongue range of motion with calipers (Fig 15-4).
  a. Total jaw opening (measured from maxillary to mandibular incisors): ______ mm
  b. Tongue tip on palate (TIP) opening: ______ mm

c. Tongue suctioned to palate (lingual palatal suction [LPS]) opening: _______ mm
d. Total jaw opening/TIP × 100: ___________%
e. Total jaw opening/LPS × 100: ___________%

Cervical range of motion

- Evaluate the cervical range of motion.
  a. Upper cervical flexion rotation test: Determine if C1 is rotated out of neutral, restricting movement opposite to the side of parallel upward sloping lines. Instruct the patient to flex their head to their chest and then rotate right to mark an imaginary line on the clavicle. Keeping the head flexed, have them rotate left to mark an imaginary line on the clavicle. Compare the difference.
     ❑ Equal rotation ❑ Right rotation greater ❑ Left rotation greater
  b. Full cervical rotation: Instruct the patient to turn their head toward each shoulder.
     Right: ❑ Not limited, no pain ❑ Limited, no pain ❑ Limited, pain
     Left: ❑ Not limited, no pain ❑ Limited, no pain ❑ Limited, pain
  c. Side bending: Instruct the patient to move their ear to their shoulder, keeping the shoulders relaxed.
     Right: ❑ Not limited, no pain ❑ Limited, no pain ❑ Limited, pain
     Left: ❑ Not limited, no pain ❑ Limited, no pain ❑ Limited, pain
  d. Flexion: Instruct the patient to look down toward the floor with their mouth closed.
     ❑ Not limited, no pain ❑ Limited, no pain ❑ Limited, pain
  e. Extension: Instruct the patient to look up to the ceiling.
     ❑ Not limited, no pain ❑ Limited, no pain ❑ Limited, pain

Facial muscles

- Instruct the patient to smile, and note right to left lip excursion.
  ❑ Even ❑ Right higher ❑ Left higher
- Instruct the patient to lift their eyebrows.
  ❑ Even ❑ Right higher ❑ Left higher

TMJ charting

Having an easy and consistent way to chart TMJ triplanar range of motion is essential for diagnosis and to track progress. Use a chart like the one shown in Fig 15-5 to mark opening, protrusion, and lateral movement, noting

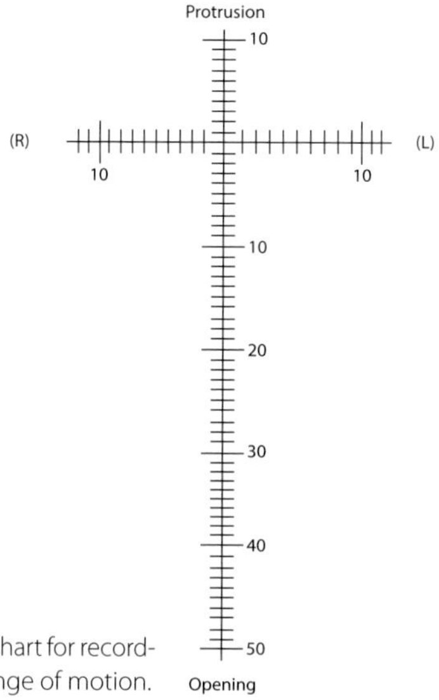

Fig 15-5 Chart for recording TMJ range of motion.

deflection, deviation, time of clicks, and the presence of pain. Normal opening is measured from the right maxillary and mandibular central incisors, as are lateral movements.

- Initial oral opening: Rotation should be the primary movement for the first 25 mm, followed by translation. Note if translation occurs early.
- Normal opening: 0 to 45 mm checked with slight overpressure. Record the total range and pain with overpressure.
- Deviations are a movement to one side and then a return to midline. Typically, they are caused by a displaced disc on the side the patient deviates toward. At the time of reduction (click), the jaw will return to midline. Record clicks at the mm of opening and the side they occur on.
- Deflections involve movement to one side without a return to midline. Typically, they are caused by a displaced disc that does not reduce or a tight joint capsule on the side of deflection. Record the range of motion and pattern.
- Lateral movement: Lateral movement is the ability of one condyle to translate while the other compresses into the posterior, superior, and medial aspect of the opposite joint. Normal left and right movement is about 10 mm or one-fourth of mouth opening capacity. Movement should be silent and without pain. Slight overpressure applied in the direction toward which the mandible is moving should not result in pain. Pain suggests that the disc is anteriorly or laterally displaced. Mark the total range of

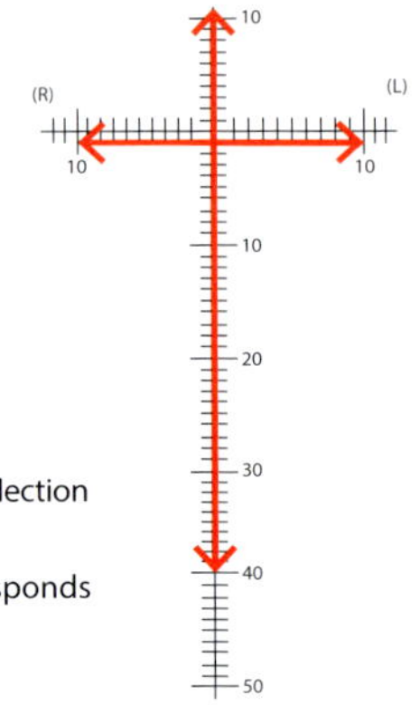

TMJ charting—Normal

Normal joint movement when palpating over the condylar poles:

- Slight translation then rotation to 25 mm
- Opens to approximately three finger widths (~40 mm) without deviation or deflection
- No clicks or pops
- Lateral movement at a 1:4 ratio with opening (ie, the 40-mm opening corresponds with 10 mm of lateral movement)
- Protrusive (straight) movements at a 1:4 ratio with opening (ie, 10 mm)

Fig 15-6 Example of a bilateral TMJ function chart.

lateral movement, the range at which any clicking is heard or palpated, and whether applying overpressure causes pain.

- Protrusion: Normal protrusion is movement that is straight ahead without deflection or deviation. Mark the total range and the click at the mm palpated/heard.
- Jaw closing: Is the patient able to close their jaw completely? Lightly place both pinkies in each ear of the patient, and note the following:
  - ❑ Full closure, no pain ❑ Pain (right ear) ❑ Pain (left ear)
  - ❑ No condylar pressure ❑ Condylar pressure (right ear)
  - ❑ Condylar pressure (left ear)

An example of a normal bilateral TMJ function chart is shown in Fig 15-6.

Facial muscle trigger points

Next, the dentist should evaluate for retrodiscitis and palpate the facial muscle trigger points (Fig 15-7). Palpate each point on the face using enough pressure to blanch the nail bed. Maintain this consistent pressure throughout the examination. Instruct the patient to raise their hand when pain is elicited and to rate the pain on a scale of 1 to 10, with 1 representing minimal pain and 10 representing the worst possible pain. Ask the patient to bite down on the teeth lightly during each palpation and then relax.

1. (R)_____(L)_____ Anterior temporalis (behind orbit of eye)
2. (R)_____(L)_____ Middle portion of temporalis
3. (R)_____(L)_____ Posterior portion of temporalis

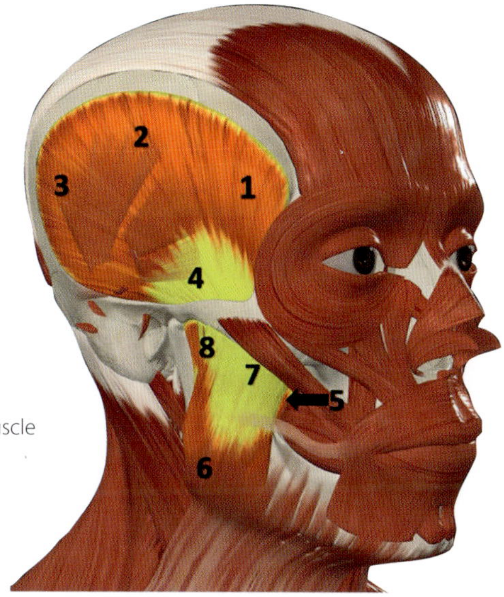

Fig 15-7 Facial muscle trigger points.

4. (R)_____(L)_____ Tendon of the temporalis muscle found above the zygomatic arch
5. (R)_____(L)_____ Temporalis tendon at its attachment to the coronoid process (Place your index fingers anteriorly, under the zygomatic arch, and have the patient open their mouth into your fingers.)
6. (R)_____(L)_____ Superficial masseter at the angle of mandible
7. (R)_____(L)_____ Aponeurosis attachment of the superficial masseter muscle found just under the zygomatic arch
8. (R)_____(L)_____ Deep masseter muscle found with strong clenching just anterior to the condyle
9. (R)_____(L)_____ Retrodiscal tissue externally (Insert your pinky in the patient's ear, and instruct them to open their mouth slightly to gain access; then have the patient close gently, and the condyle will move posteriorly.)
10. (R)_____(L)_____ Medial pterygoid (Palpate internally at the bottom of the mouth between the tongue and mandible as posteriorly as possible. You can also palpate externally just beneath and medial to the ramus of the mandible.)
11. (R)_____(L)_____ Lateral pterygoid (Use your pinky to palpate internally between the upper cheek and molars. Proceed posteriorly into the pocket.)

BOX 15-2 Symptoms that indicate referral to an ACPT

Craniofacial symptoms
- Tension in the neck and upper back that progresses into the head
- Tension in the face, head, jaw, and neck that progresses throughout the day
- Headaches/migraines
- Cranial or facial discomfort while actively undergoing orthodontic treatment

Orofacial symptoms
- Pain in one or both TMJs when talking, chewing, or upon waking
- Fatigue in the jaw with talking or chewing
- Mouth breathing, difficult nasal breathing
- Jaw discomfort while actively undergoing orthodontic treatment
- Limited/locked jaw opening or closing
- Parafunctional habits during the day or night

Cervical symptoms
- Asymmetric limitations in neck movements
- Neck pain at rest or with movement
- Referred pain down the arm with neck range of motion assessment
- Excessive cervical muscle involvement with breathing
- Neck discomfort while actively undergoing orthodontic treatment

Shoulder and thoracic symptoms
- Chest tightness while breathing
- Back and/or shoulder pain with limited range of motion

Other symptoms
- Gait and/or balance disturbances
- Poor posture and/or body mechanics
- Fatigue and shortness of breath with daily activities
- Pain and/or slow progress while undergoing orthodontic treatment

Box 15-2 lists the symptoms that should trigger a referral to an ACPT.

ACPT Evaluation

Physical therapists identify specific areas of inefficiencies during an ACPT evaluation to help determine a craniofacial airway plan of care. This evaluation includes a postural assessment to identify breakdowns in the neurologic and musculoskeletal system that may be contributing to airway insufficiencies. A breathing assessment helps determine whether a patient is using their respiratory system efficiently and will pinpoint areas of dysfunction. It is important to note that improper daytime breathing may translate into suboptimal nighttime breathing.

Many patients experience pain, clicking, and reduced range of motion in the TMJ, which can have a profound negative impact on daily living. TMJ problems can be either a symptom or a driver of an airway issue. It is important to perform consistent evaluations to properly diagnose and treat the TMJs. If not treated properly, most TMJ problems will worsen with time. Likewise, discord in the stomatognathic system will likely contribute to disharmony in the orofacial and craniomandibular regions. Proper assessment with a thorough myofunctional evaluation is essential to identify and address these problems. It is well-documented that the positioning and mechanics of the mandible are influenced by the cranium and cervical spine. A proper upper cervical examination by a physical therapist may lead to treatment solutions that have eluded other professionals. A treatment program to address the underlying structural and/or functional areas that may be contributing to an airway problem may uncover repetitive behavioral issues that may be sabotaging recovery. These behaviors may include how the patient sits at their workstation, positions themselves in bed, lifts their infant or child, sits on their bike, lifts weights, or any other daily activity.

Effective communication between the patient, physical therapist, dentist, and other health care professionals involved in treatment planning is essential for achieving positive outcomes. Addressing the complexities of airway problems typically requires a collaborative effort. Making an appropriate referral at the right time and using a common language to describe the treatment goals and plan of care are crucial for success. Additionally, any patient undergoing orthodontic treatment is going to experience changes in cranial and occlusal positioning that will impact the entire system. Working with a physical therapist while going through treatment will help to reduce symptoms from these alterations.

Improving communication between professionals requires a good understanding of how physical therapists address each area covered in the quick screen that led to referral. The following sections describe the components of evaluation and treatment strategies employed when dysfunction is identified.

Behavioral assessment

Repetitive, habitual behaviors can be detrimental to a rehabilitation program, particularly if patients are unaware of them. Habits that reinforce poor positioning under load may hinder recovery efforts, especially if they have persisted for years without being addressed. Examples of such habits include poor positioning at a workstation, biting nails when anxious, consistently leaning on one side of the body, or clenching teeth all day long. Modifying habitual behaviors is one of the most challenging aspects of rehabilitation. It is crucial for patients to understand the adverse effects of these habits, as failure to do so may compromise their progress toward recovery. An essential responsibility of a physical therapist within a collaborative team is to identify patients' habitual patterns, explain why these patterns may be detrimental to their health, and devise effective strategies that are both feasible and relevant to each patient.

Postural assessment

Maintaining proper postural alignment is crucial for ideal physical function. It helps reduce wear and tear, prevents pain and discomfort, and facilitates correct respiratory function. Furthermore, it fosters balance and core engagement, ultimately contributing to increased stability. To achieve good postural alignment, it is necessary to have effective neuromuscular control and a balanced distribution of forces between the left and right sides of the body, while avoiding excessive extension, flexion, or lateral curvature of the spine. In an ideal posture, the head is positioned over the shoulders, which are aligned above the hips, with the rib cage vertically oriented over the pelvis. This arrangement allows for unhindered access to the diaphragm and efficient respiratory function, as well as an even distribution of forces throughout the body. Although anatomical variations and past injuries may result in differences in postural alignment, maintaining proper alignment is generally associated with improved overall health and well-being. On the other hand, suboptimal alignment can cause overuse of neck and back muscles, increased energy consumption, and bodily tension, ultimately leading to stress, inflammation, and degeneration of the soft tissues and joints. Additionally, it can create increased resistance to airflow, further challenging the respiratory system.

An individual's posture is a multifactorial moving target influenced by various factors, including genetics, childhood mirroring, past injuries, and repetitive positions associated with specific activities. Because posture is a learned behavior, modifying it can prove challenging. Physical therapists employ assessments to identify postural dysfunction and use this objective data to elucidate the detrimental effects of sustained poor postural positioning, ultimately encouraging behavior modification.

The initial phase of a postural assessment involves a visual inspection to compare the right and left sides of the body in the frontal and sagittal planes (Fig 15-8). In the frontal plane, therapists examine the alignment of the eyes, tops of ears, shoulders, hips, and knees. This evaluation allows for assessing segmental rotations of each body part, as well as determining if weight is unevenly distributed by comparing head position with the midline between the feet. In the sagittal plane, therapists can analyze the alignment of the head, thorax, shoulders, pelvis, and feet. Envision placing a heavy weight atop the head and predicting where the system would collapse. This visualization is crucial for pinpointing areas requiring correction.

Once a visual inspection of static posture has been conducted, the next step is to evaluate a combination of passive and active movements to test

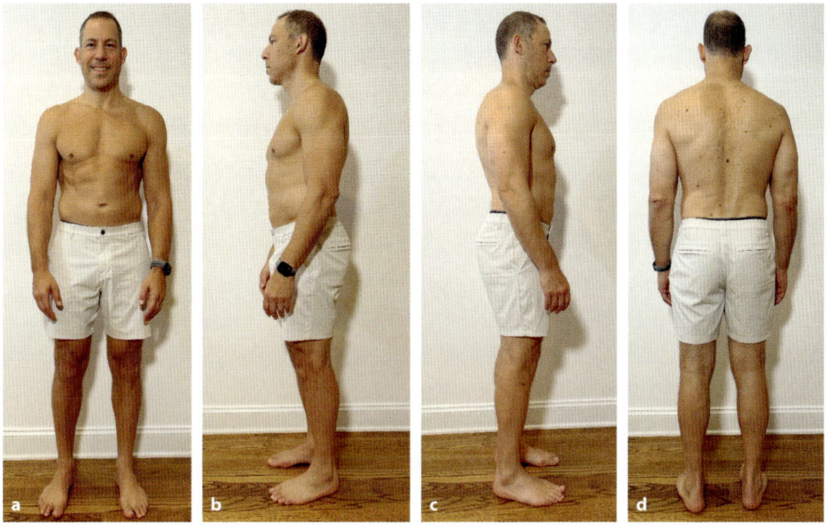

Fig 15-8 *(a to d)* Postural assessment in the frontal and sagittal planes.

neutrality, strength, and stability. Specific tests are used for each area of the body to identify patterns of dysfunction that may be contributing to postural disharmony. These tests may include the following:

- Dermatome/myotome diagnostic tests to evaluate neurologic function
- Provocative testing of joints and soft tissues to reproduce or exacerbate symptoms to diagnose possible nerve impingements, herniated discs, or joint injuries
- Gait assessment to evaluate walking pattern and identify abnormalities, compensations, or inefficient movement
- Additional functional testing to challenge balance, stability, and neuromuscular control to assess resilience of the system

Breathing and respiratory function assessment

Breathing and respiratory function are an important part of the physical therapy assessment. Efficient respiratory function ensures that the body receives adequate oxygen and eliminates excess carbon dioxide, which is critical for maintaining proper cellular function and physiologic processes. Breathing is also intricately linked to other bodily functions, such as circulation, digestion, pain management, cognition, athletic performance, and mental health. Thus, optimizing respiratory function can have a significant impact on overall well-being. There are two primary components of breathing that need to be assessed in patients.

1. Patients should be able to breathe exclusively through the nose with proper oral resting posture (tongue at the roof of the mouth, teeth slightly apart, and lips lightly sealed). They should also breathe with a diaphragm-driven respiratory pattern during static and functional activities. Tests may include the following:
   - Observation of the nasal valves, lip/jaw position, abdomen, rib cage, and sternal changes during inspiratory and expiratory phases
   - Observation of the cervical accessory muscles and postural changes to detect compensatory breathing patterns
   - Measurement of the rib cage and abdominal expansion and contraction changes using a tape measure
   - Inspiratory, expiratory, and nasal pressures to measure diaphragm and expiratory muscle strength and endurance
   - Postural cueing to see changes on breathing effort, diaphragm access, and accessory muscle activity
   - Neutrality testing to evaluate the ability to expand the right and left apical and posterior mediastinal regions of the rib cage

2. The patient's breathing pattern should facilitate maintenance of an optimal internal environment (pH) by regulating oxygen and carbon dioxide levels, thereby mitigating potential symptoms associated with hypoventilation or hyperventilation. This should be tested both at rest and under stress to test causality. Testing may include the following:
   - Timed physiologic sigh to measure carbon dioxide tolerance—large nasal breath, followed by shorter end range nasal breath, followed by a very slow exhale through pursed lips as long as possible. The longer the exhale, the greater the carbon dioxide tolerance.
   - Control Pause breath hold (also known as the BOLT Score [Breathing Oxygen Level Test]) to assess carbon dioxide tolerance—performed by taking a small nasal breath in, small nasal breath out, and then a breath hold until air hunger is felt. The time of the breath hold is recorded. The longer the breath hold, the greater the carbon dioxide tolerance.
   - Capnometry to measure the partial pressure of carbon dioxide in the exhaled breath along with breaths per minute to provide an assessment of respiratory function and efficiency. This can be performed at rest to get a baseline measurement, and then the patient can be challenged by situations in which they are symptomatic to better understand if a breathing behavior pattern is driving their symptomatology.

Cranial nerve screening

Stomatognathic function is a complex set of physiologic activities that occur around the mouth (stoma) and jaw (gnathos). Eating, breathing, speaking, and swallowing without choking necessitate intricate coordination between various cranial nerves and the stomatognathic system. The trigeminal (V), facial (VII), and glossopharyngeal (IX) nerves contribute to mastication, taste sensation, and saliva production. Simultaneously, the vagus (X) and glossopharyngeal (IX) nerves work together to control the muscles involved in swallowing, helping to prevent choking by coordinating the timing of breathing and swallowing, which temporarily closes the airway. The hypoglossal nerve (XII) enables efficient tongue movements, and the vagus nerve (X) plays a role in modulating the soft palate, pharynx, and larynx for speech production. These cranial nerves harmoniously integrate essential functions to ensure overall oral and respiratory health.

Considering the critical functions of the stomatognathic system, it is imperative for physical therapists to screen for cranial nerve and stomatognathic dysfunction during patient assessments. This screening process aids in the early identification of any anomalies or impairments that may affect essential activities such as mastication, swallowing, breathing, and speech. Furthermore, dysfunctions of the cranial nerves or stomatognathic system can lead to airway-related problems, which can significantly impact a patient's overall health and well-being. Detecting dysfunction at an early stage allows for timely intervention, which can significantly improve patient outcomes and overall quality of life. Moreover, addressing cranial nerve and stomatognathic dysfunction can also help prevent secondary complications that may arise from impaired oral and respiratory function, such as aspiration pneumonia, malnutrition, communication difficulties, or airway obstruction. Consequently, incorporating cranial nerve and stomatognathic system screening into physical therapy evaluations is vital for comprehensive patient care and management.

Craniocervical mandibular complex evaluation

Understanding the complex relationship between the cranium, cervical spine, TMJs, and mandible (the cranial cervical mandibular complex [CCMC]) is vital for accurately identifying and addressing numerous conditions that contribute to sleep disorders. Although the cranium, cervical spine, and mandible may appear distinct, they are intricately connected through their articulations, positioning, neurology, and functions. A thorough understanding of the biomechanical, neurologic, and physiologic nuances in this region is essential for identifying the root causes of various symptoms, including, but not limited to, headaches, sleep disturbances, neck pain, radiculopathies, TMDs, tinnitus, balance disorders, dysautonomia, migraines, and an array of movement disorders.

The biomechanics of the atlanto-occipital joint, which connects the occiput (base of the skull) and the first cervical vertebra (atlas), play a crucial role in determining the position of the mandible and TMJs. The atlanto-occipital joint, characterized by its unique facet joint configuration, allows for a wide range of motion, including flexion, extension, lateral bending, and rotation. Due to the anatomical proximity and interconnectedness of the cervical spine and the craniomandibular system, any misalignment or dysfunction at this joint will directly impact the position and function of the TMJs. This relationship is vital for understanding the interdependence of these structures and their influence on overall head and neck biomechanics. As a result, addressing atlanto-occipital joint dysfunction or misalignment can improve TMJ-related symptoms and contribute to better management of craniofacial and cervical pain, as well as sleep-related disorders. Figures 15-9 to 15-11 show examples of the causal relationship head position has on the position of the jaw and the muscles of mastication using electromyography (EMG) on the masseter and temporalis muscles.

The neurology of the CCMC involves an intricate network of nerves that interconnect the cranium, cervical spine, and mandible. These nerves play a vital role in sensory perception and motor function in this region. Key nerves within the CCMC include the trigeminal nerve, which innervates the facial structures and controls mastication, and the cervical plexus, which provides sensory and motor innervation to the neck and upper thoracic region. Additionally, cranial nerves such as the facial, glossopharyngeal, and vagus nerves contribute to various functions, including facial expressions, swallowing, and autonomic regulation. The interplay between these neurologic structures in the CCMC influences the overall function and coordination of head and neck movements, as well as the perception of pain and other sensations.

Understanding the neurology of the CCMC is crucial for healthcare professionals when diagnosing and treating disorders affecting the head, neck, and jaw, including craniofacial pain, TMJ disorders, and sleep-related disorders. Forward head posture results in the cranium being rotated backward onto the upper part of the neck, which results in compression of the upper cervical nerves (C1–C3). Compression of both the upper cervical nerves and joints is registered in the cervical nucleus, located next to the trigeminal nucleus in the brainstem. Sensory overflow from the upper cervical nerves into the

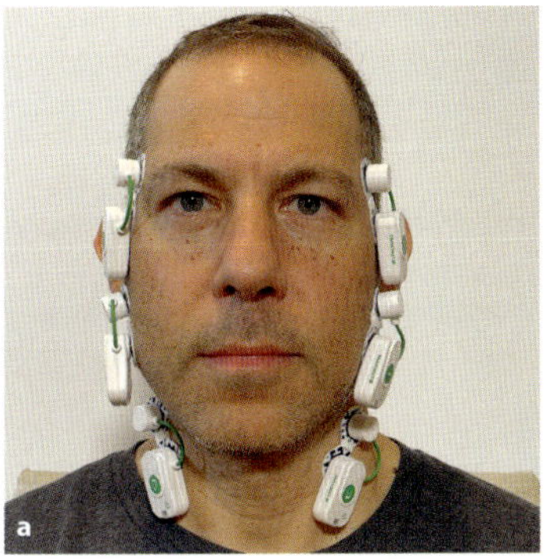

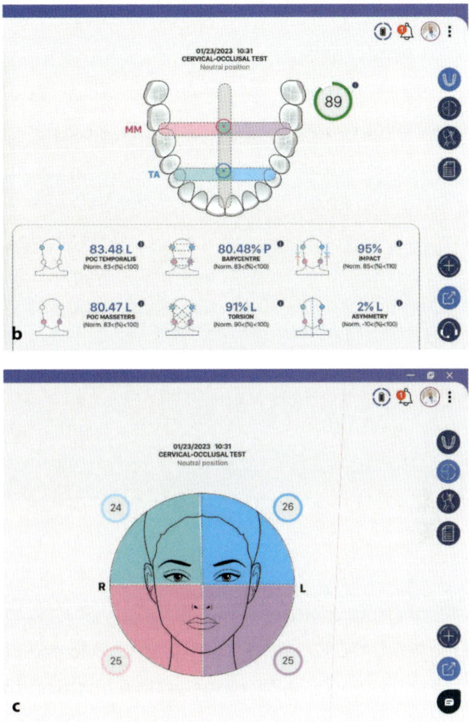

Fig 15-9 *(a)* Neutral head position with TMJ EMG electrodes on the masseter, temporalis, and sternocleidomastoid muscles during isometric clench. *(b)* EMG data in a functional model representing a neuromuscular neutral bite with equal activity across all muscles. *(c)* Pie graph representation of raw data further demonstrating neutral neuromuscular activity during clench. (Software images courtesy of Teethan. All rights reserved.)

trigeminal sensory system is considered a common factor in neck-generated symptomatology and sensory complaints present in the ophthalmic, maxillary, and mandibular sensory branches of the trigeminal nerve. Mariano Rocabado, DPT, uses a simple palpation technique to check for adequate space between the base of the skull and C2. In a normal sitting position, you should be able to place your index and middle finger between the occipital base and the C2 spinous process, which is the first palpable bone beneath the occiput. On radiograph, this space should be about 20 mm wide from the base of the occiput to C2.

SAGITTAL PLANE

The function of the CCMC should be assessed across all three planes of movement. In the sagittal plane, the impact of a forward head position on the TMJ, airway, and growth and development is multifaceted. As the head moves forward, tension increases in the supra- and infrahyoid soft tissues, as well as in the fascia extending from the chin to the chest. This increased tension elongates the face and causes it to become narrower. EMG studies demonstrate that as the head extends forward, the mandible is pulled into a retruded position, potentially harming the TMJs

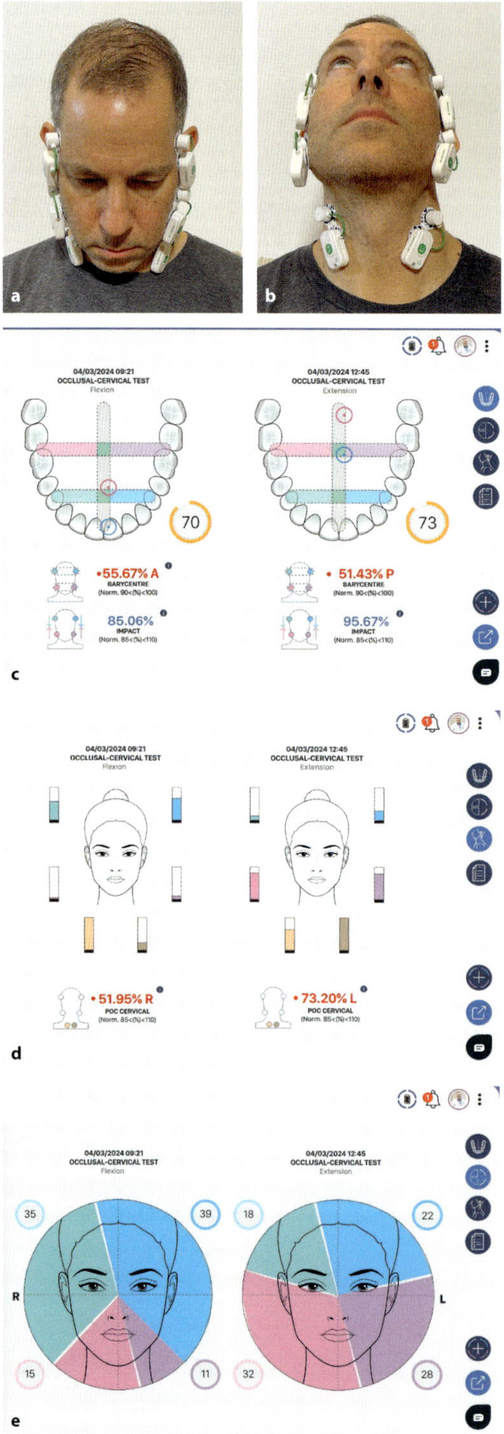

Fig 15-10 *(a)* Flexed head position with TMJ EMG electrodes on the masseter, temporalis, and sternocleidomastoid muscles during isometric clench. *(b)* Extended head position with TMJ EMG electrodes on the masseter, temporalis, and sternocleidomastoid muscles during isometric clench. *(c)* EMG data showing changes in force concentration points and tooth contacts with flexion and extension. *(d)* EMG data showing differences in muscle activity between flexion and extension. *(e)* Pie graph representation of raw data demonstrating anterior muscle activity during cervical flexion and extension with clench. (Software images courtesy of Teethan. All rights reserved.)

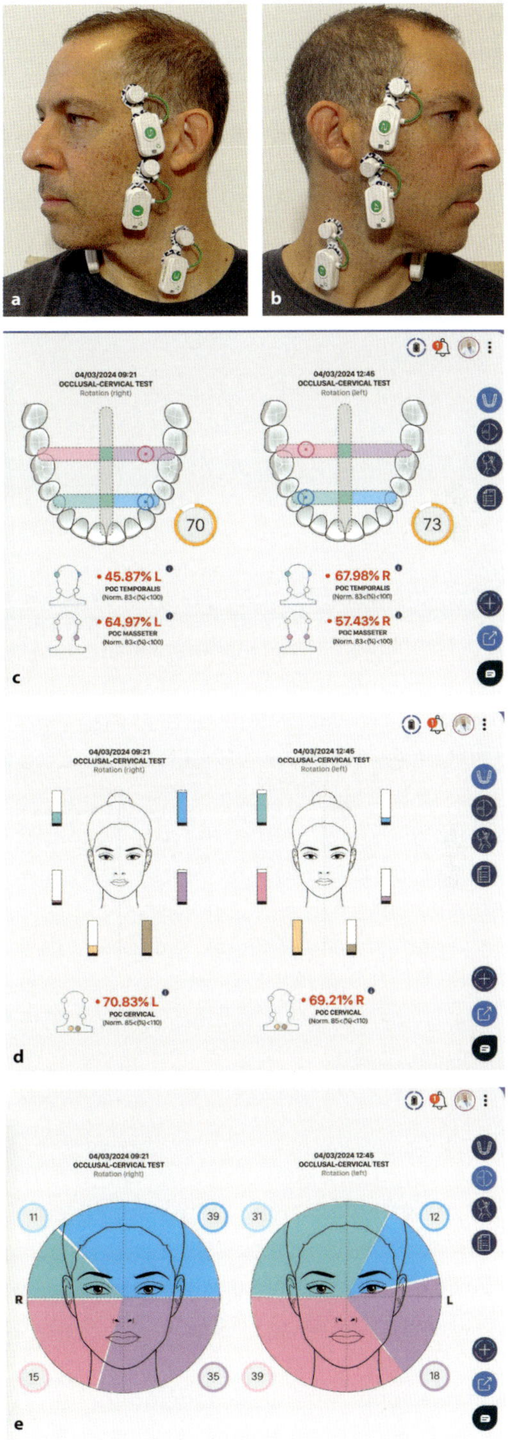

Fig 15-11 *(a)* Right rotated head position with TMJ EMG electrodes on the masseter, temporalis, and sternocleidomastoid muscles during isometric clench. *(b)* Left rotated head position with TMJ EMG electrodes on the masseter, temporalis, and sternocleidomastoid muscles during isometric clench. *(c)* Graphic showing shift in point of concentrated muscle force depending on head position. *(d)* EMG data showing different muscle activity as the head is rotated right and left. *(e)* Pie chart showing shift of EMG activity during head rotation. (Software images courtesy of Teethan. All rights reserved.)

and contributing to the development of an open bite malocclusion due to the traction on submandibular structures. Distalizing the mandibular condyles can also negatively affect airway function. Biomechanically, a forward head position moves the occiput closer to the atlas (C1), compressing the occipital nerves and joints, which can lead to occipital neuralgias. Forward head position is reported to be present in at least 75% of the TMD population.

In an ideal posture, as observed on a sagittal radiograph, the cervical vertebrae exhibit a gentle curve when a line is traced along their posterior aspect. The cranium is positioned centrally in the sagittal plane, minimizing the muscle effort required to support the head on the vertebral column. This posture results in minimal retrusive tension on the mandible from the anterior neck muscles and fascia. A balanced head position positively affects the airway. When a cephalometric analysis is conducted, the CVA typically measures around 101 ± 5 degrees, ensuring minimal obstruction to the exit pathways of the greater and lesser occipital nerves. The hyoid bone is situated inferior to a line connecting the mandibular symphysis and the inferior body of C3, indicative of normal tension levels in the supra- and infrahyoid musculature, which facilitates easier mandibular closure.

A typical presentation for TMD and cervical-related problems is the loss of the cervical curve (straight cervical spine) and a marked decrease in the CVA. Additionally, McGregor's plane (a line drawn from the posterior nasal sinus posteriorly along the base of the occiput) may not be horizontal but rather posteriorly rotated, indicating a posteriorly rotated position of the cranium, with the space between the base of the occiput and C1 significantly decreased. As mentioned earlier, the posterior compression of the suboccipital space and irritability of the nerves and tissue in this region is common. Often the lightest palpation in this area causes a reproduction of headache complaints.

FRONTAL PLANE

Looking at the patient in the frontal plane allows you to view how head position affects occlusion and the muscle function of the face, head, neck, and mandible. Start by drawing a horizontal line through the pupils of the eyes and across the lips. There are two common presentations that will be seen in this view. One pattern that is observed is convergence, in which the lines on one side of the face are closer together. Often on the side of convergence, you will find partial or complete disc displacement. Convergence is highly correlated with previous injury to the side of convergence during growth and development. The second pattern seen is where lines drawn across the pupils and lips are parallel and upward sloping to one side. When matching upward-sloping parallel lines are present, often there is a cervical dysfunction at C1/C2. Upward-sloping parallel lines are often indicative of an atlas rotation to the high side, with atlas position confirmed by palpation and motion restrictions to the opposite side of the elevation. It is also important to note that an atlas rotation elevates the occlusion on the side opposite the rotation.

Does body positioning impact the occlusion?

A 2007 study[3] examined the relationship between mandibular position and body posture. Various sizes of heel lifts up to 10 mm were placed under the foot. Consistent changes in occlusal contact were measured using a T-Scan. A heel lift placed under the left side resulted in early occlusal contact on the left side, and a heel lift on the right side resulted in early occlusal contact on the right side. Looking at what is occurring with the head position in relation to the ground coming up under one heel reveals that the atlas rotates to the opposite direction of the longer leg. The longer leg elevates the pelvis, which effectively creates spinal compensations all the way up the chain. A heel lift under the right side elevates the right pelvis, causing the lumbar spine to tilt left. To compensate for the lumbar tilt, the lower and mid thoracic area tilt to the right. Continued compensations are seen moving cranially, with a shift of the cervical area to the left, and finally, the head tilts to the right in an attempt to level the system. In this situation, we have induced a functional head tilt down on the right side secondary to the biomechanical shapes of the skull, atlas (C1), and C2 and associated ligament restraints in the craniovertebral area and atlas rotation to the left. We now know this will create an early occlusion on the right side. This long list of compensatory changes due to a leg length discrepancy can contribute to conditions such as scoliosis, malocclusion, balance problems, and neck and back disorders. This exemplifies the importance of a proper postural evaluation and treatment planning to minimize the effects of poor posture on the entire body.

Sleep hygiene

Sleep hygiene plays a pivotal role in allowing for restorative sleep each night. It encompasses a range of practices and habits that contribute to the promotion of healthy sleep patterns. Adequate sleep is integral to overall well-being and has a direct impact on various aspects of health, including cognitive function, emotional regulation, joint and tissue recovery, and cardiovascular health. We spend at least one-third of our life in bed—roughly 25 years. The cumulative stress of gravity over time if the body is not supported properly can contribute to fragmented or shorter sleep. Shorter sleep leads to a shorter life! If your body is well supported by a quality mattress and pillows are placed

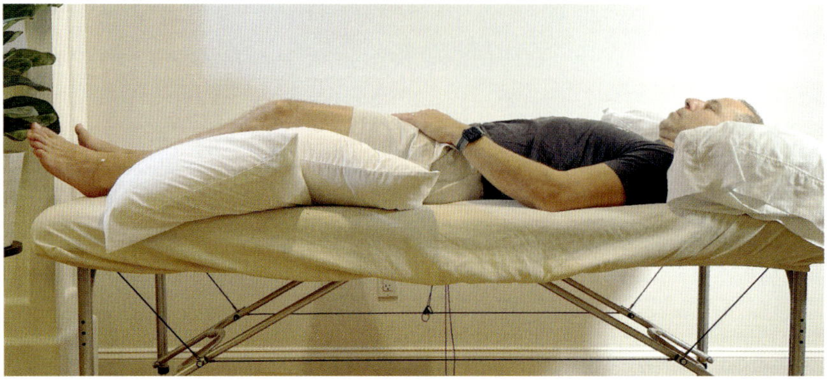

Fig 15-12 Proper support for a supine sleeping position.

in the proper supportive positions, you will be more comfortable and have a much better opportunity to achieve longer and deeper sleep with fewer interruptions. I always tell my patients, "If you go to sleep at night without pain in your back, neck or hips, and wake up with pain in any of these three areas, there is a good chance your sleeping position is contributing to your pain and lack of restorative sleep."

Principles to achieve well-supported sleep in each of the three primary sleeping positions are presented here:

1. Position the head and spine in a neutral and pain-free position to reduce tissue tension.
2. Support any unsupported areas by filling in any gaps so the body can completely relax.
3. Reduce torque on the system by supporting from proximal to distal.

SUPINE POSITION

Back sleeping should be used only if the patient doesn't snore. Gravity pulls the jaw and tongue back if not properly stabilized, which increases the chance for obstruction. The following areas should be supported (Fig 15-12):

- The head and neck should be supported from the base of the neck to the top of the head. Make sure the shoulders are not resting on the pillow
- Use a pillow under the "sit bones," running to either the knees or ankles depending on preference. This helps to reduce excessive lumbar flexion and hip flexor activity.

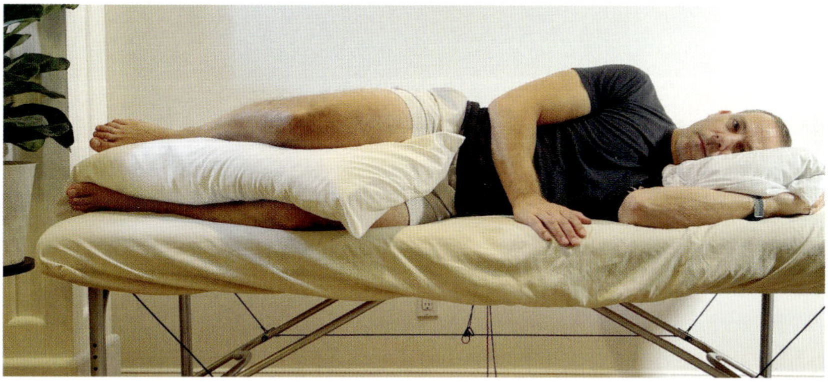

Fig 15-13 Proper support for a side sleeping position.

SIDE POSITION

Sleeping on the side is the most desirable position for somebody with sleep-related issues. The following areas should be supported (Fig 15-13):

- Support the head and neck in a comfortable position by ensuring that the pillow is deep into the neck, supporting the head in a horizontal or slightly upward tilted position.
- Run a pillow from the groin to between the ankles to allow the hips and spine to remain aligned.
- If there is a large differential between the hips and the abdomen, a small towel or pillow can be placed between the rib cage and the hips.
- A pillow supporting the upper arm can be used to remove tension from the shoulder and neck.

PRONE POSITION

This is the least desirable position for sleeping because it places the head and spine in an excessively extended and rotated position, which can lead to neck and back pain. Reduced tension on the spine in stomach sleepers can be achieved with the partial prone position shown here (Fig 15-14):

- Use a very thin pillow under the head and neck. A thick pillow will increase side bending, which may lead to neck pain and headaches.
- Place a pillow under the abdomen and knee to flex the hip up on the same side the head is rotated toward. Place another pillow lengthwise under the same knee extending down to the ankle.

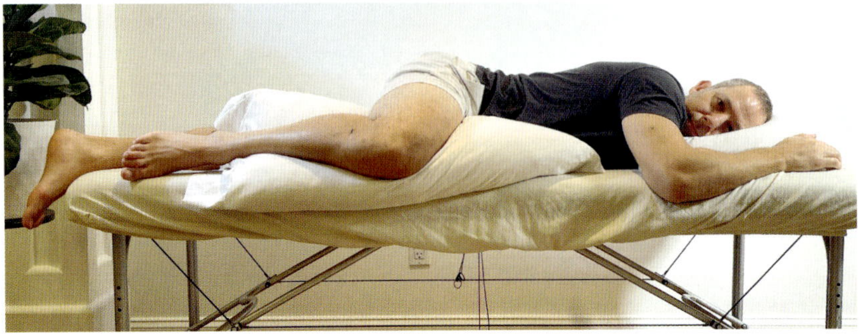

Fig 15-14 Proper support for a prone sleeping position.

Intervention

After conducting a comprehensive physical therapy assessment, any identified behavioral patterns contributing to poor posture or inefficient movement patterns that may exacerbate airway disorders are outlined. Additionally, musculoskeletal mobility or strength deficits are also outlined. Based on the clinical findings, dentists and physical therapists collaboratively devise an integrative plan of care to address these issues. Interventions may include the following:

- Manual therapy—a "hands on technique" such as soft tissue or joint mobilization to address myofascial or joint restrictions that are preventing efficient movement and may be pain-provoking.
- Therapeutic exercises targeted at establishing new movement patterns to inhibit poor muscular patterning, strengthen weakened muscles, and reinforce proper alignment in both static and dynamic activities.
- Home exercises. Reinforcement learning is a crucial component in establishing new behaviors. It involves a system of rewards and feedback that incentivizes and encourages patients to adopt and maintain positive changes in their behavior. A well-designed home exercise program can promote changes in behavior that reduce patient symptoms and aid in establishing healthy habits.
- Collaborative communication. Orthotics plays a crucial role in supporting both the neurologic and musculoskeletal systems. Oral splints, for instance, can provide significant occlusal support that can enhance postural stability, respiratory function, and pain management throughout the body. To ensure optimal outcomes, it is essential for the physical therapist to maintain open communication with the dentist regarding the fitting and use of any oral device. Changes in postural positioning and function should be communicated to the dentist and patient.

Locating an ACPT

Now that you have an appreciation for the important role physical therapists play in a collaborative care model, finding the appropriate physical therapist to work with may prove challenging. The following guidelines can help you locate potential physical therapists to add to your team.

1. Physical therapists, like dentists and medical doctors, do not receive foundational education on airway or TMJ dysfunction during their graduate programs, necessitating further postgraduate education and a strong passion for self-directed learning in this specialized area. A variety of certification programs exist to equip therapists with diverse training approaches suitable for treating patients with craniofacial and airway disorders. The following is a list of programs that can help physical therapists develop the skills and knowledge needed for effective collaboration with dentists and comprehensive patient care. This list would be a valuable place to begin searching:
   - Postural Restoration Institute: posturalrestoration.com
   - Institute of Physical Art: instituteofphysicalart.com
   - The Barral Institute: iahp.com
   - American Academy of Physiological Medicine & Dentistry: aapmd.org
   - American Academy of Orofacial Pain: https://aaop.org
   - Physical Therapy Board of Craniofacial & Cervical Therapeutics (PTBCCT): ptbcct.org/members/
2. Once you find a therapist that meets the credentials you are searching for, you should set up a meeting either over the phone or in person. There are some basic questions you should ask the therapist to determine if they are a good fit.
   - Is the therapist comfortable treating patients with craniofacial, TMJ, and airway disorders? If not, are they willing to take some additional coursework to improve their diagnosis and treatment skills? Sometimes, you may need to develop a therapist in your area if there is nobody with experience available.
   - Is the therapist open to observing in the office with patients? The best learning experiences are when dentists and physical therapists are learning from one another in a treatment setting.
   - Is the therapist open to taking continuing education courses or doing a mini-airway residency with the dentist? (There is no better way to develop a working relationship than learning together.)
   - Have the therapist in question treat you. This way, you will have a full understanding of their skills and treatment paradigm. Knowing the therapist's specific set of skills will boost your confidence when referring patients.

Forms

The following forms may be useful to you as customizable templates for assessing patients for physical therapy referral.

Screening for ACPT Referral Form

Screening for ACPT Referral

Patient: ______________________ **Date:** ______________________

1. Facial symmetry

( ) Convergent (R) ( ) Mandible (R)

( ) Convergent (L) ( ) Mandible (L)

( ) Upward parallel (R)

( ) Upward parallel (L)

( ) Class I ( ) Class II ( ) Class III

( ) Top one-third = > <

( ) Mid one-third = > <

( ) Bottom one-third = > <

( ) Scar on chin ( ) L ( ) R

( ) Forward head: ______ inches

2. Airway

( ) History of breathing problems

( ) Breathes with mouth open

( ) Breathes with mouth closed

( ) Upper ( ) Lower, diaphragmatic

( ) Does not wake refreshed

( ) Dry mouth/throat upon waking

( ) Snores/gasps/fragmented sleep

( ) Shortness of breath/dyspnea

3. Upper lip

( ) Covers one-fourth maxillary front teeth

( ) Short anatomical lip

( ) Short but functional upper lip

( ) Short, non-functional upper lip

4. Lower lip

( ) Covers one-fourth maxillary incisors

( ) Covers > one-fourth maxillary incisors

( ) Excessive mentonian groove

( ) Elastic lower frenulum

5. Upper/lower lip frenulum

( ) Upper/lower aligned

( ) Lower shifted right

( ) Lower shifted left

( ) Elastic lower frenulum

6. Vertical/Horizontal overlap

( ) Vertical overlap ________mm

( ) Horizontal overlap ________mm

7. Tongue

( ) Scalloped

( ) Microglossia

( ) Macroglossia

( ) On palate

( ) On bottom of mandible

( ) Can produce suction/cluck sound

( ) Short lingual frenulum

8. Maxillomandibular relationship

( ) Teeth apart at rest

( ) Teeth touching at rest

( ) Anterior teeth wear

9. Clench lines

( ) Absent

( ) Present

( ) Mandibular tori present

( ) Maxillary tori present

10. Mandibular mechanics

( ) Rotation then translation

( ) Early translation ( ) L ( ) R

11. Joint sounds

( ) Right open at ________mm

( ) Left open at ________mm

( ) Right close at ________mm

( ) Left close at ________mm

( ) Crepitus ( ) R ( ) L

12. Resisted test (✔) = painful

( ) Resisted R = left pterygoid

( ) Resisted L = right pterygoid

( ) Resisted opening

Resisted closure/protected ( ) L ( ) R

13. Cervical ROM/atlas

Upper Cervical flexion _____

Rotation (R) _________%

Rotation (L) _________%

1

Screening for ACPT Referral *(cont)*

14. Muscle palpation

1. Anterior temporalis ( ) R ( ) L ____________
2. Middle temporalis ( ) R ( ) L ____________
3. Posterior temporalis ( ) R ( ) L ____________
4. Temporalis tendon ( ) R ( ) L ____________
5. Temporalis tendon insertion ( ) R ( ) L ____________
6. Masseter insertion ( ) R ( ) L ____________
7. Masseter origin ( ) R ( ) L ____________
8. Deep masseter ( ) R ( ) L ____________
9. Retrodiscal tissue ( ) R ( ) L ____________
10. Medial pterygoid ( ) R ( ) L ____________
11. Lateral pterygoid ( ) R ( ) L ____________

15. Palpation/joint

1. Anterior inferior synovium ( ) R ( ) L ____________
2. Anterior superior synovium ( ) R ( ) L ____________
3. Lateral capsule ( ) R ( ) L ____________
4. Temporomandibular ligament ( ) R ( ) L ____________
5. Posterior inferior synovium ( ) R ( ) L ____________
6. Posterior superior synovium ( ) R ( ) L ____________
7. Posterior ligament ( ) R ( ) L ____________
8. Retrodiscal tissue ( ) R ( ) L ____________

2

Craniofacial Airway Physical Therapy Referral Form

Craniofacial Airway Physical Therapy Referral

Dentist information
- Name: ______________________________
- Practice: ______________________________
- Address: ______________________________
- Phone: ______________________________
- Email: ______________________________

Patient information
- Name: ______________________________
- Date of Birth: ______________________________
- Address: ______________________________
- Phone: ______________________________
- Email: ______________________________

Diagnosis
- Primary: ______________________________
- Secondary (if applicable): ______________________________

Treatment goals (check all that apply):

( ) Postural reeducation and correction
( ) Airway-focused myofunctional therapy
( ) TMJ dysfunction management
( ) Cervical spine mobility and stabilization
( ) Thoracic spine mobility and stabilization
( ) Upper airway muscle strengthening
( ) Breathing pattern retraining
( ) Orofacial pain management
( ) Sleep hygiene education
( ) Myofunctional therapy
( ) Other: ______________________________

Referral instructions
- Frequency: ____ sessions per week
- Duration: ____ weeks
- Evaluation and treatment of airway and sleep disorders as deemed appropriate by the physical therapist

Additional notes (if applicable):

Dentist's signature: ______________________________ **Date:** ______________

Airway and Cervical Spine Quick Screen for Dentists

Airway and Cervical Spine Quick Screen

Patient: ______________________ **Date:** ______________________

Questionnaire

- Do you generally breathe through your mouth? Yes / No
- When you swallow, is the tip of your tongue anywhere else than behind your top teeth? Yes / No
- Do you have difficulty swallowing saliva, food, or pills? Yes / No
- Do you have frontal, temporal, or occipital headaches? Yes / No
- Do you have pain or decreased neck range of motion? Yes / No
- Do you have pain or symptoms in your arms? Yes / No
- Have you experienced trauma to your head or neck? Yes / No
- Do you feel rested when you wake up in the morning? Yes / No
- Do you snore or gasp for air at any point during sleep? Yes / No

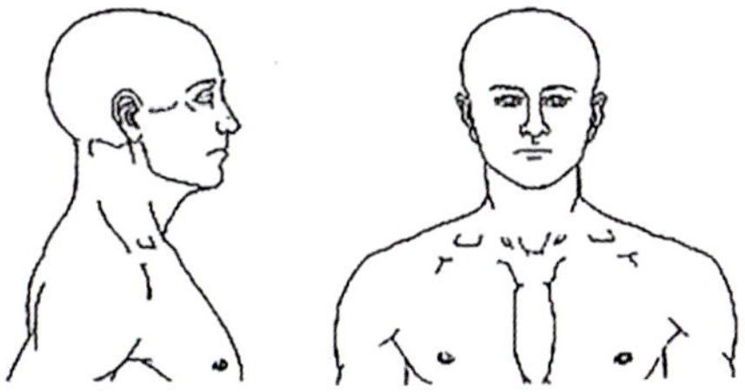

Observation

Forward head posture? Yes / No

Head tilt: R / L

Rotation: R / L

Cervical spine range of motion

Flexion (45 degrees): Normal / Decreased / Pain

Extension (45 degrees): Normal / Decreased / Pain

Rotation (60 degrees): R: Normal / Decreased / Pain; L: Normal / Decreased / Pain

Palpation	**R**	**L**
Upper trapezius	Pain / No pain	Pain / No pain
Sternocleidomastoids	Pain / No pain	Pain / No pain
Suboccipital muscles	Pain / No pain	Pain / No pain

References

1. Gesch D, Bernhardt O, Kirbscheus A. Association of malocclusion and functional occlusion with TMD in adults: A systematic review of population-based studies. Quintessence Int 2004;35:211–221.
2. Zaghi S, Shamtoob S, Peterson C, et al. Assessment of posterior tongue mobility using lingual-palatal suction: Progress towards a functional definition of ankyloglossia. J Oral Rehabil 2021;48:692–700.
3. Sakaguchi K, Mehta NR, Abdallah EF, et al. Examination of the relationship between mandibular position and body posture. Cranio 2007;25:237–249.

He lives most life whoever breathes most air.

—Elizabeth Barrett Browning

16

Rhinomanometry

Karen Parker Davidson | Klaus Vogt

Nasal function is of paramount significance in dentistry. The nose plays an essential role in maintaining optimal oral health and contributes to craniofacial development. The nasal and oral structures are in close proximity and intricately connected, influencing everything from the alignment of teeth and the maintenance of a healthy oral environment to the overall balance of facial features. Beyond its impact on oral health, nasal function profoundly influences overall well-being. Thus, understanding nasal function not only enhances diagnostic capabilities but also empowers dental professionals to provide more personalized and comprehensive care tailored to the individual needs of each patient. Assessing nasal function depends on both patient report and objective measurements.

Subjective questionnaires used in the medical community for assessing nasal breathing and congestion reflect the evolution of tools to capture patient experiences and perceptions.[1] Asking patients how they see themselves and how they understand their medical state helps dentists obtain critical information to supplement the diagnostic data gathered during an office or telehealth visit. We see this in sleep medicine with validated forms such as the STOP-BANG questionnaire and the Epworth Sleepiness Scale. In contemporary medical practice, subjective questionnaires also complement objective measures to provide a more holistic approach to patient care.

The Nasal Obstruction Symptom Evaluation (NOSE) scale was introduced in the early 2000s as a patient-reported measure designed to assess nasal obstruction and its impact on quality of life. It includes questions related to nasal congestion, breathing difficulty, and overall satisfaction with nasal function. The Rhinoconjunctivitis Quality of Life Questionnaire (RQLQ) is another option and focuses on how nasal and ocular symptoms impact daily life.[1]

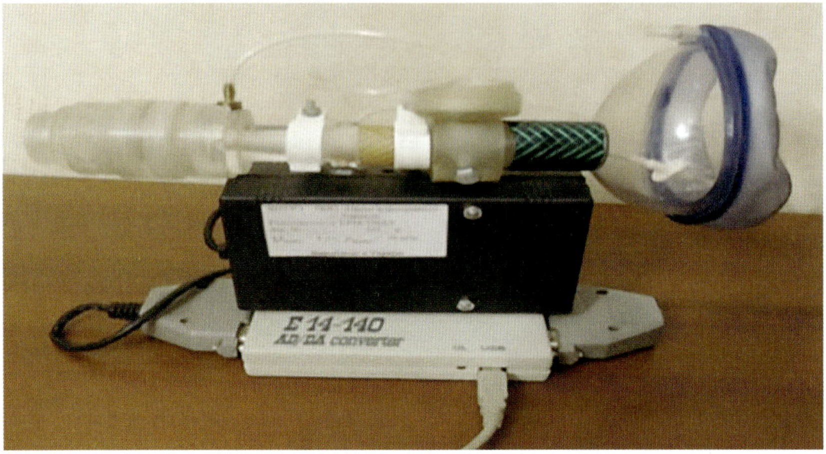

Fig 16-1 One of the first prototypes of a rhinomanometry machine (1966–1970s).

These questionnaires have facilitated a more comprehensive understanding of patient experiences and serve as standardized assessments in clinical trials and research studies. The integration of patient-reported outcomes in nasal assessments helps clinicians tailor interventions based on both objective data and subjective patient experiences, ultimately improving quality of care and patient satisfaction.[2] These concepts have now reached dental and orthodontic offices across the globe.

History of Nasal Function Testing

The history of nasal function testing can be traced back to the early 20th century, when researchers and medical professionals began to recognize the importance of understanding the nasal airway and its impact on respiratory function. In the mid 1900s, advancements in technology led to the development of objective nasal function testing. Rhinomanometry emerged as a valuable tool, allowing for the quantification of nasal airflow and resistance in 1958. Semarak described the first "Nasal Patency Assessment Device" that enabled simultaneous measurement of both the nasal respiratory flow and the pressure difference between the nasal entrance and choanae.[3] This technique provided valuable insights into the mechanical aspects of nasal function.

Later, frustrated by the subjective reports from patients after nasal surgery, ENT surgeon, former dentist, and maxillofacial surgeon Dr Klaus Vogt introduced four-phase rhinomanometry (4PR) in 1966 (Fig 16-1).[3] By the 1980s, new sensor techniques, data processing, and fluid physics were helping Vogt to analyze

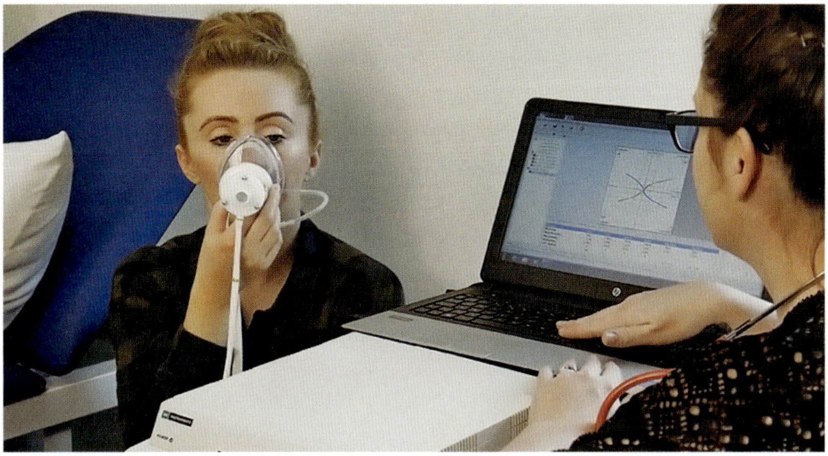

Fig 16-2 Four-phase rhinomanometer (2017–present; GM Instruments).

any errors of the rhinomanometer and create a practical method for functional diagnostics of nasal airflow. Vogt's work was presented in Stockholm during the European Rhinologic Society meeting in 1982,[3] and in 1983, the International Standardization Committee on the Objective Assessment of the Nasal Airway was reestablished after being created by Peter Clement in Nancy, France.[3] In 1989, Vogt was introduced to Dr Christian Guilleminault in Riga, Latvia. Their work in the field of rhinomanometry continues under the direction of this chapter's co-author Dr Davidson. Figure 16-2 shows the modern-day version of the rhinomanometer created by Dr Vogt. In 2015, Vogt and his team studied more than 36,000 rhinomanometry tracings to discover how they correlated with subjective symptoms reported by patients.[3] This was the birth of the updated system we know today, which is used around the world.

Rhinomanometry in Medicine and Dentistry

As the interdisciplinary landscape of oral health care expands, the intricate relationship between nasal function and orofacial development is taking center stage. In the ever-evolving field of dentistry and orthodontics, the pursuit of holistic patient care has led to the integration of various diagnostic and treatment methods that extend beyond traditional oral health. 4PR is designed to objectively and quantitatively measure and analyze nasal airflow and resistance and offers deep insights into how air moves through the nasal passages against pressure gradients that equate to nasal resistance. This sheds light on any obstructions, deviations, or imbalances that may affect a person's ability to breathe through their nose efficiently. This invaluable tool is widely used in otolaryngology, pulmonology, and related medical specialties, and its popularity is rapidly growing in airway dentistry and orthodontics.

Rhinomanometry offers several key advantages and is recognized in many countries around the globe as a standard of care for accurate diagnosis, individualized treatment planning, and monitoring of treatment progress, as well as for its research applications. Rhinomanometry is widely used in the diagnosis of a range of nasal conditions, from allergies to anatomical abnormalities. The data it provides guides health care professionals in formulating personalized treatment plans that may include medical interventions, myofunctional therapy, orthodontic treatment, or surgical procedures.

How Rhinomanometry Works

Rhinomanometry is a specialized diagnostic technique for measuring nasal airflow and resistance. The adoption of Pascals (Pa) to standardize pressure measurements within the nasopharyngeal area, including the nasal cavity, retroglossal area, and retropalatal areas, has been crucial for diagnostics and research with rhinomanometry. Measurements are based on the principle of pressure differential (ΔP), which describes the amount of pressure gradient required to move a certain amount of air through the nose. It can also be calculated based on the airflow that can travel through the nasal passages at a certain given pressure.[3–5]

The setup for rhinomanometry involves specialized equipment to accurately measure pressure and airflow within the nasal passages. The procedure begins with patient preparation. First a brief explanation of the test is provided to the patient, and then a nasal decongestant spray is applied to ensure unimpeded airflow. The patient is then positioned comfortably, usually in a seated position, and the catheter is carefully inserted. Typically, a small, flexible catheter is inserted into one nostril, while the other nostril remains unobstructed for breathing. The catheter is connected to a pressure transducer (or pneumotachometer or flow head) and an airflow sensor, which together capture the dynamic changes in pressure and airflow during the breathing cycle. Throughout the test, the patient is instructed to keep their mouth closed and to breathe normally or follow specific breathing patterns. The pressure and airflow measurements are continuously recorded by a data acquisition system, providing real-time information on nasal resistance and airflow dynamics. After the test, the recorded data is analyzed to assess various parameters, including nasal resistance and airflow patterns (Fig 16-3).

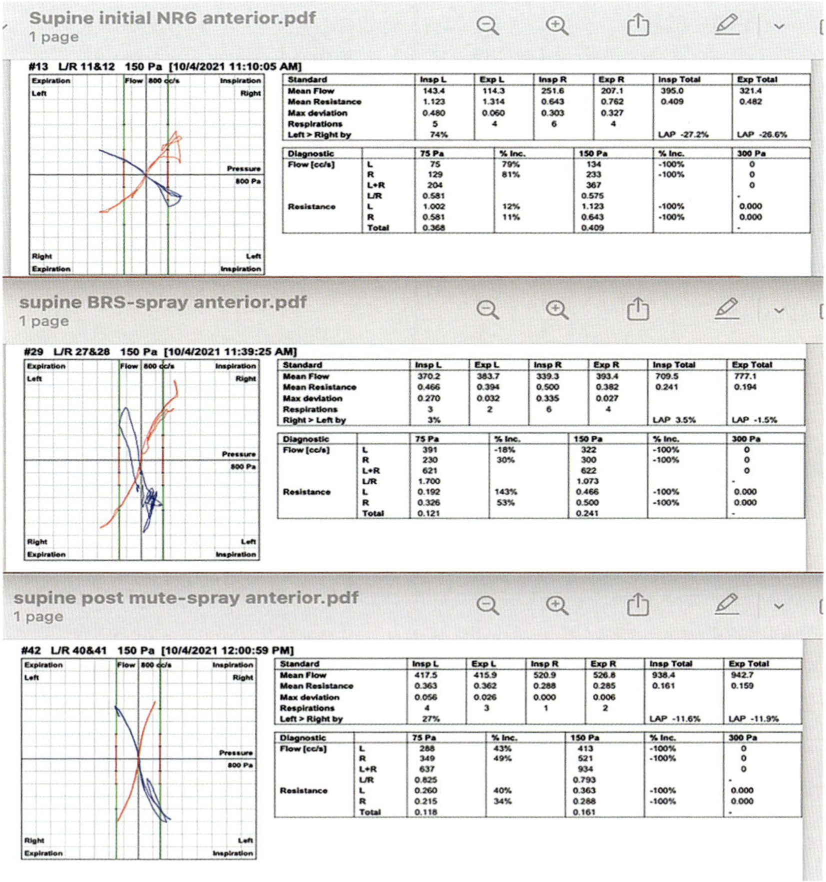

Standard	Insp L	Exp L	Insp R	Exp R	Insp Total	Exp Total
Mean Flow	143.4	114.3	251.6	207.1	395.0	321.4
Mean Resistance	1.123	1.314	0.643	0.762	0.409	0.482
Max deviation	0.480	0.060	0.303	0.327		
Respirations	5	4	6	4		
Left > Right by	74%				LAP -27.2%	LAP -26.6%

Diagnostic		75 Pa	% Inc.	150 Pa	% Inc.	300 Pa
Flow [cc/s]	L	75	79%	134	-100%	0
	R	129	81%	233	-100%	0
	L+R	204		367		0
	L/R	0.581		0.575		-
Resistance	L	1.002	12%	1.123	-100%	0.000
	R	0.581	11%	0.643	-100%	0.000
	Total	0.368		0.409		-

Standard	Insp L	Exp L	Insp R	Exp R	Insp Total	Exp Total
Mean Flow	370.2	383.7	339.3	393.4	709.5	777.1
Mean Resistance	0.466	0.394	0.500	0.382	0.241	0.194
Max deviation	0.270	0.032	0.335	0.027		
Respirations	3	2	6	4		
Right > Left by	3%				LAP 3.5%	LAP -1.5%

Diagnostic		75 Pa	% Inc.	150 Pa	% Inc.	300 Pa
Flow [cc/s]	L	391	-18%	322	-100%	0
	R	230	30%	300	-100%	0
	L+R	621		622		0
	L/R	1.700		1.073		-
Resistance	L	0.192	143%	0.466	-100%	0.000
	R	0.326	53%	0.500	-100%	0.000
	Total	0.121		0.241		-

Standard	Insp L	Exp L	Insp R	Exp R	Insp Total	Exp Total
Mean Flow	417.5	415.9	520.9	526.8	938.4	942.7
Mean Resistance	0.363	0.362	0.288	0.285	0.161	0.159
Max deviation	0.056	0.026	0.000	0.006		
Respirations	4	3	1	2		
Left > Right by	27%				LAP -11.6%	LAP -11.9%

Diagnostic		75 Pa	% Inc.	150 Pa	% Inc.	300 Pa
Flow [cc/s]	L	288	43%	413	-100%	0
	R	349	49%	521	-100%	0
	L+R	637		934		0
	L/R	0.825		0.793		-
Resistance	L	0.260	40%	0.363	-100%	0.000
	R	0.215	34%	0.288	-100%	0.000
	Total	0.118		0.161		-

Fig 16-3 Rhinomanometry numeric data output and tracings of a normal test in the supine position after nasal provocation with xylitol-containing saline spray and a nasal dilator.

Nasal resistance is a key parameter that rhinomanometry quantifies (Fig 16-4). It reflects the ease or difficulty with which air moves through the nasal passages. Elevated nasal resistance is often a sign of obstruction and can be categorized as structural or functional. Causes of structural obstructions may include a deviated septum, enlarged turbinates, or nasal polyps. Functional obstructions can result from problems like muscle imbalances and improper tongue posture.

Flow rate, the rate at which air flows through the nostrils, is another essential aspect of rhinomanometry. Measuring the flow rate provides critical data on the volume of air that passes through the nose, as well as the patterns of

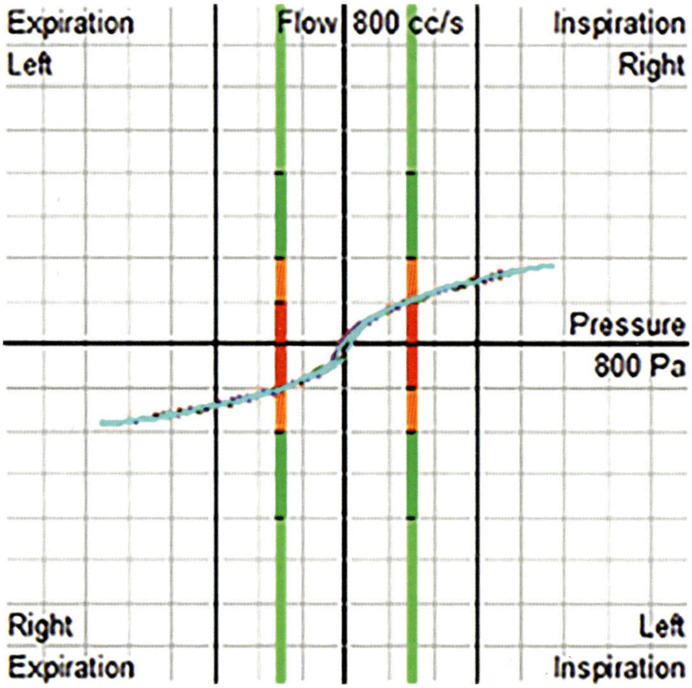

Fig 16-4 Recorded curves in a patient's file will show a series of colored sections on the vertical lines on either side of the y-axis. These lines are designed to aid in categorizing results using a "traffic light" system: Light green signifies normal resistance, dark green signals mild resistance, orange shows moderate resistance, and red denotes severe resistance.

inhalation and exhalation. Additionally, pressure gradients are assessed to identify pressure differences within the nasal passages, which helps clinicians pinpoint areas of constriction or turbulence that might hinder smooth airflow. Finally, measurement of the nasopharyngeal passages at various points is also crucial for diagnosing potential anatomical variations and assessing the adequacy of the nasal airway.

Dentists and other health care providers using rhinomanometry must be trained to interpret findings for clinical decision-making. A software platform called DAFNE (Davidson Airway Function and Nasal Evaluation) Score (Fig 16-5) can be used to identify patterns using artificial intelligence. DAFNE uses an algorithm of evidence-based parameters to help clinicians better understand what the data means and gives health care providers insight into how current interventions are affecting transnasal pressure changes. DAFNE

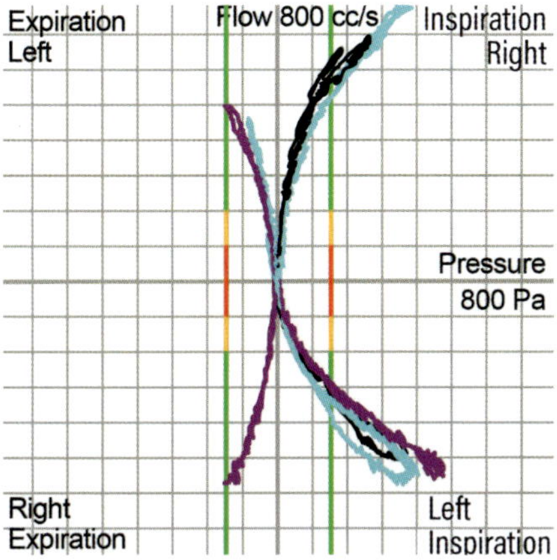

a

Severe range

Rhinomanometry tracing will intersect on the y-axis in the red area of the graph. This signifies that certain conditions will require further diagnosis or treatment.

Severe nasal obstruction/hypoventilation.

Studies show that this range indicates severe sleep apnea with a high AHI.

Therapeutic options:

ENT surgery candidate.

May consider maxillary expansion after surgery.

May consider CPAP therapy when nasal resistance does not interfere with the mask interface and patient can tolerate the CPAP therapy for optimal outcomes.

b

Fig 16-5 *(a and b)* DAFNE software predicts a high Apnea-Hypopnea Index (AHI) prior to a sleep study.[6]

also determines the amount of mucosal membrane involvement and offers recommendations for adjunct therapies, as well as the resistance changes to expect with therapies such as maxillary expansion. DAFNE also includes an algorithm for suggesting collaboration with the most effective specialty and provider to improve patient outcomes.

Rhinomanometry in Diagnosis

Rhinomanometry plays a crucial role in diagnosing airway obstructions, whether they are anatomical in nature (such as deviated septa or turbinate hypertrophy) or functional (involving muscular imbalances). Precise measurements provide a comprehensive assessment of the nasal passages to help clinicians understand how the mechanical or physiologic deficits affect the soft tissue and skeletal structures. The relationship between nasal function, the mandible, and the tongue is integral to understanding the interconnected dynamics of orofacial development. Efficient nasal breathing plays a crucial role in guiding proper jaw growth and influences the positioning of the tongue within the oral cavity. Efficient nasal breathing contributes to a well-developed maxilla with ample space for the tongue within the oral cavity. Conversely, nasal obstruction may result in a constricted maxilla, potentially leading to issues such as a high arched palate or a compromised airway. The tongue's resting position against the palate, facilitated by nasal breathing, also influences the growth and alignment of the mandible. This harmonious interplay ensures that the maxilla and mandible develop in a balanced manner that results in facial symmetry and optimal occlusion.

Chronic nasal congestion or obstruction can lead to a shift from nasal to oral breathing, with the tongue resting lower in the mouth and impacting the natural growth process of the mandible. This altered tongue posture may contribute to malocclusions, such as open bites or crossbites, and influence the overall structure of the face. Individuals who predominantly breathe through their mouths may exhibit signs such as a dry mouth, increased susceptibility to oral health issues, and altered facial development. Mouth breathing can be a compensatory mechanism in response to nasal congestion or obstruction, and identifying the root cause is essential for effective intervention. By assessing the resistance levels, dental professionals can pinpoint areas of obstruction or dysfunction. This information can then be used to develop targeted treatment plans. Rhinomanometry provides the objective data to identify and quantify nasal obstructions or dysfunctions contributing to mouth breathing. At a certain level of Pascals, breathing changes from nasal to oral. Left unaddressed, mouth breathing affects treatment progress and outcomes and contributes to the relapse of invasive therapies such as frenectomies and orthognathic surgery.

Rhinomanometry and Myofunctional Therapy

Rhinomanometry plays a crucial role in treatment planning for myofunctional therapy (see chapter 13). Objectively measuring nasal airflow and resistance assists healthcare professionals in identifying any nasal obstructions or dysfunctions that may be contributing to myofunctional issues, such as mouth breathing or improper tongue posture (Fig 16-6). If nasal resistance is elevated due to structural issues or chronic congestion, myofunctional therapy may include exercises to improve nasal breathing, strengthen the muscles involved in proper tongue posture, and address any compensatory habits developed as a result of nasal obstructions. The precision offered by rhinomanometry enables a tailored and evidence-based approach to ensure that therapeutic interventions align with the specific nasal dynamics of the individual.

Moreover, the collaboration between rhinomanometry and myofunctional therapy underscores the interconnectedness of nasal and orofacial functions. By addressing nasal issues through myofunctional therapy, health care professionals aim to optimize overall respiratory health, enhance facial muscle function, and contribute to the harmonious development of the orofacial complex. This integrative approach highlights nasal function as an integral component in the comprehensive treatment planning of myofunctional therapy, ultimately promoting holistic well-being for individuals seeking improvement in orofacial muscle function.

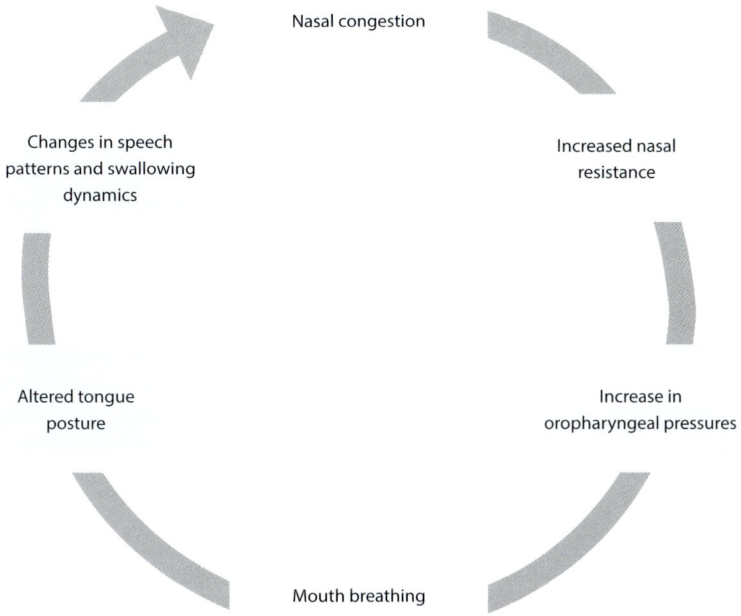

Fig 16-6 How the orofacial complex compliments nasal function.

Incorporating rhinomanometry into treatment planning in airway dentistry and orthodontics is pivotal for devising effective interventions. It allows for individualized myofunctional therapy strategies to optimize nasal breathing, correct oral posture, and improve overall oral and facial development. The effect of poor tongue posture and/or tone can be seen in rhinomanometry tracings (see Fig 16-8). Patients can be referred for myofunctional therapy, and results can be assessed with repeat tracings.

Other Objective Tests

In addition to functional testing, visual techniques and plot points with acoustic pulse waves are used in acoustic rhinometry (not to be confused with rhinomanometry). These methods made their way into the market based on the work of Dr Ole Hilburg.[3,4] Acoustic rhinometry uses sound waves to measure the cross-sectional area of the nasal cavity, thus offering a noninvasive and quick evaluation.[5] Nasal endoscopy enables direct visualization of the nasal passages to identify anatomical abnormalities and assess mucosal health.

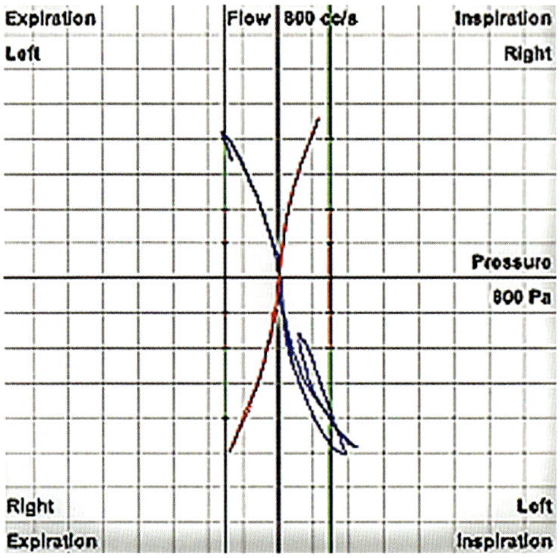

Fig 16-7 Upper airway resistance revealed with rhinomanometry.

More recent advancements in nasal function testing include computational fluid dynamics (CFD) modeling, which allows for a detailed analysis of airflow patterns within the nasal cavity. This has furthered our understanding of the complex interactions between anatomy and airflow. CFD used in the airway does not look at transnasal pressure changes but uses fluid changes in the tissue to simulate nasal airflow patterns. It requires sophisticated software and 3D imaging. As of this writing, it is not yet FDA cleared for clinical use.

Case Studies

A 5-year-old boy presented with snoring and behavior suggesting attention deficit hyperactivity disorder (ADHD). No diagnosis of ADHD was noted, but the following symptoms were present: inattentiveness, trouble focusing in school, outbursts, decline in grades, requiring redirection to stay on task. The child was not taking any medications for ADHD, and no in-lab sleep study was conducted. Rhinomanometry was used to diagnose ineffective breathing patterns by assessing nasal airflow and resistance, providing valuable information about the upper airway (Fig 16-7).

The measurement of upper airway resistance with rhinomanometry can yield insights into the efficiency of nasal breathing and potential obstructions. Increased upper airway resistance in a 5-year-old child may indicate nasal issues that can impact breathing patterns. Common factors contributing to elevated resistance in the upper airway include nasal congestion, adenoid hypertrophy, or anatomical abnormalities. Children in this age group may not always express

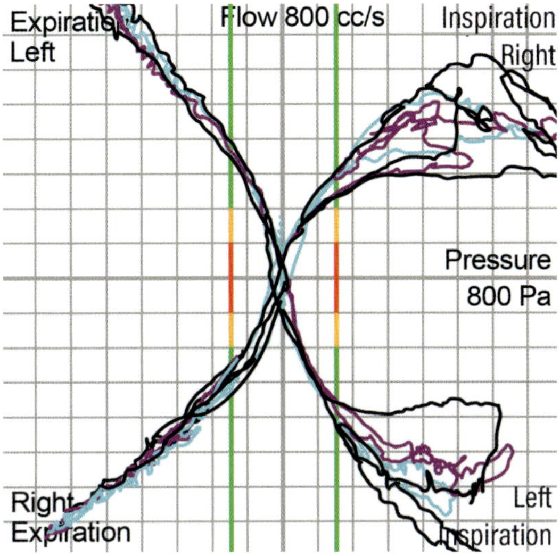

Fig 16-8 Results of rhinomanometry in a patient with poor tongue posture and mouth breathing.

their discomfort, making objective assessments like rhinomanometry crucial for identifying potential respiratory issues. If rhinomanometry reveals elevated resistance, health care professionals can tailor interventions to address the specific nasal dynamics of the child. This may include targeted treatments to alleviate congestion or manage allergies, or in some cases, an otolaryngologist may be consulted to assess adenoid or tonsil conditions. The dental community may also play an important role if maxillary expansion is required.

Using rhinomanometry to understand upper airway resistance in children allows for early intervention to optimize respiratory function. Addressing nasal issues at this stage is particularly important because it can influence overall health, sleep quality, and orofacial development. In another case, a 17-year-old girl presented post-frenectomy with an Apnea-Hypopnea Index (AHI) of 2 on a sleep study. Rhinomanometry tracings showed nasal flow limitations and resistance (Fig 16-8). Four respirations acquired clear data (ie, "a good test") showing category 3 upper airway resistance, nasal resistance (0.395 to 0.567 on the chart), and nasal cycling, with L > R. The divergent tracings seen on the right side indicate movement of soft tissue on inspiration due to increased negative pressure in the oropharyngeal space. I call it "crazy tongue" because the tongue base is pulled into the lumen of the oropharynx and is unstable in the changing pressure of active breathing.

Conclusion

Today, nasal function testing plays a vital role in the diagnosis and management of various nasal conditions, including nasal congestion, rhinitis, sinus disorders, and sleep problems.[6,7] These tests provide valuable information for clinicians to tailor treatment plans, whether through medical interventions, surgical procedures, or other therapeutic approaches. As technology continues to advance, the field of nasal function testing is likely to see further refinement and innovation, contributing to enhanced diagnostic precision and improved patient outcomes.

References

1. Percodani J. Functional investigations of the nose. In: Anniko M, Bernal-Sprekelsen M, Bonkowsky V, Bradley P, Iurato S (eds). Otorhinolaryngology, Head and Neck Surgery. European Manual of Medicine. Springer, 2010.
2. Camacho M, Chang ET, Song SA, et al. Rapid maxillary expansion for pediatric obstructive sleep apnea: A systematic review and meta-analysis. Laryngoscope 2017;127:1712–1719.
3. Pevernagie DA, Gnidovec-Strazisar B, Grote L, et al. On the rise and fall of the apnea-hypopnea index: A historical review and critical appraisal. J Sleep Res 2020;29:e13066.
4. Toh ST, Lin CH, Guilleminault C. Usage of four-phase high-resolution rhinomanometry and measurement of nasal resistance in sleep-disordered breathing. Laryngoscope 2012;122:2343–2349.
5. Hilberg O, Jackson AC, Swift DL, Pedersen OF. Acoustic rhinometry: Evaluation of nasal cavity geometry by acoustic reflection. J Appl Physiol (1985) 1989;66:295–303.
6. Hoel HC, Kvinnesland K, Berg S. Impact of nasal resistance on the distribution of apneas and hypopneas in obstructive sleep apnea. Sleep Med 2020;71:83–88.
7. Vogt K, Wernecke KD, Behrbohm H, Gubisch W, Argale M. Four-phase rhinomanometry: A multicentric retrospective analysis of 36,563 clinical measurements. Eur Arch Otorhinolaryngol 2016;273:1185–1198.

RECOMMENDED MATERIALS

Disclaimer: Neither author has any financial or other connection to the materials and resources listed below; they are what we find useful in our practices. Because both authors are frequent lecturers, it is possible that one or more of the companies listed have supported events where we have presented, but neither author has any compensation-for-sales relationship. Home company websites are provided, but may many of these materials are widely available.

Screening patients for risk of SRBDs and titrating patients in therapy	
Nonin 3150 pulse oximeter	www.nonin.com
SleepImage CPC	www.sleepimage.com
GEMPro sleep wellness monitor	www.ddmeonline.com
Positional therapy	
SlumberBUMP	www.slumberbump.com
Night Shift	www.nightshifttherapy.com
Impression and bite registration materials	
Silginat, Panasil, and Futar	www.kettenbachusa.com
ThermAcryl Plus beads	www.tapintosleep.com
TRIOS intraoral scanner	www.3shape.com
3D bite-recording devices	
George Gauge	www.greatlakesdentaltech.com
ProGauge	www.tapintosleep.com
Airway Metrics	www.kettenbachusa.com
Appliance cleaning	
Stain Away Plus	widely distributed
Additional aids	
Max-Air Nose Cones	www.maxairnosecones.com
Xlear nasal spray	www.xlear.com
3M Micropore Surgical Tape	www.3m.com

SLEEP MEDICINE TERMINOLOGY

Abdominal movement In diagnostic sleep studies, abdominal movement is recorded to diagnose central sleep apnea.

Actigraphy Devices measure body position and movement to distinguish wakefulness, NREM, and REM sleep.

Adenosine An essential molecule found in all cells and involved in the initiation of sleep. Caffeine use promotes wakefulness by blocking the actions of adenosine.

Antihistamines Drugs that block the action of histamine, lessening the effect of allergic reactions. Antihistamines have a sedative side effect and are often found in many over-the-counter sleep medications.

Apnea A cessation of breathing. Events are scored when airflow is reduced 90% from normal for at least 10 seconds.

Apnea index A measure of the severity of sleep apnea; the number of apnea events per hour.

Apnea-Hypopnea Index (AHI) The number of apneas and hypopneas per hour.

Arousal Abrupt change from a "deeper" stage of NREM sleep to a "lighter" stage.

Arousal threshold Ease with which a sleeping person is awakened.

Arrhythmia Irregularity or absence of the heart rhythm caused by disturbances in the transmission of electrical impulses through cardiac tissue.

Auto-adjusting continuous positive airway pressure device (SmartPAP) A type of CPAP machine that monitors changes in breathing and compensates automatically by making appropriate adjustments in pressure.

Benzodiazepines Developed in the 1950s, this class of compounds tranquilizes and sedates.

Bilevel PAP The "bi" refers to two pressures provided to open the airway: a lower pressure for exhalation and a higher pressure for inhalation. Some patients tolerate it better because they can exhale more comfortably against the lowered pressure. (Sometimes called BiPAP, but that is a trademark name of one system.)

Body mass index (BMI) An estimation of an individual's relative body fat calculated from his or her height and weight. The formula for calculating BMI is weight (in kilograms) divided by height squared (in meters).

Bruxism Teeth grinding during sleep.

Cataplexy An abnormal, sudden, dramatic loss of muscle tone and deep reflexes that leads to muscle weakness, paralysis, or postural collapse. Sudden paralysis of some or all skeletal muscles brought on by strong emotions such as laughter, startle, anger, or sudden physical exercise. Cataplexy is a hallmark of narcolepsy.

Central apnea (central sleep apnea) A cessation of breathing attempts for at least 10 seconds during sleep caused by irregularity in the brain's control of breathing.

Circadian rhythm A day/night pattern in many physiologic and behavioral functions, including sleep and waking, that is generated internally by a circadian pacemaker and persists under constant environmental conditions. It is generally tied to the 24-hour day/night cycle but sometimes to a different periodicity (eg, 23 or 25 hours) when light/dark and other time cues are removed.

Compliance Adhering to or conforming with a regimen of treatment, such as CPAP.

Consumer sleep technology Devices used by patients to monitor their various biosignals, such as overnight oximetry. These are *not* FDAcleared medical devices and should be used with caution for medical decision-making. Examples include FitBit, watches, rings, and phone apps.

Continuous positive airway pressure (CPAP) A treatment for OSA in which a continuous stream of air under pressure is delivered through a mask worn over the nose, or the nose and mouth, to keep the sleeper's airway open. The positive pressure can range from 5 to 25 cmH_2O.

Cortisol A steroid hormone released by the outer part of the adrenal glands that is thought to prepare the body for the stresses of the day. Cortisol release may inhibit sleep and is one reason that stressful activities before bedtime are not recommended.

Craniofacial respiratory complex Term describing the entire area of a dentist's focus from a growth and development perspective.

Diagnostic sleep study Monitoring of several physiologic activities in a sleeping individual. Usually performed to determine the absence or presence of a specific sleep disorder. The sleep study can occur in a sleep disorders center or in the patient's home with portable recording equipment.

Diaphragm The large, concave muscle attached to the rib cage at the bottom of the chest (top of the abdomen). Inhalation occurs when the diaphragm contracts. Exhalation is passive as the muscle relaxes.

Durable medical equipment (DME) A term used to describe any medical equipment used in the home to facilitate better quality of living. DME, including devices for OSA, must be prescribed by a physician.

Ear, nose, and throat (ENT; otolaryngologist) A doctor specializing in diseases of the ear, nose, and throat. Otolaryngologists may become board certified in sleep medicine with additional training.

Electrocardiography (ECG) A method of measuring the electrical activity of the heart.

Electroencephalogram (EEG) A recording through the scalp of electrical potentials from the brain. The EEG is one of the three basic variables (along with the EOG and EMG) used to score sleep stages and waking.

Electromyogram (EMG) A recording of electrical activity from the muscular system. In sleep recording, a chin EMG is one of the three basic variables used to score sleep stages and waking, along with EEG and EOG. Surface electrodes are also used to record sleep bruxism.

Electrooculogram (EOG) Human sleep recordings using surface electrodes placed near the eyes to record the movement of the eyeballs to distinguish between REM and NREM sleep.

Enuresis (bed wetting) Urinating while asleep.

Epoch A standard 30-second duration segment of the sleep recording.

Epworth Sleepiness Scale Index of the likelihood of feeling drowsy in eight common situations.

Esophageal pressure Measurement of pressure changes in the upper airway as a result of respiratory effort. Can help predict which therapy might be most effective for the patient.

Excessive daytime sleepiness (EDS) or somnolence Difficulty in staying awake during the daytime when a person intends to be alert.

Expiratory positive airway pressure (EPAP) Pressure prescribed for the expiratory (breathing out) phase of an individual on bilevel PAP therapy for OSA. There are also EPAP devices used by patients to restrict expiration through the nose and maintain pressure in the oropharynx.

Fatigue Feeling of tiredness or weariness usually associated with performance decrements. It is possible that it is not accompanied by sleepiness.

Fiberoptic nasopharyngoscope Flexible fiberoptic scope used for examination of the nasal passages, oropharynx, hypopharynx, and larynx.

Flow limitation Partial closure of the upper airway, impeding the flow of air into the lungs. Seen on airflow waveforms from flow signals of sleep tests.

Fragmentation (pertaining to sleep architecture) Interruption of a sleep stage as a result of the appearance of a lighter stage or the occurrence of wakefulness, which leads to disrupted NREM/REM sleep cycles.

Gastroesophageal reflux disease (GERD) Flow of stomach acid upward into the esophagus that can cause arousals and disrupt sleep.

Ghrelin A hormone produced in the stomach that stimulates appetite. The body's production of ghrelin may be influenced by the amount of sleep a person gets.

Growth hormone A hormone secreted by the pituitary gland that promotes growth of the body and influences the metabolism of proteins, carbohydrates, and lipids. The secretion of growth hormone peaks during N3 sleep.

Histamine A substance released by cells in the brain promoting arousal. Antihistamine medication can promote sleep.

Histogram (sleep) Graph indicating sleep stages throughout the night.

Hypercapnia Excessive or elevated carbon dioxide in the blood.

Hypersomnia Excessive, prolonged sleep.

Hypertension High blood pressure.

Hypnogram A graph that summarizes the pattern of sleep stages throughout a night as recorded in the sleep laboratory.

Hypnotics In sleep medicine, hypnotics are agents that promotes sleep—sleep-inducing drugs.

Hypopharynx Lowermost portion of the pharynx, below the base of the tongue and above the larynx and esophagus.

Hypopnea Shallow breathing in which the airflow in and out of the airway is reduced 30% from normal. The definition may or may not include specific levels of oxygen desaturation, depending on which institution or organization is publishing the guideline.

Hypoventilation Reduced rate and depth of breathing.

Hypoxemia Abnormal lack of oxygen in the arterial blood.

Hypoxia Deficiency of oxygen reaching the tissues of the body.

Hypoxic Burden Describes the area under the desaturation curve of overnight oximetry. A more precise measure of the physiologic risk of SDB.

Imidazopyridines New class of compounds inducing sleepiness. Zolpidem (Ambien, Sanofi) is in this class.

Insomnia Trouble falling asleep, staying asleep, or waking up earlier than planned. This is a common complaint describing difficulty in sleeping.

Leptin A hormone that stimulates satiety and thus decreases appetite. Reduced sleep duration may lead to a reduction in leptin, thereby stimulating appetite.

Letter of medical necessity (LOMN) Certification by a physician that the prescribed item(s) is/are medically indicated, reasonable, and necessary with reference to the standards of medical practice and treatment of a patient's condition.

Macroglossia Large tongue; usually a congenital disorder (present at birth).

Mallampati score A scoring system for visibility of the oropharynx when the mouth is open. Used to assess whether a crowded upper airway increases the risk of OSA.

Mandibular maxillary osteotomy and advancement (MMOA) Jaw surgery to reposition skeletal structures to decrease collapsibility of the upper airway. Often coordinated with orthodontic therapy.

Melatonin A hormone produced by the pineal gland to assist with sleep onset in humans.

Microarousal Partial awakening from sleep.

Microsleep A brief period of sleep, lasting only a few seconds. Microsleeps occur most frequently when a very sleepy person is trying to stay awake. Thought to be a component of "sleepy driving."

Mixed (sleep) apnea Flow changes during sleep, beginning as a central apnea and then becoming an obstructive apnea.

Modafinil A central nervous system stimulant that promotes wakefulness. Modafinil is primarily used to treat the symptoms of EDS in people with narcolepsy.

Multiple sleep latency test (MSLT) A sleep laboratory test that consists of a series of 20-minute nap opportunities during the daytime to measure a patient's sleepiness. Patients who fall asleep in less than 10 minutes or who enter REM sleep rather than NREM sleep may suffer from EDS.

Nadir Lowest point. Used in sleep testing to note lowest oxygen saturation.

Narcolepsy A rare sleep disorder marked by sudden sleep attacks. Narcolepsy is characterized by an abnormal tendency to pass directly from wakefulness into REM sleep. May include cataplexy.

Nasal airflow/nasal ventilation Recording of the complete respiratory cycle by measuring inspiratory and expiratory airflow.

Neurology Branch of medicine referring to the nervous system and its diseases.

Neurotransmitters Endogenous chemical components that are released from axon terminals of one neuron and transmit the signal to the next neuron.

Nocturia Excessive, often frequent, urination during the night.

NREM or non-REM sleep Sleep stage characterized by slower and larger brainwave activity, comprising approximately 75% to 80% of sleep. The stages of sleep that do not include rapid eye movement patterns. According to current guidelines for sleep stage classification, NREM consists of three stages: N1, N2, and N3.

N1 The lightest stage of NREM sleep. Slow eye movements are often present.

N2 The second stage of NREM sleep. EEGs during N2 sleep show sleep spindles and K-complexes on a background of relatively low-voltage, mixed-frequency EEG activity.

N3 The deepest stage of NREM sleep, characterized by a larger amount of synchronized slow-wave EEG (brainwave) activity than in other stages. The brain is less responsive to external stimuli, and it is difficult to awaken a person during slow-wave sleep.

Obesity hypoventilation syndrome Obese individuals hypoventilating during wakefulness.

Obstructive apnea (obstructive sleep apnea [OSA]) Sleep apnea is usually due to complete or partial obstruction of the airway. Obstructions lasting 10 seconds or more are counted as apnea events. Efforts to breathe accompany OSA.

Obstructive hypopnea Periodic and partial closure of the throat during sleep resulting in reduced airflow (at least a 30% reduction) with an accompanying 3% to 4% reduction in oxygen saturation.

Optimum sleep Average amount of sleep needed every night by an individual.

Orexin A neurotransmitter that promotes wakefulness by stimulating the brainstem arousal center.

Oximeter (pulse oximentry) Gives estimates of arterial oxyhemoglobin saturation by using selected wavelengths of light to noninvasively determine the saturation of oxyhemoglobin.

Oxygen desaturation Less than normal amount of oxygen carried by hemoglobin in the blood; values below 90% are considered abnormal.

Oxygen saturation Measure of oxygen carried by hemoglobin in the blood. Normal values are 90% to 100%. Measured with oximetry and labeled SaO_2.

Parasomnia Troubling or undesirable behaviors that intrude during sleep, such as sleepwalking or sleep talking. They often are associated with abnormal or partial arousal and typically disrupt normal sleep.

Periodic limb movements of sleep (PLMS) Leg movements or jerks that typically occur every 20 to 40 seconds during sleep. The term periodic limb movement disorder is used if the leg movements produce daytime sleepiness. Often the patient is unaware but the bed partner complains. Can be effectively measured only during in-lab sleep studies.

Pharynx Area posterior to the nares and the oral cavity; passageway for air from the nasal cavity and/or the mouth to the lungs via the larynx and the trachea, and for food and liquids from the mouth to the esophagus.

PLMD arousal index Number of sleep-related periodic leg movements per hour of sleep that are associated with an EEG arousal.

Polysomnographic technologist Health care professional trained in performing diagnostic sleep studies. An RPSGT is a registered PSG technologist.

Polysomnography (PSG) Continuous and simultaneous recording of physiologic variables during sleep, including EEG, EOG, EMG (the three basic stage scoring parameters), ECG, respiratory air flow, respiratory excursion, lower limb movement, and other electrophysiologic variables. In-lab PSG can have up to 20 data signals; home sleep apnea testing usually includes 4 signals.

REM latency The length of time from sleep onset to the first appearance of stage REM.

REM rebound or recovery Lengthening and increase in frequency and density of REM periods, which results in an increase in REM percent above baseline. REM rebound follows REM deprivation once the inhibitory influence is removed.

REM sleep The stage of sleep characterized by a period of intense brain activity often associated with dreams. It is named for the rapid eye movements that occur during this time. REM sleep is additionally characterized by flitting motions of the eyes and weakness of the muscles; vivid dreaming occurs in this stage, which accounts for about 20% of sleep in adults. Also called paradoxical or dreaming sleep.

REM sleep behavior disorder (RBD) Disorder in which REM motor atonia is partially or completely absent and the individual acts out the ongoing dream.

RERA (respiratory effort–related arousal) A sequence of breaths (lasting 10 seconds or longer) characterized by increasing respiratory effort and leading to an arousal from sleep but not meeting the criteria for an apnea or hypopnea.

Respiratory disturbance index (RDI) Includes all respiratory events per hour. A record of the number and duration of apnea episodes, both obstructive, central, mixed, hypopneas, and RERAs, per hour of sleep.

Restless legs syndrome (RLS) A condition characterized by achy or unpleasant feelings in the legs associated with a need to move. Most prominent in the evening, making it hard to fall asleep or stay asleep. This is a disease of wakefulness, not the same as periodic limb movements of sleep.

Sedatives Compounds tending to calm and reduce nervousness or excitement and foster sleep.

Septoplasty Surgery on the nasal septum (dividing the nasal passage).

Serotonin Neurotransmitter in the brain that modulates mood, appetite, sexual activity, aggression, body temperature, and sleep.

Sleep A state marked by lessened consciousness, lessened movement of the skeletal muscles, and slowed-down metabolism.

Sleep apnea A cessation of breathing during sleep. In adults, the episode must last 10 seconds; in children, these events last at least the duration of two breath cycles.

Sleep architecture NREM/REM stage and cycle infrastructure of sleep understood from the vantage point of the quantitative relationship of these components to each other.

Sleep cycle Synonymous with NREM/REM cycle.

Sleep debt An individual's accumulated sleep loss from insufficient sleep, regardless of cause.

Sleep deprivation Acute or chronic lack of sufficient sleep.

Sleep efficiency (SE) Proportion of sleep in the period potentially filled by sleep; ratio of total sleep time to time in bed.

Sleep episode Interval of sleep that may be voluntary or involuntary.

Sleep fragmentation Brief arousals occurring throughout the night, reducing the total amount of time spent in the deeper levels of sleep.

Sleep hygiene Conditions and practices that promote continuous and effective sleep, including regularity of bedtime and arise time; conforming time spent in bed to the time necessary for sustained and individually adequate sleep (ie, the total sleep time sufficient to avoid sleepiness when awake); restriction of alcohol and caffeine in the period prior to bedtime;

employment of exercise, nutrition, and environmental factors so that they enhance, rather than disturb, restful sleep.

Sleep inertia Feelings of grogginess and/or sleepiness that persist longer than 10 to 20 minutes after waking up.

Sleep latency Time period measured from "lights out," or bedtime, to the beginning of sleep. How long it takes a person to fall asleep from the onset of the potential sleep period.

Sleep log (diary) Daily written record of an individual's sleep-wake pattern containing such information as time of retiring and arising, time in bed, estimated total sleep period, number and duration of sleep interruptions, quality of sleep, daytime naps, use of medications or caffeine, nature of waking activities, and other data.

Sleep maintenance insomnia Disturbance in maintaining sleep once achieved; persistently interrupted sleep without difficulty initially falling asleep.

Sleep onset insomnia Difficulty with transition from wake to sleep.

Sleep talking Talking in sleep takes place during stage REM, representing a motor breakthrough of dream speech, or during transitory arousals from NREM sleep and other stages. Full consciousness is not achieved, and no memory of the event remains.

Sleepwalker or sleepwalking Individual subject to somnambulism (one who walks while sleeping). Sleepwalking typically occurs in the first third of the night, during N3.

Snoring Noise produced primarily with inspiratory respiration during sleep owing to vibration of the soft palate and the pillars of the oropharyngeal inlet. Many snorers have incomplete obstruction of the upper airway and may develop OSA.

Soft palate Membranous and muscular fold suspended from the posterior margin of the hard palate and partially separating the oral cavity from the pharynx.

Somatic complaints Awareness of pain or problems in the body.

Suprachiasmatic nucleus (SCN) Also referred to as circadian clock, circadian pacemaker, or internal biologic clock. A small group of nerve cells located in the hypothalamus that controls the circadian cycles and influences many physiologic and behavioral rhythms occurring over a 24-hour period, including the sleep/wake cycle.

Tachycardia Rapid heart rate, usually defined by a pulse rate of over 100 beats per minute (bpm).

Thermocouples Small devices placed near the nostrils or mouth to measure airflow by sensing temperature changes; expired air is warmer than inspired air.

Tidal volume Amount of air that passes in and out of the lungs in an ordinary breath; usually expressed in liters.

Titration Progressive, stepwise increase in CPAP pressure to establish the optimal treatment pressure. Mandibular advancement devices are titrated by changing the position of the mandible and testing for effectiveness.

Tonsillectomy Surgical removal of the tonsils.

Tonsils Pair of prominent masses of lymphoid tissue that are located opposite each other in the throat between the anterior and posterior pillars of the fauces (the narrow passage from the mouth to the pharynx situated between the soft palate and the base of the tongue). Composed of lymph follicles grouped around one or more deep crypts. Tonsils are sized and graded 0 to 4.

Total recording time Duration of time from the start of the test until the system is shut off at the end of the test. In addition to total sleep time, it comprises the time taken up by wake periods and movement time until wake-up.

Total sleep time (TST) Amount of actual sleep time in a sleep period; equal to total sleep period less movement and awake time. Total sleep time is the total of all REM and NREM sleep in a sleep period.

Tricyclic antidepressants Medications for depression. Most tricyclic antidepressants also reduce REM sleep. Also used to control cataplectic attacks, hypnagogic hallucinations, and sleep paralysis.

Turbinate Small, shelf-like, cartilaginous structures covered by mucous membranes, which protrude into the nasal airway to help warm, humidify, and cleanse inhaled air on its way to the lungs.

Upper airway Part of the respiratory anatomy that includes the nose, nostrils, sinus passages, septum, and turbinates; the tongue, jaws, hard and soft palate; and the muscles of the tongue and throat—every part of the anatomy over which air passes above the larynx.

Upper airway resistance syndrome (UARS) Part of the spectrum of obstructive SRBDs in which repetitive increases in resistance to airflow in the upper airway lead to brief arousals and daytime fatigue. Apneas and hypopneas may be totally absent. Blood oxygen levels can be in the normal range.

Uvula Small, soft structure hanging from the bottom of the soft palate in the midline above the back of the tongue.

Uvulopalatopharyngoplasty (UPPP) An operation performed on the throat to treat snoring and sleep apnea.

Zeitgeber Environmental time cue that regulates biologic rhythms to a specific periodicity. Known zeitgebers are light, melatonin, and physical activity. To be effective, these signals must occur when the biologic clock is in a responsive phase. If they occur out of phase, they can inhibit sleep quality.

Index

Page numbers followed by "f" denote figures, those followed by "t" denote tables, and those followed by "b" denote boxes.

B

E

F

N